C0-AMS-920

Health Information Systems

Second Edition

Alfred Winter • Reinhold Haux
Elske Ammenwerth • Birgit Brigl
Nils Hellrung • Franziska Jahn

Kathryn J. Hannah • Marion J. Ball
(Series Editors)

Health Information Systems

Architectures and Strategies

Second Edition

With a Foreword by Reed M. Gardner

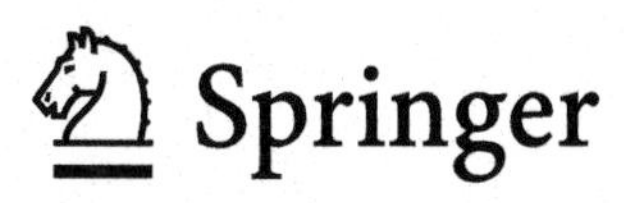

Authors
Alfred Winter, PhD
Professor of Medical Informatics
Institute for Medical Informatics, Statistics and Epidemiology
University of Leipzig, Germany
Alfred.Winter@imise.uni-leipzig.de

Reinhold Haux, PhD
Professor of Medical Informatics
Peter L. Reichertz Institute for Medical Informatics
University of Braunschweig – Institute of Technology and Hannover Medical School, Germany
Reinhold.Haux@plri.de

Elske Ammenwerth, PhD
Professor of Medical Informatics
Institute for Health Information Systems
University for Health Sciences, Medical Informatics and Technology (UMIT), Austria
Elske.Ammenwerth@umit.at

Birgit Brigl, PhD
Friedrichsdorf, Germany
Birgit.Brigl@t-online.de

Nils Hellrung, PhD
Peter L. Reichertz Institute for Medical Informatics,
University of Braunschweig – Institute of Technology and Hannover Medical School, Germany
Nils.Hellrung@plri.de

Franziska Jahn, Dipl.-Inf.
Institute for Medical Informatics, Statistics and Epidemiology
University of Leipzig, Germany
Franziska.Jahn@imise.uni-leipzig.de

ISBN 978-1-84996-440-1 e-ISBN 978-1-84996-441-8
DOI 10.1007/978-1-84996-441-8
Springer London Dordrecht Heidelberg New York

British Library Cataloguing in Publication Data
A catalogue record for this book is available from the British Library

Library of Congress Control Number: 2010933608

Cover design: eStudioCalamar Figueres/Berlin

Printed on acid-free paper

Springer is part of Springer Science+Business Media (www.springer.com)

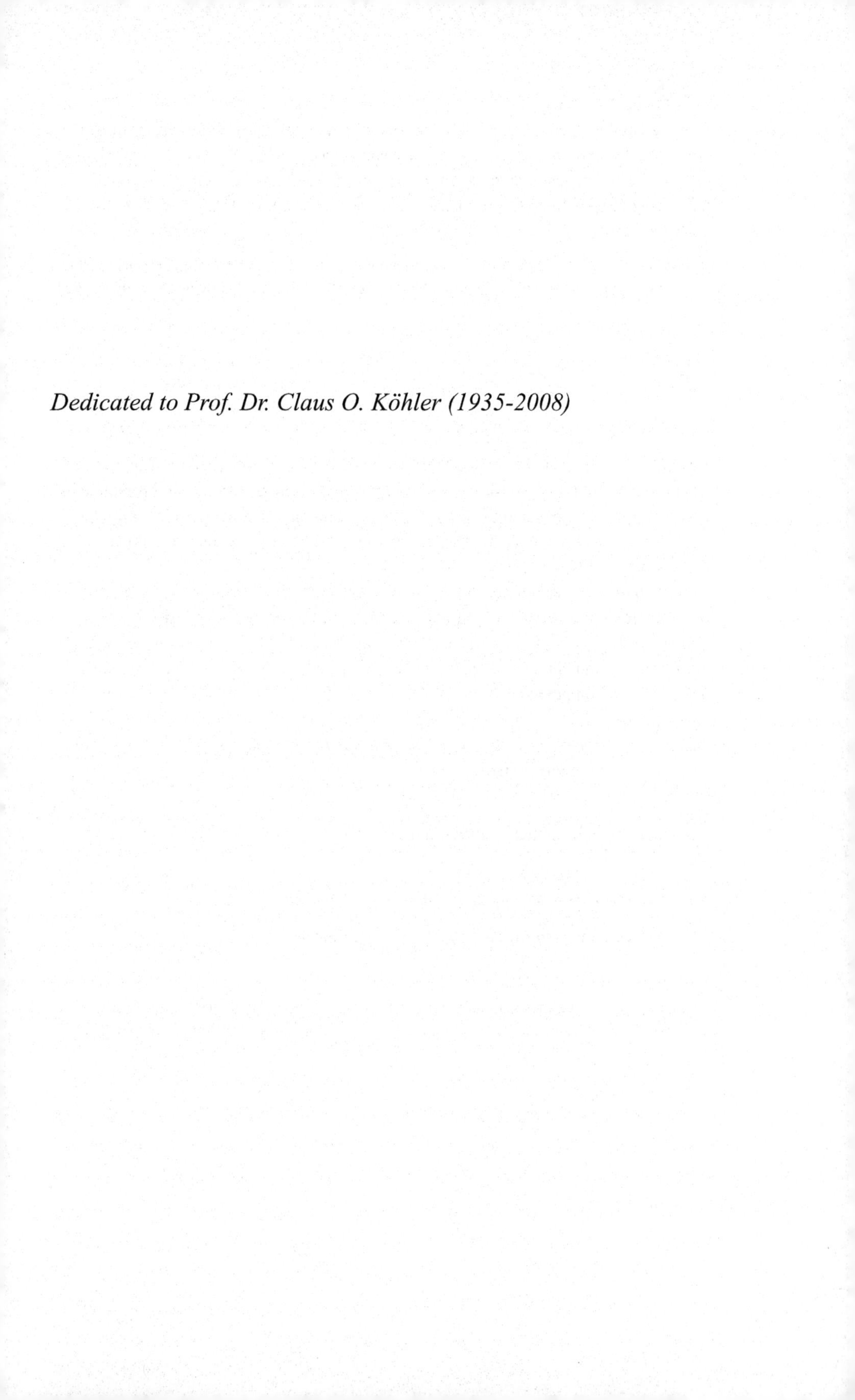

Dedicated to Prof. Dr. Claus O. Köhler (1935-2008)

"Any technology sets a relationship between human beings and their environment, both physical and human. No technology can be seen as merely instrumental. This is especially relevant when dealing with large automatic information systems, developed to contribute to the management and integration of large organizations, such as hospitals."

Jean-Marie Fessler and Francois Grémy (first recipient of the IMIA Award of Excellence). Ethical Problems with Health Information Systems. Methods of Information in Medicine 2001; 40: 359-61.

"1.1 Why Do We Need Biomedical and Health Informatics [BMHI] Education?

Despite the documented benefits, there are still barriers to HIT [health information technology] in clinical settings, including a mismatch of return on investment between those who pay and those who benefit, challenges to ameliorate workflow in clinical settings, lack of standards and interoperability, and concerns about privacy and confidentiality … .
Another barrier, lesser studied and quantified but increasingly recognized, is the lack of characterization of the workforce and its training needed to most effectively implement HIT systems … This has led to calls for BMHI to become a professional discipline … and for it to acquire the attributes of a profession, such as a well-defined set of competencies …

…

Table 2: Recommended ... learning outcomes in terms of levels of knowledge and skills for professionals in healthcare ...

…

1.6 Characteristics, functionalities and examples of information systems in health-care …

1.7 Architectures of information systems in healthcare …

1.8 Management of information systems in healthcare …

…"

Recommendations of the International Medical Informatics Association (IMIA) on Education in Biomedical and Health Informatics - 1st Revision. Methods of Information in Medicine 2010; 49: 105-120.

Foreword from the 1st Edition in 2004

Healthcare management is a complex and ever-changing task. As medical knowledge increases, as clinical management strategies or administrative management strategies change, and as patients move from one city to another or from one country to another, the challenges of managing healthcare have changed and will continue to change. Central to all of these changes is a need to store and process administrative and clinical records for the patient. For the reasons listed above, computerization of record systems in hospitals and clinics has been and continues to be a slow and complex process. Developing a strategy to provide the best healthcare service at the lowest possible cost is a common goal of almost every healthcare system in the world. Care given in the hospital is typically the most advanced, the most complex, and the most expensive. As a consequence, understanding and managing healthcare in hospitals is crucial to every healthcare delivery system. This book provides a wonderful overview for students and medical informatics professionals. It also provides the background that every medical informatics specialist needs to understand and manage the complexities of hospital information systems.

This book deals primarily with the underlying administrative systems that are in place in hospitals throughout the world. These systems are fundamental to the development and implementation of the even more challenging systems that acquire, process, and manage the patient's clinical information. Hospital information systems provide a major part of the information needed by those paying for healthcare, be they hospital administrators, health insurance companies, public health authorities, or local or national political leaders. As a consequence an important and complex set of strategies has been implemented to document medical problems and procedures that hospitals are dealing with. Problems are usually coded with International Classification of Diseases (ICD-9 or ICD-10) coding systems while medical procedures are designated using Current Procedural Terminology (CPT) codes. Typically, these codes are used to generate bills to an insurance company or governmental unit. As a consequence, these data must be generated, transmitted, and processed accurately and promptly. Computer technology enhances the ability of hospital clinical and administrative staff to provide these data.

Because of the complexities and changing needs of medical information, the field of medical informatics is in need of a growing number of professionals who understand how to use computers and are familiar with the administrative requirements of the healthcare field and clinical medicine. Having a person who has knowledge in all of these fields is unusual. However, I am convinced that the rate at which medicine is able to better use computer technology is limited by the lack of a sufficient number of well-trained professionals who have an understanding of all of these fields. As a consequence, I congratulate each of you who is studying hospital information systems and encourage you to take what you will learn from this book and move the field forward.

After you have an understanding of what is presented in this text, I encourage you to take on the challenge of clinical informatics. Study and learn how computers can be used to advantage by those providing clinical care – physicians, nurses, pharmacists, therapists, and other caregivers. In the future we must all work toward developing computer and communications systems that will enhance the acquisition of clinical data so that the data can be used to provide better patient care and more efficient and better administrative documentation.

Enjoy this book. Its clearly written materials and exercises should give every reader a challenge and opportunity to learn. I found Appendix A, the thesaurus, a treasure of important information. The thesaurus will be very handy for everyone for years to come. I congratulate the authors for their knowledge, skillfulness, and dedication in writing and publishing this book.

Salt Lake City, Utah, USA Reed Gardner

Series Preface

This series is directed to healthcare professionals leading the transformation of healthcare by using information and knowledge. For over 20 years, Health Informatics has offered a broad range of titles: some address specific professions such as nursing, medicine, and health administration; others cover special areas of practice such as trauma and radiology; still other books in the series focus on interdisciplinary issues, such as the computer-based patient record, electronic health records, and networked healthcare systems. Editors and authors, eminent experts in their fields, offer their accounts of innovations in health informatics. Increasingly, these accounts go beyond hardware and software to address the role of information in influencing the transformation of healthcare delivery systems around the world. The series also increasingly focuses on the users of the information and systems: the organizational, behavioral, and societal changes that accompany the diffusion of information technology in health services environments.

Developments in healthcare delivery are constant; in recent years, bioinformatics has emerged as a new field in health informatics to support emerging and ongoing developments in molecular biology. At the same time, further evolution of the field of health informatics is reflected in the introduction of concepts at the macro or health systems delivery level with major national initiatives related to electronic health records (EHR), data standards, and public health informatics.

These changes will continue to shape health services in the twenty-first century. By making full and creative use of the technology to tame data and to transform information, Health Informatics will foster the development and use of new knowledge in healthcare.

Kathryn J. Hannah
Marion J. Ball

Preface for the 2nd Edition

In 2004, the textbook "Strategic Information Management in Hospitals – An Introduction to Hospital Information Systems" appeared in this Health Informatics Series of Springer. The book was received well and belongs – according to the publishing house – to the top selling books of this series.

Five years after its appearance, both Springer and we as authors felt the need to prepare a 2nd edition. In this 2nd edition we wanted to consider the progress in our field and also the lessons learned from our students, when using the book in our lectures, e.g. in the international "Frank van Swieten Lectures on Strategic Information Management in Hospitals" (International Journal of Medical Informatics 2004; 73, 97-100 and 807-15). Also, due to the changed perception of information systems in healthcare, which are no longer limited to single institutions like hospitals, but can embrace several healthcare institutions within healthcare networks, this revision has become necessary.

With this book on "Health Information Systems – Architectures and Strategies" we have prepared a substantially revised and elaborated 2nd edition.

What are the major differences from the 1st edition, which appeared in 2004? We shifted the focus from hospital information systems and their strategic management to strategic information management of health information systems. However, information systems in hospitals still play a major role in the book. All contents have been carefully updated. The book has been restructured in order to improve the use as a textbook for lectures on health information systems.

In addition to the four authors of the 1st edition, two new authors (N.H., F.J.) have also contributed to this edition. For the 2nd edition we also invited an international board of experts – CIOs and researchers in the field of health information systems – to give us their advice and comments, including examples and use cases.

All authors have been either directly or indirectly influenced by the visionary views on health information systems of Claus O. Köhler. Dr. Köhler was Professor of Medical Informatics at the German Cancer Research Center in Heidelberg, Germany, and long-term faculty member at the Heidelberg/Heilbronn Medical Informatics Program. His book on the 'integrated hospital information system', which appeared in Germany in 1973, significantly influenced the development of health information systems at least in Germany. Claus passed away in 2008. We want to dedicate this book to him.

Alfred Winter
Reinhold Haux
Elske Ammenwerth
Birgit Brigl
Nils Hellrung
Franziska Jahn

Acknowledgements for the 2nd Edition

Also for this 2nd edition we want to express our cordial thanks to all colleagues, contributing to this book, in particular to Bakheet Aldosari, Carl Dujat, Christopher Duwenkamp, Marco Eichelberg, Gert Funkat, Mowafa Househ, Alexander Hörbst, Florian Immenroth, Hagen Kosock, Michael Marschollek, Bassima Saddik, Paul Schmücker, Claudia Siemers-Marschollek, and Thomas Wendt.

We are grateful to the members of the book's International Advisory Board – leading CIOs and researchers in the field of health information systems – for spending their time in commenting on this book and giving us significant advice. It is our hope that we could well include these comments.

The members of the book's International Advisory Board are Dominik Aronsky (Nashville, USA), Willem Jan ter Burg (Amsterdam, The Netherlands), Young Moon Chae (Seoul, Korea), Andrew Grant (Sherbrooke, Canada), Rada Hussein (Cairo, Egypt), Georg Lechleitner (Innsbruck, Austria), Christoph U. Lehmann (Baltimore, USA), Dirk May (Hannover, Germany), Fernán González Bernaldo de Quirós (Buenos Aires, Argentina), Christoph Seidel (Braunschweig, Germany), Amnon Shabo (Haifa, Israel), Jan Erik Slot (Amsterdam, The Netherlands), Katsuhiko Takabayashi (Chiba, Japan), and Majid Al Tuwaijri (Riyadh, Saudi Arabia).

Again, our students helped us a lot by evaluating our lectures and by providing us with many constructive ideas and helpful comments. In addition, we thank Ulrike Weber who designed a lot of the figures in this book.

Acknowledgements for the 1st Edition

We would like to express our thanks to all of our colleagues who contributed to this book, especially Reed Gardner, who commented on it and wrote the Foreword. Thanks also to many other people who helped to produce this book, especially Frieda Kaiser and Gudrun Hübner-Bloder.

We would also like to thank the following colleagues for helping to obtain figures and screen shots: Marc Batschkus, Thomas Bürkle, Andrew Grant, Torsten Happek, Marianne Kandert, Thomas Kauer, Georg Lechleitner, Otwin Linderkamp, André Michel, Gerhard Mönnich, Oliver Reinhard, Christof Seggewies, Pierre Tetrault, Raimund Vogl, and Immanuel Wilhelmy. In particular, we are grateful to Ursula and Markus Beutelspacher for allowing us to take a picture of their Heidelberg quintuplets for the cover (quintuplet picture by Bernd Krug).

Not least, we want to thank our students, who kept asking critical questions and drew our attention to incomplete and indistinct arguments.

Annotation to the Figures

All persons shown in the photos have given their permission. With the exception of the Heidelberg quintuplets, no real patients are shown. The patients in the figures are mostly the authors, their families, or medical informatics VIPs. We have partly used screen shots from commercial software products in this book. This use cannot be regarded as a recommendation for those products. We only want to illustrate typical functionality and typical user interfaces of software products that support specific hospital functions. Therefore, we did not mention the product names.

Contents

1 Introduction 1

2 Health Institutions and Information Processing 3
2.1 Introduction 3
2.2 Significance of Information Processing in Health Care 3
2.2.1 Information Processing as Quality Factor 3
2.2.2 Information Processing as Cost Factor 4
2.2.3 Information as Productivity Factor 6
2.2.4 Holistic View of the Patient 6
2.2.5 Hospital Information System as Memory and Nervous System 7
2.3 Progress in Information and Communication Technology 8
2.3.1 Impact on the Quality of Health Care 8
2.3.2 Impact on Economics 10
2.3.3 Changing Health Care 11
2.4 Importance of Systematic Information Management 12
2.4.1 Affected People and Areas 12
2.4.2 Amount of Information Processing 13
2.4.3 Sharing the Same Data 14
2.4.4 Integrated Information Processing to Satisfy Information Needs 15
2.4.5 Raising the Quality of Patient Care and Reducing Costs 16
2.4.6 Basis of Systematic Information Processing 16
2.5 Examples 17
2.5.1 Knowledge Access to Improve Patient Care 17
2.5.2 Nonsystematic Information Processing in Clinical Registers 18
2.5.3 The WHO eHealth Resolution 19
2.5.4 Estimated Impact of eHealth to Improve Quality and Efficiency of Patient Care 21
2.6 Exercises 22
2.6.1 Amount of Information Processing in Typical Hospitals 22
2.6.2 Information Processing in Different Areas 22
2.6.3 Good Information Processing Practice 23
2.7 Summary 23

3 Information System Basics ... 25
- 3.1 Introduction ... 25
- 3.2 Data, Information, and Knowledge ... 25
- 3.3 Information Systems and Their Components ... 26
  - 3.3.1 Systems and Subsystems ... 26
  - 3.3.2 Information Systems ... 26
  - 3.3.3 Components of Information Systems ... 27
  - 3.3.4 Architecture and Infrastructure of Information Systems ... 29
- 3.4 Information Management ... 30
- 3.5 Exercises ... 30
  - 3.5.1 On the Term Information System ... 30
  - 3.5.2 On Enterprise Functions ... 31
  - 3.5.3 On Application Components ... 31
  - 3.5.4 On Architectures and Infrastructures ... 31
  - 3.5.5 On Information Management ... 31
- 3.6 Summary ... 31

4 Health Information Systems ... 33
- 4.1 Introduction ... 33
- 4.2 Hospital Information Systems ... 33
- 4.3 Transinstitutional Health Information Systems ... 36
- 4.4 Electronic Health Records as a Part of Health Information Systems ... 38
- 4.5 Challenges for Health Information Systems ... 38
- 4.6 Example ... 40
  - 4.6.1 Architecture of a Hospital Information System ... 40
- 4.7 Exercises ... 41
  - 4.7.1 Hospital Information System as a System ... 41
  - 4.7.2 Buying a Hospital Information System ... 41
  - 4.7.3 Transinstitutional Health Information Systems ... 41
- 4.8 Summary ... 42

5 Modeling Health Information Systems ... 43
- 5.1 Introduction ... 43
- 5.2 On Models and Metamodels ... 43
  - 5.2.1 Definitions ... 43
  - 5.2.2 Types of Models ... 45
- 5.3 A Metamodel for Modeling Health Information Systems on Three Layers: 3LGM² ... 51
  - 5.3.1 UML Class Diagrams for the Description of 3LGM² ... 52
  - 5.3.2 3LGM²-B ... 55
  - 5.3.3 3LGM²-M ... 66
  - 5.3.4 3LGM²-S ... 67
- 5.4 On Reference Models ... 68
- 5.5 A Reference Model for the Domain Layer of Hospital Information Systems ... 70

5.6 Exercises 71
5.6.1 Typical Implementation of Hospital Functions 71
5.6.2 3LGM² as a Metamodel 71
5.6.3 Modeling with 3LGM² 72
5.7 Summary 73

6 Architecture of Hospital Information Systems 75
6.1 Introduction 75
6.2 Domain Layer: Data to be Processed in Hospitals 75
6.2.1 Entity Types Related to Patient Care 76
6.2.2 Entity Types About Resources 77
6.2.3 Entity Types Related to Administration 78
6.2.4 Entity Types Related to Management 78
6.3 Domain Layer: Hospital Functions 79
6.3.1 Patient Care 79
6.3.2 Supply and Disposal Management, Scheduling, and Resource Allocation 93
6.3.3 Hospital Administration 96
6.3.4 Hospital Management 104
6.3.5 Research and Education 104
6.3.6 Clinical Documentation: A Hospital Function? 106
6.3.7 Domain Layer: Exercises 107
6.3.8 Domain Layer: Summary 108
6.4 Logical Tool Layer: Application Components 110
6.4.1 Patient Administration System 111
6.4.2 Medical Documentation System 113
6.4.3 Nursing Management and Documentation System 115
6.4.4 Outpatient Management System 116
6.4.5 Provider or Physician Order Entry System (POE) 118
6.4.6 Patient Data Management System (PDMS) 120
6.4.7 Operation Management System 122
6.4.8 Radiology Information System 124
6.4.9 Picture Archiving and Communication System (PACS) 125
6.4.10 Laboratory Information System 127
6.4.11 Enterprise Resource Planning System 128
6.4.12 Data Warehouse System 129
6.4.13 Document Archiving System 131
6.4.14 Other Computer-Based Application Components 133
6.4.15 Clinical Information System and Electronic Patient Record System as Comprehensive Application Components 134
6.4.16 Typical Non-Computer-Based Application Components 135
6.5 Logical Tool Layer: Integration of Application Components 137
6.5.1 Taxonomy of Architectures at the Logical Tool Layer 138
6.5.2 Integrity 144
6.5.3 Types of Integration 146

6.5.4 Standards ... 149
6.5.5 Integration Technologies ... 155
6.5.6 Logical Tool Layer: Example ... 161
6.5.7 Logical Tool Layer: Exercises ... 163
6.5.8 Logical Tool Layer: Summary ... 167
6.6 Physical Tool Layer: Physical Data-Processing Systems ... 168
6.6.1 Servers and Communication Networks ... 169
6.6.2 Clients ... 169
6.6.3 Storage ... 170
6.6.4 Typical Non-Computer-Based Physical Data-Processing Systems 170
6.6.5 Infrastructure ... 171
6.7 Physical Tool Layer: Integration of Physical Data-Processing Systems ... 172
6.7.1 Taxonomy of Architectures at the Physical Tool Layer ... 172
6.7.2 Physical Integration ... 174
6.7.3 Computing Centers ... 175
6.7.4 Physical Tool Layer: Example ... 176
6.7.5 Physical Tool Layer: Exercises ... 177
6.7.6 Physical Tool Layer: Summary ... 177
6.8 Summarizing Example ... 178
6.8.1 Health Information Systems Supporting Clinical Business Processes ... 178
6.9 Summarizing Exercises ... 181
6.9.1 Hospital Functions and Processes ... 181
6.9.2 Application Components and Hospital Functions ... 181
6.9.3 Multiprofessional Treatment Teams ... 182
6.9.4 Information Needs of Different Health Care Professionals ... 182
6.9.5 HIS Architectures ... 182
6.9.6 Communication Server ... 182
6.9.7 Anatomy and Physiology of Information Processing ... 182
6.10 Summary ... 183

7 Specific Aspects for Architectures of Transinstitutional Health Information Systems ... 185
7.1 Introduction ... 185
7.2 Domain Layer ... 186
7.2.1 Specific Aspects for Hospital Functions ... 186
7.2.2 Additional Enterprise Functions ... 188
7.3 Logical Tool Layer ... 188
7.3.1 Integration of Application Components ... 188
7.3.2 Strategies for Electronic Health Record Systems ... 190
7.4 Physical Tool Layer ... 192
7.5 Examples ... 193
7.5.1 "Gesundheitsnetz Tirol (GNT)": The Tyrolean Health Care Network ... 193
7.5.2 Veterans Health Information Systems and Technology Architecture (VISTA) ... 196

7.5.3 The Hypergenes Biomedical Information Infrastructure 196
7.5.4 The National Health Information System in Korea 197
7.6 Exercises 198
7.6.1 Challenges of Transinstitutional Health Information Systems 198
7.6.2 Strategies for Transinstitutional Electronic Health Records 198
7.6.3 The Term "Electronic Health Record" 199
7.6.4 Transinstitutional Information Systems in Other Sectors 199
7.7 Summary 199

8 Quality of Health Information Systems 201
8.1 Introduction 201
8.2 Quality of Structures 202
8.2.1 Quality of Data 202
8.2.2 Quality of Computer-Based Application Components and Their Integration 203
8.2.3 Quality of Physical Data Processing Systems 205
8.2.4 Quality of the Overall HIS Architecture 206
8.2.5 Exercises 206
8.2.6 Summary 207
8.3 Quality of Processes 208
8.3.1 Single Recording, Multiple Usability of Data 208
8.3.2 No Transcription of Data 208
8.3.3 Leanness of Information Processing Tools 208
8.3.4 Efficiency of Information Logistics 210
8.3.5 Patient-Centered Information Processing 210
8.3.6 Exercises 211
8.3.7 Summary 212
8.4 Quality of Outcome 212
8.4.1 Fulfillment of Hospital's Goals 213
8.4.2 Fulfillment of the Expectations of Different Stakeholders 213
8.4.3 Fulfillment of Information Management Laws 215
8.4.4 Exercises 216
8.4.5 Summary 216
8.5 Balance as a Challenge for Information Management 216
8.5.1 Balance of Homogeneity and Heterogeneity 217
8.5.2 Balance of Computer-Based and Non-Computer-Based Tools 217
8.5.3 Balance of Data Security and Working Processes 218
8.5.4 Balance of Functional Leanness and Functional Redundancy 219
8.5.5 Balance of Documentation Quality and Documentation Efforts 219
8.5.6 Exercises 220
8.5.7 Summary 220
8.6 Evaluation of Health Information Systems Quality 221
8.6.1 Typical Evaluation Phases 221
8.6.2 Typical Evaluation Methods 224
8.6.3 Exercises 227
8.6.4 Summary 228

8.7 Summarizing Examples 228
8.7.1 The Baldrige Health Care Information Management Criteria 228
8.7.2 Information Management Standards of the Joint Commission 229
8.7.3 The Baby CareLink Study 230
8.7.4 In-Depth Approach: The Functional Redundancy Rate 230
8.8 Summarizing Exercises 235
8.8.1 Evaluation Criteria 235
8.8.2 Joint Commission Information Management Standards 235
8.9 Summary 235

9 Strategic Information Management in Hospitals 237
9.1 Introduction 237
9.2 Strategic, Tactical and Operational Information Management 238
9.2.1 Information Management 238
9.2.2 Information Management in Hospitals 241
9.2.3 Strategic Information Management 242
9.2.4 Tactical Information Management 243
9.2.5 Operational Information Management 244
9.2.6 Relationship Between IT Service Management and Information Management 246
9.2.7 Example 248
9.2.8 Exercises 248
9.2.9 Summary 249
9.3 Organizational Structures of Information Management 249
9.3.1 Chief Information Officer 249
9.3.2 Information Management Department 251
9.3.3 Example 251
9.3.4 Exercises 252
9.3.5 Summary 253
9.4 Strategic Planning 254
9.4.1 Tasks 254
9.4.2 Methods 256
9.4.3 The Strategic Information Management Plan 257
9.4.4 Example 261
9.4.5 Exercises 261
9.4.6 Summary 263
9.5 Strategic Monitoring 263
9.5.1 Tasks 264
9.5.2 Methods 267
9.5.3 Examples 268
9.5.4 Exercises 272
9.5.5 Summary 272
9.6 Strategic Directing 273
9.6.1 Tasks 273
9.6.2 Methods 273

9.6.3 Example ... 274
9.6.4 Exercise ... 274
9.6.5 Summary ... 274
9.7 Last But Not Least: Education! ... 275
9.8 Summarizing Examples ... 275
9.8.1 Deficiencies in Information Management ... 275
9.8.2 Computer Network Failures ... 276
9.8.3 Information Management Responsibilities ... 277
9.8.4 Safely Implementing Health Information and Converging Technologies ... 278
9.8.5 Increased Mortality After Implementation of a Computerized Physician Order Entry System ... 279
9.9 Summarizing Exercises ... 279
9.9.1 Management of Other Information Systems ... 279
9.9.2 Beginning and End of Information Management ... 279
9.9.3 Cultivating Hospital Information Systems ... 280
9.9.4 Hospital Information System Failure ... 280
9.9.5 Increased Mortality ... 280
9.9.6 Relevance of Examples ... 280
9.9.7 Problems of Operational Information Management ... 280
9.10 Summary ... 281

10 Strategic Information Management in Health Care Networks ... 283
10.1 Introduction ... 283
10.2 Description of Health Care Networks ... 284
10.3 Organizational Structures of Information Management in Health Care Networks ... 284
10.3.1 Centrality of Information Management in Health Care Networks . 284
10.3.2 Intensity of Information Management in Health Care Networks ... 286
10.4 Types of Health Care Networks ... 286
10.5 Example ... 287
10.5.1 Regional Health Information Organizations ... 287
10.6 Exercise ... 288
10.6.1 The Plötzberg Health Care Network ... 288
10.7 Summary ... 288

11 Final Remarks ... 291

Thesaurus ... 293

Recommended Further Readings ... 327

Index ... 331

List of Figures

Fig. 2.1 Radiological conference in a radiodiagnostic department 4

Fig. 2.2 The office of a senior physician 6

Fig. 2.3 An example of the patient summary within an electronic patient record 7

Fig. 2.4 A paper-based patient record archive as one information storing part of the hospital's memory and nervous system 8

Fig. 2.5 Snapshot in a server room of a hospital showing the computer-based nerve cords of the hospital's memory and nervous system 9

Fig. 2.6 Physician using a picture archiving and communication system for diagnostics... 10

Fig. 2.7 A mobile computer on a ward to support medical documentation and information access...................................... 12

Fig. 2.8 A study nurse in an outpatient unit dealing with a multitude of paper-based forms.. 13

Fig. 2.9 Regular clinical round by different health care professionals on a ward... 14

Fig. 2.10 During a ward round: Health care professionals jointly using information processing tools 15

Fig. 2.11 Prof. L., Head of the Department of Pediatrics, working with a literature server... 17

Fig. 2.12 The Heidelberg quintuplets 18

Fig. 3.1 An example for forms and folders for nursing documentation, representing a physical data processing system. The rules that describe who may use these forms, and how they should be used, make up the application component 28

Fig. 3.2 Typical physical data processing systems in an outpatient unit (e.g., printer, telephone, and non-computer-based patient record) 29

Fig. 4.1 A health care professional accessing patient information 35

Fig. 4.2 A general practitioner accessing documents of a hospital information system 37

Fig. 5.1 An extract of a technical HIS model with some physical data processing systems and their data transmission links of the hospital information system of the Plötzberg Medical Center and Medical School (PMC) 47

Fig. 5.2 An extract of a technical HIS model with some application components and their communication links of the hospital information system of the Plötzberg Medical Center and Medical School (PMC) 47

Fig. 5.3 An extract from the organizational model of Plötzberg Medical Center and Medical School (PMC) 48

Fig. 5.4 A simplified data model (UML class diagram), describing the relationships between the entity types patient, case, and procedure, as extract from the data model of the HIS of the Plötzberg Medical Center and Medical School (PMC) 49

Fig. 5.5 Example of a business process model, based on a UML activity diagram, describing a part of the *admission* process in the Department of Child and Juvenile Psychiatry at Plötzberg Medical Center and Medical School (PMC) 50

Fig. 5.6 Abstract classes and subclasses in a UML class diagram 53

Fig. 5.7 Associations between classes in a UML class diagram 53

Fig. 5.8 Association classes in a UML class diagram 53

Fig. 5.9 Decomposition as one type of association between one class and itself in a UML class diagram 54

Fig. 5.10 Specialization as another type of association between one class and itself in a UML class diagram 54

Fig. 5.11 Concepts of the $3LGM^2$ Domain Layer 57

Fig. 5.12 Example of a $3LGM^2$ Domain Layer 58

Fig. 5.13 Concepts of the $3LGM^2$ logical tool layer. Lines denote interlayer relationships between logical tool layer and domain layer 59

Fig. 5.14 Example of a $3LGM^2$ logical tool layer 60

Fig. 5.15 Concepts of the $3LGM^2$ physical tool layer. Dotted lines denote interlayer relationships between logical tool layer and physical tool layer 61

Fig. 5.16 On the top, the concept of a cluster virtualizing several physical data processing systems is illustrated. At the bottom, there is one physical data processing system which is virtualized into several virtual machines 62

Fig. 5.17 Example of a $3LGM^2$ physical tool layer 63

Fig. 5.18 Complete UML diagram of the $3LGM^2$-B metamodel showing all concepts, intra- and interlayer relationships 64

Fig. 5.19 Example of three $3LGM^2$ layers and their interlayer relationships 66

Fig. 5.20 Concepts of $3LGM^2$-M. The diagram only contains the new concepts message type and communication standard and their relationships with other concepts 67

Fig. 5.21 Concepts of $3LGM^2$-S. The diagram only contains the new concepts service, service class, invoking interface and providing interface and their relationships with other concepts 68

Fig. 5.22 Hospital functions of the Reference Model for the Domain Layer of Hospital Information Systems (presented until second hierarchy level) 70

Fig. 6.1 A patient being admitted in a patient admission department 80

Fig. 6.2 Extract of the domain layer of the $3LGM^2$-based reference model describing the enterprise function *patient admission*, its subfunctions, and interpreted and updated entity types 80

Fig. 6.3 Typical organizational media: a magnetic card and stickers with patient identification data 82

Fig. 6.4 Informing patients' relatives on a ward........ 84

Fig. 6.5 Extract of the domain layer of the $3LGM^2$-based reference model describing the enterprise function *decision making, planning and organization of patient treatment*, its subfunctions, and interpreted and updated entity types........ 84

Fig. 6.6 Paper-based nursing documentation on a ward........ 85

Fig. 6.7 Extract of the domain layer of the $3LGM^2$-based reference model describing the enterprise function order entry, its subfunctions, and interpreted and updated entity types........ 86

Fig. 6.8 A paper-based order entry form for laboratory testing........ 87

Fig. 6.9 Clinical examination conducted by a pediatrician 88

Fig. 6.10 Extract of the domain layer of the $3LGM^2$-based reference model describing the enterprise function *execution of diagnostic, therapeutic and nursing procedures*, its subfunctions, and interpreted and updated entity types........ 89

Fig. 6.11 Extract of the domain layer of the $3LGM^2$-based reference model describing the enterprise function *coding of diagnoses and procedures*, its subfunctions, and interpreted and updated entity types 90

Fig. 6.12 Preparing for the *discharge* of a *patient* from a ward 91

Fig. 6.13 Extract of the domain layer of the $3LGM^2$-based reference model describing the enterprise function *patient discharge and transfer to other institutions*, its subfunctions, and interpreted and updated entity types 92

Fig. 6.14 Extract of the domain layer of the $3LGM^2$-based reference model describing the enterprise function *supply and disposal management*, its subfunctions, and interpreted and updated entity types........ 94

Fig. 6.15 The stock of drugs on a hospital ward........ 94

Fig. 6.16 Extract of the domain layer of the $3LGM^2$-based reference model describing the enterprise function *scheduling and resource allocation*, its subfunctions, and interpreted and updated entity types 95

Fig. 6.17 Extract of the domain layer of the $3LGM^2$-based reference model describing the enterprise function *human resources management*, its subfunctions, and interpreted and updated entity types 96

Fig. 6.18 Extract of the domain layer of the $3LGM^2$-based reference model describing the enterprise function *archiving of patient information*, its subfunctions, and interpreted and updated entity types 97

Fig. 6.19 A paper-based hospital archive with a robot system for storing and gathering boxes filled with patient records 98

Fig. 6.20 Extract of the domain layer of the $3LGM^2$-based reference model describing the enterprise function *quality management*, its subfunctions, and interpreted and updated entity types 99

Fig. 6.21 Extract of the domain layer of the $3LGM^2$-based reference model describing the enterprise function *cost accounting*, its interpreted and updated entity types 100

Fig. 6.22 Extract of the domain layer of the $3LGM^2$-based reference model describing the enterprise function *controlling* and its interpreted and updated entity types 101

Fig. 6.23 Excerpt from a DRG scorecard, which is an important part of a hospital's controlling report (in German). The left column lists a set of key performance indicators (KPIs) to be controlled (e.g., "Verweildauer (Mittel)": patients' average length of stay). The next columns contain for some time periods values as recorded (e.g., "Ist Monat 12 2009": values recorded in December 2009) or as planned (e.g., "Plan Monat 12 2009": values planned for December 2009) 102

Fig. 6.24 Extract of the domain layer of the $3LGM^2$-based reference model describing the enterprise function *financial accounting*, its interpreted and updated entity types 103

Fig. 6.25 Extract of the domain layer of the $3LGM^2$-based reference model describing the enterprise function *facility management*, its subfunctions, and interpreted and updated entity types 103

Fig. 6.26 Extract of the domain layer of the 3LGM²-based reference model describing the enterprise function *information management*, its subfunctions, and interpreted and updated entity types 103

Fig. 6.27 Extract of the domain layer of the 3LGM²-based reference model describing the enterprise function *hospital management*, its interpreted and updated entity types 105

Fig. 6.28 Extract of the domain layer of the 3LGM²-based reference model describing the enterprise function *research and education*, its subfunctions, and interpreted and updated entity types 105

Fig. 6.29 Reference model of the hospital functions on the domain layer 109

Fig. 6.30 Screenshot of a *patient administration system* showing the patient list of a department of neurosurgery in the background and a window for assigning an appointment to a patient in the front 111

Fig. 6.31 A screenshot of a *medical documentation system* showing a list of patient-related documents on the left and an opened discharge letter on the right 113

Fig. 6.32 Screenshot of a nursing documentation system. On the left, it shows the selected nursing pathways for the given *patient*. On the right, it shows the corresponding open tasks that now have to performed 115

Fig. 6.33 Screenshot of an application component for scheduling in an outpatient unit 117

Fig. 6.34 Screenshot of a lab order entry system. An order set of electrolyte has been chosen to see details (lower right). If available, results can already be reviewed (lower left) 119

Fig. 6.35 Screenshot of a *patient data management system* showing a patient's vital parameters and given drugs during a day 120

Fig. 6.36 Screenshot of an operation management system, showing the surgeons as well as the *patients* that are assigned to them. For each *patient*, the planned *procedure* and the status of the operation is displayed. The status can also be displayed for each operation room using a time line (not shown) 122

Fig. 6.37 Screenshot of a *radiology information system* (RIS) showing all radiologic documents of one patient 124

Fig. 6.38 Screenshot from a *Picture Archiving and Communication System* (*PACS*) application component, presenting different images of a *patient* 126

Fig. 6.39 In a laboratory unit. The laboratory information system (LIS; running on the PC in the front) manages the analysis of *samples* by laboratory devices (in the background) 127

Fig. 6.40 Screenshot of a *data warehouse system*. The diagram shows a target/actual comparison for the bed occupation of a university hospital 130

Fig. 6.41 Screenshot of a document archiving system. Besides text documents like findings from the laboratory, operation reports, letters, anamneses, etc., it also contains radiological images 132

Fig. 6.42 The patient chart 136

Fig. 6.43 The paper-based patient record 136

Fig. 6.44 DB^n style with multiple computer-based application components, each with its own database system, using 3LGM2 symbols. The cloud in the center indicates that some as yet unknown means is needed to link the components 140

Fig. 6.45 (DB^1, AC^1) architecture using $3LGM^2$ symbols. The gray rectangle denotes the computer-based application component that contains a database system (denoted by the cylinder) 141

Fig. 6.46 (DB^1, AC^n) architecture with multiple computer-based application components, using $3LGM^2$ symbols. Only one computer-based application component (in the center) contains a database system 141

Fig. 6.47 (DB^n, AC^n, V^n, CP^n) architecture with multiple computer-based application components, using $3LGM^2$ symbols, with several bidirectional communication interfaces. This representation is also called a "spaghetti" architectural style 143

Fig. 6.48 (DB^n, AC^n, V^n, CP^1) architecture with multiple computer-based application components connected by a specific application component, using $3LGM^2$ symbols. This representation is also called a "star" architectural style 143

Fig. 6.49 Assignment of findings to orders and to cases, and of those cases to a particular patient, in a UML-based data model ... 145

Fig. 6.50 Event-driven communication with HL7 ... 150

Fig. 6.51 DB^n architectural style with multiple computer-based application components, each with its own database system, using 3LGM symbols. A communication server links the components ... 158

Fig. 6.52 An integrated *clinical information system* (*CIS*) as an example for a (DB^1, V^1) architecture. The CIS often contains the *medical documentation system*, the *nursing management and documentation system*, the *outpatient management system*, and the *physician or provider order entry system* (POE) as modules ... 162

Fig. 6.53 A (DB^1, V^1)-styled subinformation system at Chiba University Hospital, Japan. The central electronic medical record (EMR) system has a database which can also be accessed by other application components ... 162

Fig. 6.54 A typical situation in German University Hospitals: the enterprise resource planning (ERP) system includes a component for *patient administration*. 163

Fig. 6.55 At an ophthalmology unit (1) ... 164

Fig. 6.56 At an ophthalmology unit (2) ... 164

Fig. 6.57 At an ophthalmology unit (3) ... 165

Fig. 6.58 At an ophthalmology unit (4) ... 165

Fig. 6.59 A ward in a "paperless" hospital ... 166

Fig. 6.60 A health care professional accessing patient information ... 170

Fig. 6.61 Typical paper-based physical data processing systems ... 171

Fig. 6.62 A modern server room in a computing center of a university hospital ... 176

Fig. 7.1 *Patient admission* in the office of a general practitioner ... 187

Fig. 7.2 Overview of sense Architecture based on several IHE Integration Profiles. Actors are depicted as boxes and transactions as lines ... 194

Fig. 8.1 Example of a transcription (1) 209

Fig. 8.2 Example of a transcription (2) 209

Fig. 8.3 Extract from the business process "meal ordering" 212

Fig. 8.4 A stylish client at a patient admission unit 218

Fig. 8.5 The major steps of an evaluation study. Boxes comprise activities; arrows into a box from top are input; arrows out from a box are output. Feedback loops indicate that earlier steps may have to be redone or refined 222

Fig. 8.6 Matrix SUP: rectangles denote enterprise functions, rounded rectangles denote application components, and connecting lines illustrate a "1" in the respective position of the matrix, that is, that a certain enterprise function is supported by a certain application component. For example, enterprise function E *decision making* can be supported by application component 5 *decision support system* or 7 *pathology information system* alternatively 232

Fig. 9.1 Relationship between planning, directing, and monitoring during *strategic, tactical*, and *operational information management*. For explanation see paragraph before 240

Fig. 9.2 Three-dimensional classification of information management activities 240

Fig. 9.3 *Strategic, tactical*, and *operational information management* in hospitals, HIS operation, and their relationships 241

Fig. 9.4 Typical phases of *tactical information management projects* 243

Fig. 9.5 Monitoring of the server of a hospital information system 245

Fig. 9.6 An immediate support center for third-level support of a vendor 247

Fig. 9.7 An information management board meeting at a university hospital. Participants in this meeting are (from the *left*): the director of procurement, the chair of the staff council, the assistant of the information management department's director, the director of the information management department, a senior physician as chair of the board, a medical informatics professor as vice-chair of the board, a director of a medical research department as representative of the medical faculty and medical school, the director of nursing. The director of finance and vice-director of administration took the photo 250

Fig. 9.8 Organization of information management at the Plötzberg Medical Center and Medical School (PMC) 252

Fig. 9.9 Strategic information management planning of hospitals. A strategic information management plan gives directives for the construction and development of a hospital information system. It describes the recent and the intended hospital information system's architecture. (Details are explained in the following sections) 258

Fig. 10.1 Types of health care networks 287

Figure Credits

- A Specialist Practice in Bammental, Germany: Figure 6.9, Figure 7.1
- A Specialist Practice in Innsbruck, Austria: Figure 4.2
- Braunschweig Medical Center, Braunschweig, Germany: Figure 6.41
- Cerner Corporation: Figure 2.3, Figure 6.33, Figure 6.34, Figure 6.36
- Cerner Immediate Support Services, Kansas City, Missouri, USA: Figure 9.6
- Chiba University Hospital, Chiba, Japan: Figure 6.19
- Diakonissehjemmets Sykehus Haraldsplass, Bergen, Norway: Figure 8.2
- German Cancer Research Center, Heidelberg, Germany: Figure 8.1
- ITH icoserve technology for healthcare GmbH, Innsbruck, Austria: Figure 2.6, Figure 6.38
- LDS Hospital, Salt Lake City, Utah, USA: Figure 2.9
- One of the author's former home office, Meckesheim, Germany: Figure 6.61
- Selayang Hospital, Kuala Lumpur, Malaysia: Figure 2.7, Figure 6.12, Figure 6.59, Figure 9.5
- University Medical Center Erlangen, Germany: Figure 4.1, Figure 6.6
- University Medical Center Heidelberg, Germany: Figure 2.2, Figure 2.4, Figure 2.11, Figure 2.12, Figure 6.1, Figure 6.3, Figure 6.15, Figure 6.55, Figure 6.56

- University Medical Center Innsbruck, Austria: Figure 2.1, Figure 2.7, Figure 2.10, Figure 3.1, Figure 3.2, Figure 6.32, Figure 6.39, Figure 6.43, Figure 6.57, Figure 6.58

- University Medical Center Leipzig, Germany: Figure 2.5, Figure 2.8, Figure 6.8, Figure 6.23, Figure 6.30, Figure 6.31, Figure 6.35, Figure 6.37, Figure 6.40, Figure 6.42, Figure 6.62, Figure 9.7

- Weinberg Cancer Center Johns Hopkins, Baltimore, Maryland, USA: Figure 6.4

List of Tables

Table 2.1 Example of Simpson's paradox – Success rates of Novum and Verum treatments for patients with diagnosis Δ, treated during the years δ at the Plötzberg Medical Center and Medical School (PMC) 19

Table 5.1 An extract from the functional HIS model, describing hospital functions relevant for patient care and hospital administration at the Plötzberg Medical Center and Medical School (PMC) 46

Table 6.1 Typical supported hospital functions and related features of the *patient administration system* 112

Table 6.2 Typical supported hospital functions and related features of the *medical documentation system* 114

Table 6.3 Typical supported hospital functions and related features of the *nursing management and documentation system* 116

Table 6.4 Typical supported hospital functions and related features of the *outpatient management system* 118

Table 6.5 Typical supported hospital functions and related features of the *provider/physician order entry* (*POE*) *system* 119

Table 6.6 Typical supported hospital functions and related features of the *patient data management system* 121

Table 6.7 Typical supported hospital functions and related features of the *operation management system* 123

Table 6.8 Typical supported hospital functions and related features of the "radiology information system" (RIS) 125

Table 6.9 Typical supported hospital functions and related features of the "radiology information system" (RIS) 126

Table 6.10 Typical supported hospital functions and related features of the *laboratory information system* (*LIS*) 128

Table 6.11 Typical supported hospital functions and related features of the *enterprise resource planning system* 129

Table 6.12 Typical supported hospital functions and related features of the *data warehouse system* 131

Table 6.13 Typical supported hospital functions and related features of the *document archiving system* 133

Table 6.14 Further specific application components in hospital information systems (HIS) 134

Table 8.1 The matrix SUP for EF and AC. The matrix is illustrated in Fig. 8.6 231

Table 8.2 $isup_p$ 232

Table 8.3 Vector $\overrightarrow{ISUP}^{min}$ 235

Table 9.1 Dimensions to be considered for *operational information management* of the computer-based part of hospital information systems 246

Table 9.2 Structure of the strategic information management plan (2010–2015) of the Plötzberg Medical Center and Medical School (PMC) 262

Table 9.3 Extract from the PMC HIS benchmarking report 2010 (KPI = key performance indicator) 269

Table 9.4 Examples of CCHIT functional criteria for medication ordering 271

Table 10.1 Attributes for the description of health care networks 285

About the Authors

Alfred Winter

Alfred Winter is Professor for Medical Informatics at the Institute for Medical Informatics, Statistics, and Epidemiology of the University of Leipzig, Germany.

He studied informatics at the Technical University in Aachen, Germany, and received his Ph.D. and a license for lecturing (German "Habilitation") for medical informatics from the Faculty of Theoretical Medicine at the University of Heidelberg.

His research focuses on methods and modeling tools for the management of health information systems. He teaches information management in healthcare in a medical informatics masters course at Leipzig University and in master programs for health care management and for health information management at the private Dresden International University in Dresden. He works as a consultant and is responsible for coordinated strategic information management at Leipzig University Hospital and Leipzig University Medical Faculty. He is member of the board of the German professional association of medical informaticians (BVMI), member of the board of the joint medical informatics division of the German Association of Medical Informatics, Biometry and Epidemiology (GMDS) and the German Association of Informatics (GI) and chair of their working group "Methods and tools for the management of hospital information systems."

Reinhold Haux

Reinhold Haux is Professor for Medical Informatics and Director of the Peter L. Reichertz Institute for Medical Informatics of the University of Braunschweig – Institute of Technology and of Hannover Medical School, Germany.

He studied Medical Informatics at the University of Heidelberg/University of Applied Sciences Heilbronn, Germany, where he graduated as M.Sc. (German "Diplom") in 1978. He received a Ph.D. from the Faculty for Theoretical Medicine, University of Ulm, in 1983 and a Postdoctoral Lecture Qualification (German "Habilitation") for Medical Informatics and Statistics from the Medical Faculty of RWTH Aachen University in 1987.

His current research fields are health information systems and management and health-enabling technologies. Since its start in 2001, the international Frank-van Swieten-Lectures on Strategic Information Management in Hospitals are part of his teaching activities. Reinhold Haux was and is chairperson or member of IT strategy boards of various hospitals in Germany and Austria, among others of the Heidelberg (1989–2001) and Erlangen

University Medical Centers (1999–2001), of TILAK (2002–2004), of Braunschweig Medical Center (since 2005), and of Hannover Medical School (since 2007). He is Editor of *Methods of Information in Medicine* and, for the term 2007–2010, President of the International Medical Informatics Association (IMIA).

Elske Ammenwerth

Elske Ammenwerth is professor for health informatics and head of the Institute for Health Information Systems at the University for Health Sciences, Medical Informatics and Technology (UMIT) in Hall in Tyrol, Austria.

She studied medical informatics at the University of Heidelberg/University of Applied Sciences Heilbronn, Germany. Between 1997 and 2001, she worked as a research assistant at the Institute for Medical Biometry and Informatics at the University of Heidelberg, Germany. In Heidelberg, her work comprised the evaluation of hospital information systems, nursing informatics, and requirements analysis for hospital information systems. In 2000, she received her Ph.D. from the Medical Faculty of the University of Heidelberg for her work on requirements modeling.

At UMIT, she works on the electronic health record, electronic medication systems, evaluation methods, nursing informatics, and on process modeling and optimization. She regularly lectures on hospital information systems and their management, on evaluation of information systems, and on project management.

Elske Ammenwerth is Austrian representative within EFMI, the European Federation for Medical Informatics, and within IMIA, the International Medical Informatics Association. She is also heading the EFMI working group "Assessment of Health Information Systems."

Birgit Brigl

Birgit Brigl is currently responsible for the service management of the IT full service provider of the German Federal Ministry of Finance. Earlier, she worked as a research scientist at the Institute of Medical Informatics, Statistics, and Epidemiology of the University of Leipzig, Germany. Her research interests cover the management of hospital information systems, with a special focus on hospital information systems modeling and IT service management.

She studied medical informatics at the University of Heidelberg/University of Applied Sciences, Heilbronn, Germany. Between 1992 and 1998 she worked as a research assistant at the Institute for Medical Biometry and Informatics at the University of Heidelberg, focusing on the integration of decision support systems in hospital information systems. In 1997, she received her Ph.D. from the Faculty of Theoretical Medicine at the University of Heidelberg for her work on knowledge acquisition.

Nils Hellrung

Nils Hellrung is senior researcher at the Peter L. Reichertz Institute for Medical Informatics of the University of Braunschweig – Institute of Technology and of Hannover Medical School, Germany.

He studied industrial engineering at the Berlin – Institute of Technology, Germany, where he graduated as a degreed engineer in 2003 and Medical Informatics at the Health and Life Science University Hall/Tyrol, Austria, where he graduated as M.Sc. in 2005. He received a Ph.D. from Peter L. Reichertz Institute for Medical Informatics of the University of Braunschweig – Institute of Technology and of Hannover Medical School in 2009.

His current research fields are health information systems and management with a focus on transinstitutional information management and health care networks. Since its start in 2008 he is coordinator for the publicly funded project PAGE (Platform for Integration of Health Enabling Technologies in Health Care Networks).

Franziska Jahn

Franziska Jahn is research assistant at the Institute for Medical Informatics, Statistics and Epidemiology of the University of Leipzig, Germany.

She studied computer science with medical informatics as main subject at the University of Leipzig and graduated in 2008. Her research focuses on hospital information system architectures and their management. She currently works on her Ph.D. thesis about process benchmarking of hospital information systems. She teaches medical informatics students and coordinates their education at the University of Leipzig.

She organizes annual Ph.D. students' symposia of the German Association of Medical Informatics, Biometry and Epidemiology (GMDS).

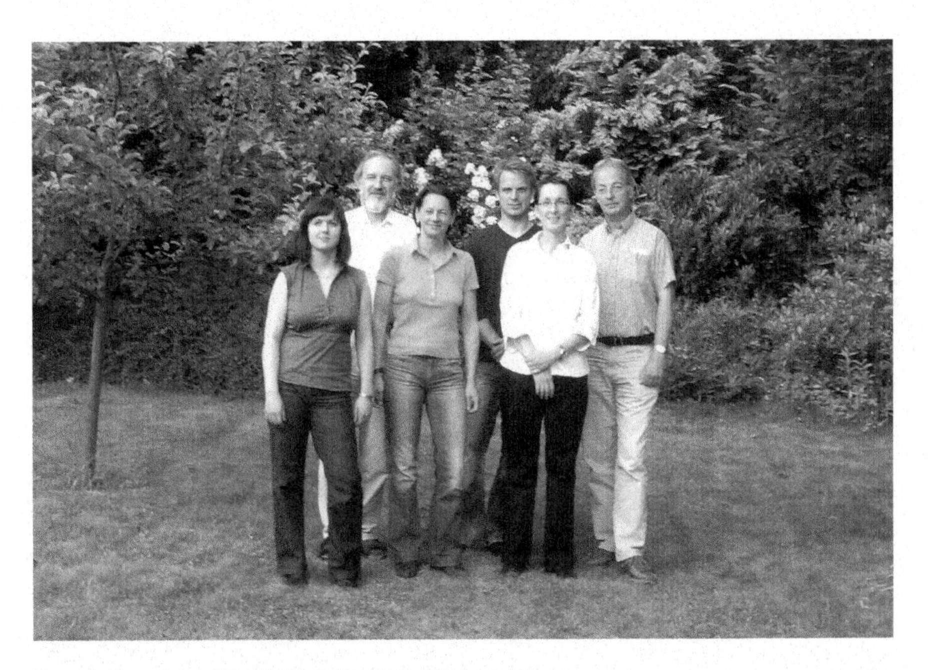

From left to right: F.J., R.H., B.B., N.H., E.A., A.W.

1 Introduction

What is a health information system? The literature defines health information systems (HIS) in many different ways and presents various views. Some articles focus on the organizational aspects of information processing, while others focus on the technology used. To begin with, we understand a health information system as the information processing and information storing subsystem of a health care organization, which may be a single institution, for example, a hospital, or a group of health care institutions like a health care network.

This book discusses the significance of information processing in health care, with an emphasis on information processing in hospitals, the progress in information and communication technology, and the importance of systematic information management. Nearly all people working in health care institutions have an enormous demand for information, which has to be fulfilled in order to achieve high-quality and efficient patient care. For example, physicians and nurses need information concerning the health status of patients from different departments of their hospital. They also need current medical knowledge as a basis for their clinical decisions. In addition, the management of a hospital needs up-to-date information about the hospital's costs and services. Of course, the quality of information processing is important for the competitiveness of a hospital. Consequently, this system of information processing can be regarded as the memory and nervous system of the respective health care institution.

The subject of information processing is quite complex. Nearly all groups and all areas in a health care institution depend on the quality of information processing. The amount of information processing is tremendous. Additionally, the information needs of the different groups are often based on the same data. Therefore, integrated information processing is necessary. If health information systems are not systematically managed and operated, they tend to develop chaotically. This, in turn, leads to negative consequences such as low data quality, resulting in low quality of patient care and increasing costs. Systematic information management can help to prevent such HIS failures and contribute to a high-quality and efficient patient care.

Well-educated specialists in health informatics/medical informatics, with the knowledge and skills to systematically manage and operate health information systems are therefore needed to appropriately and responsibly apply information and communication technology to the complex information processing environment of health care settings.

This book discusses the typical architectures of health information systems and their systematic strategic management. A lot of examples will show how certain methods and

A. Winter et al., *Health Information Systems*,
DOI: 10.1007/978-1-84996-441-8_1,

tools can be used to describe and assess architectures of health information systems and to support the various information management tasks in an integrated fashion.

This textbook addresses you as a health care and health/medical informatics professional as well as a student in health/medical informatics and health information management. It should be regarded as an introduction to this complex subject. For a deeper understanding, you will need additional knowledge and, foremost, practice in this field.

If you are not familiar with patient care and medical research, you can find an introductory chapter to health institutions and their respective information processing tasks. If you are not familiar with information systems, you can find an introductory chapter to information system basics.

We want to provide you with a terminology about health information systems which is as complete and sound as possible. To support this, we compiled a catalog of the most important terms as a thesaurus at the end of the book. The terms cataloged are underlined in the text, where they are explained. If you find terms which are printed in italics, these terms will refer to

- actions to be undertaken in health care in order to process data and information and to thereby contribute to the mission of health care (i.e., hospital functions).
- computer-based tools to support professionals in health care to undertake these actions (i.e., application components).

You will find explanations of the respective terms in Sects. 6.3, 6.4.

After reading this book, you should be able to answer the following questions:

- Why is systematic information processing in health care institutions important?
- What are appropriate models for health information systems?
- How do health information systems look like and what architectures are appropriate?
- How can we assess the quality of health information systems?
- How can we strategically manage health information systems?

In the end, we are confident that you will be able to answer the question "How can good information systems be designed and maintained?"

If you are a lecturer, we would like to support you by some supplementary materials based on the book which can be downloaded from http://www.3lgm2.de/en/Publications/Materials/HealthInformationSystems.jsp."

Health Institutions and Information Processing

2

2.1 Introduction

Health information systems strongly influence quality and efficiency of health care, and technical progress offers advanced opportunities to support health care. In this chapter, we will discuss the interrelation between health information systems on one side and health care on the other side.
After reading this chapter, you should be able to answer the following questions:

- What is the significance of information systems for health care?
- How does technical progress affect health care?
- Why is systematic information management important?

2.2 Significance of Information Processing in Health care

2.2.1 Information Processing as Quality Factor

Decisions of health care professionals are based on vast amounts of information about the patient's health state. It is essential for the quality of patient care and for the quality of hospital management to fulfill these information needs.

When a patient is admitted to a hospital, a physician or nurse first needs information about the reason for patient admission and the patient history. Later, she or he needs results from services such as laboratory and radiology (Fig. 2.1), which are some of the most frequent diagnostic procedures. In general, clinical patient-related information should be available on time, and it should be up-to-date and valid. For example, the recent laboratory report should be available on the ward within 2 h after the request. If this is not the case, if it comes too late, or is old or even wrong, quality of care and patient safety is at risk. An incorrect laboratory report may lead to erroneous and even harmful treatment decisions. Additionally, if examinations have to be repeated or lost findings have to be searched for, the costs of health care may increase. Information should be documented adequately, enabling health care professionals to access the information needed and to make sound decisions.

A. Winter et al., *Health Information Systems*,
DOI: 10.1007/978-1-84996-441-8_2, © Springer-Verlag London Limited 2011

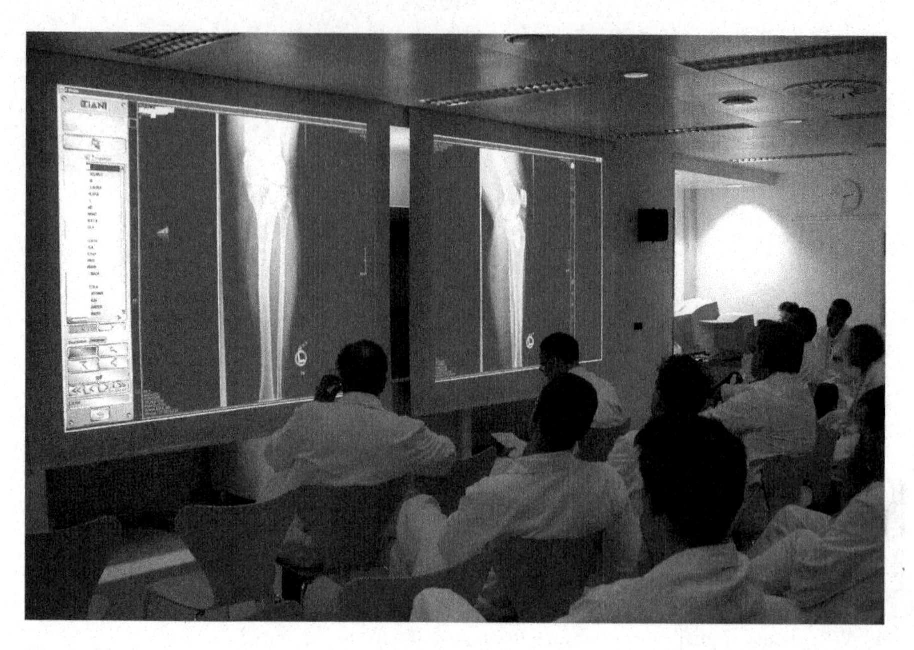

Fig. 2.1 Radiological conference in a radiodiagnostic department

People working in hospital administration also must be well informed in order to carry out their tasks. They should be informed timely and receive current information. If the information flow is too slow, bills are written days or even weeks after the patient's discharge. If information is missing, payable services cannot be billed, and the hospital's income will be reduced. For example, under certain circumstances, the amount payable by the health insurance is reduced, if the invoice from the hospital arrives after a certain deadline.

Hospital management also has an enormous information need. Up-to-date information about costs and proceeds are necessary as a basis for controlling the enterprise. Information about the quality of patient care is equally important, for example, about the form and severity of patients' illnesses, about nosocomial infections, or about complication rates of therapeutic procedures. If this information is not accurate, not on time, or incomplete, the hospital's work cannot be controlled adequately, increasing the risks of management errors.

Thus, information processing is an important quality factor in health care and, in particular, in hospitals.

2.2.2 Information Processing as Cost Factor

In 2007, member states of the Organization for Economic Cooperation and Development (OECD) spent between 6 and 15% of their total gross domestic product (GDP) on health care.[1]

[1] Organization for Economic Co-operation and Development (OECD). OECD Health Data 2008. Statistics and Indicators for 30 countries. http://www.oecd.org

In 2006, the costs for the approximately 2,100 German hospitals with their 510,000 beds amounted to €60 billion; 1.1 million people worked in these organizations in Germany, and 17 million inpatients were treated.[2] In the USA, hospital spending was nearly $600 billion. The overall US national health expenditure reached $2.2 trillion in 2007, and accounted for 16.2% of the Gross Domestic Product.[3]

A relevant percentage of those costs is spent on information processing. However, the total percentage of information processing can only be estimated. Already in the 1960s, studies observed that 25% of a hospital's costs are due to (computer-based and non-computer-based) information processing.[4] However, such an estimate depends on the definition of information processing. In general, the investment costs (including purchase, adaptation, introduction, and training) must be distinguished from the operating costs (including continued maintenance and support as well as staff), and the costs for computer-based from the costs for non-computer-based information processing (which still are often much higher in hospitals).

Looking at computer-based information processing, the annual budget that health care institutions spend on information and communication technology (ICT) (including computer systems, computer networks, and computer-based application components) was in 2006 between 2.5% and 3.3% of the total hospital operating expense, depending on the number of beds.[5] In many hospitals, the annual budget is even lower. Most hospital chief information officers (CIOs) expect an increasing budget.[6]

When looking at non-computer-based information processing (see Fig. 2.2, for example), the numbers become increasingly vague. However, we can expect that, for example, the annual operating costs (including personnel costs) for a non-computer-based archive, storing about 300,000–400,000 new patients records each year, may easily amount to more than €500,000. A typical, standardized, machine-readable form, including two carbon copies (a radiology order, for example) costs approximately €0.50. A typical inpatient record at a university hospital consists of about 40 documents.

Based on these figures, it becomes apparent that information processing in health care is an important cost factor and considerably significant for a national economy. It is clear that, on the one hand, efficient information processing offers vast potential for cost reductions. On the other hand, inefficient information processing leads to cost increases.

---

[2]Federal Statistical Office. Statistical Yearbook 2008 for the Federal Republic of Germany. http://www.destatis.de

[3]US Department for Health and Human Services. National Health Expenditure Data 2007. http://www.cms.hhs.gov/NationalHealthExpendData

[4]Jydstrup R, Gross M. Cost of information handling in hospitals. Health Services Research 1966; 1:235–71.

[5]Healthcare Information and Management Systems Society (HIMSS): 2007 Annual Report of the US Hospital IT Market. http://marketplace.himss.org

[6]Healthcare Information and Management Systems Society (HIMSS). The 19th Annual 2008 HIMSS Leadership Survey CIO Results Final Report. 2000. http://www.himss.org

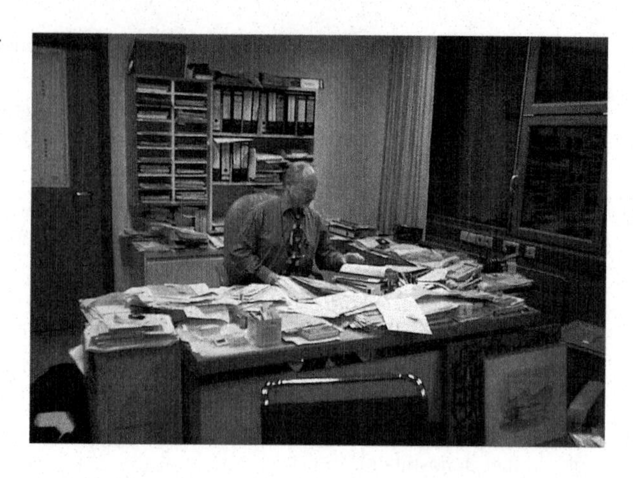

Fig. 2.2 The office of a senior physician

2.2.3 Information as Productivity Factor

In the nineteenth century, many societies were characterized by rising industry and industrial production. By the second half of the twentieth century, the idea of communicating and processing data by means of computers and computer networks was already emerging. Today we speak of the twenty-first century as the century of information technology, or of an "information society." Informatics and information and communication technology (ICT) are playing a key role. Information, bound to a medium of matter or energy, but largely independent of place and time, shall be made available to people at any time and in any place imaginable. Information shall find its way to people, not vice versa.

Today, information belongs to the most important productivity factors of a hospital. Productivity is defined as a ratio of output and input. All resources like personnel, medical devices, etc. are part of the input. Therefore, from an economic point of view, productivity of a hospital might be defined as the ratio of the number of cases and full-time employees. If, however, output is considered as quality of patient care, it is much more difficult to calculate productivity. Therefore, a lot of reliable clinical data are needed. For high-quality patient care and economic management of a hospital, it is essential that the hospital information system can make correct information fully available on time. This is also increasingly important for the competitiveness of hospitals.

2.2.4 Holistic View of the Patient

Information processing in a hospital should offer a comprehensive, holistic view of the patient and of the hospital. "Holistic" in this context means to have a complete picture of the care of a patient available, independent of the health care institutions

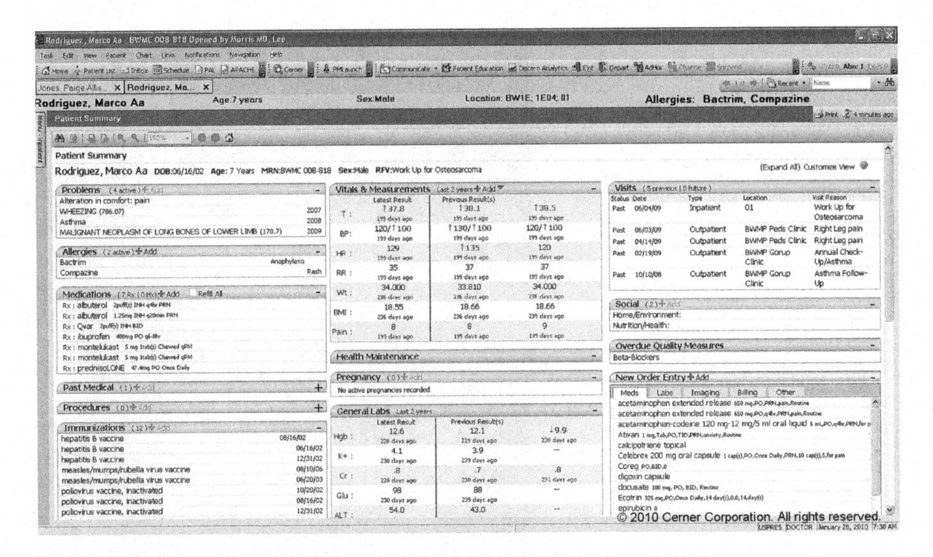

Fig. 2.3 An example of the patient summary within an electronic patient record

and hospital departments in which the patient has been or will be treated. This holistic view on the patient can reduce undesired consequences of highly specialized medicine with various departments and health care professionals involved in patient care. Despite highly differentiated diagnostics and therapy, and the multitude of people and areas in a hospital, adequate information processing (and a good hospital information system) can help to make information about a patient available completely (Fig. 2.3). As specialization in medicine and health care increases, so does the fragmentation of information, which makes combining information into such a holistic view more and more necessary. However, it must be clearly ensured that only authorized personnel can access patient data and data about the hospital as an enterprise.

2.2.5 Hospital Information System as Memory and Nervous System

Figuratively speaking, a hospital information system might be regarded as the memory and the nervous system of a hospital. A hospital information system, comprising the information processing and storage in a hospital (Figs. 2.4 and 2.5), to a certain extent can be compared to the information processing of a human being. The hospital information system also receives, transmits, processes, stores, and presents information. The quality of a hospital information system is essential for a hospital, again figuratively, in order to be able to adequately recognize and store facts, to remember them, and to act on them.

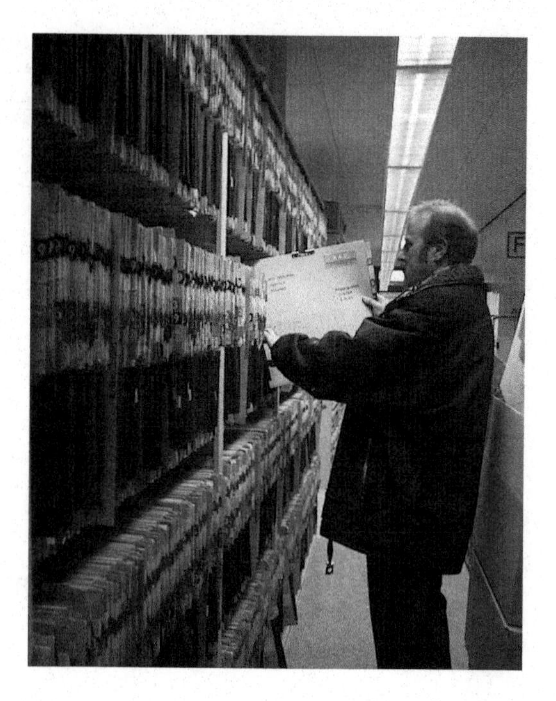

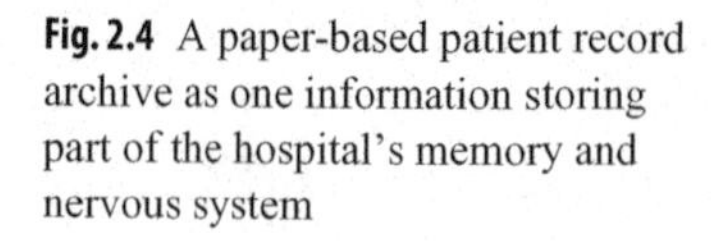

Fig. 2.4 A paper-based patient record archive as one information storing part of the hospital's memory and nervous system

2.3 Progress in Information and Communication Technology

2.3.1 Impact on the Quality of Health Care

Progress in information and communication technology (ICT) changes societies and affects the costs and quality of information processing in health care. It is thus useful to take a look at the world of information and communication technology.

Tremendous improvements in diagnostics have been made available by modern technology, for example, in the area of medical signal and image processing. Magnetic resonance imaging and computer tomography, for example, would not have been possible without improvements in information processing and information methodology and without modern information and communication technology (see Fig. 2.6). Improved diagnostics then lead to an improvement in therapy. Some therapies, for example, in neurosurgery or radiotherapy, are possible mainly due to the progress in ICT. The same is true in the field of medical biotechnology: the development of new drug agents, research in molecular principles of diseases, and the resulting new patient-specific therapeutic option enable a better treatment of patients.

Nowadays, clinical research can to an increasing degree be conducted with success, and be internationally competitive, only if carried out on an interdisciplinary, often also

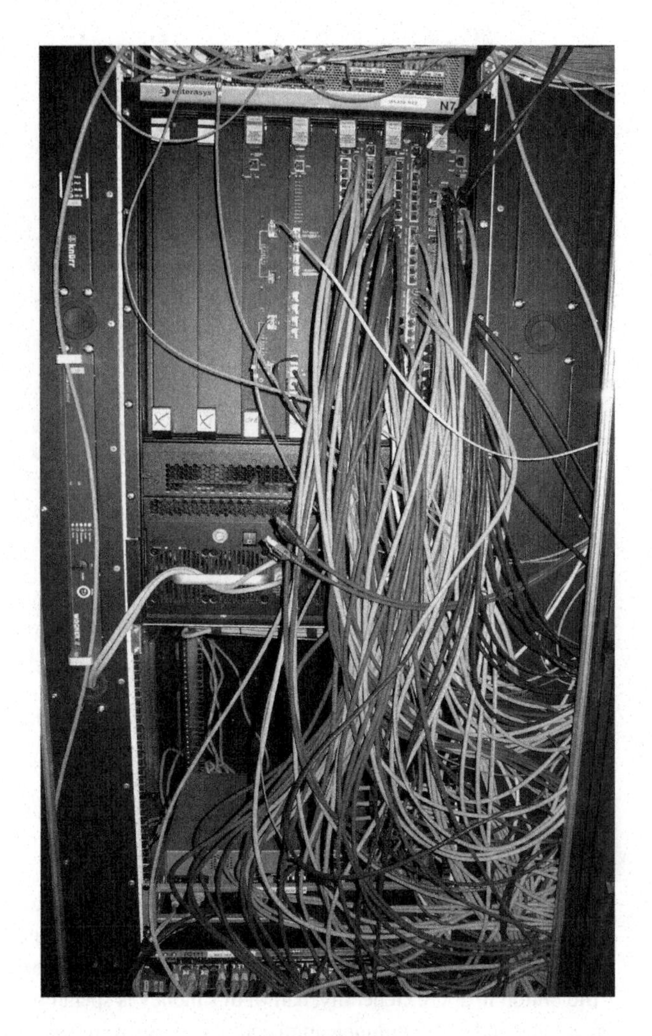

Fig. 2.5 Snapshot in a server room of a hospital showing the computer-based nerve cords of the hospital's memory and nervous system

inter-regional or international, and collaborative basis. This collaboration has been and is fostered by integrated systems of information technology. The translation of medical research outcomes into new therapies needs tight information exchange from "bench" to "bed", that is, from research to patient care. Vice versa information about experiences with therapies is collected by computer-based tools within clinical trials and is resent to and carefully analyzed at research institutions.

Important progress due to improvements in modern ICT can also be observed in information systems of health care organizations. The role of computer-based information systems, together with clinical documentation and knowledge-based decision support systems, can hardly be overestimated in respect to the quality of health care, as the volume of data available today is much greater than it was a few years ago.

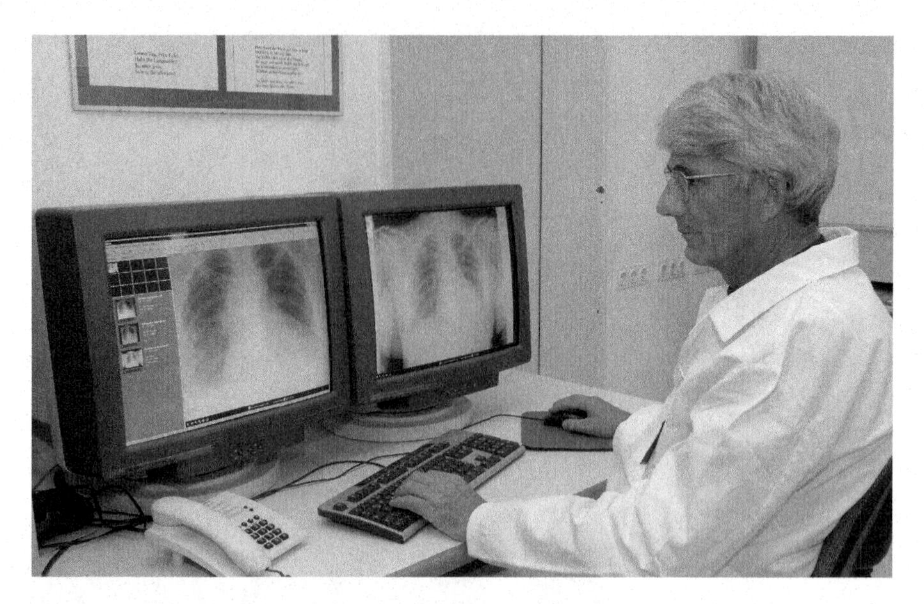

Fig. 2.6 Physician using a picture archiving and communication system for diagnostics

2.3.2 Impact on Economics

For many countries, the vision of an "information society" has become a reality. Nearly every modern economic branch is shaped by information processing and information and communication technology.

The worldwide information and communication technology market volume is estimated at nearly €2.5 trillion in 2009 with a growth rate of about 5% per year.[7] Germany's expected total annual turnover on information and communication technology was approximately €146 billion in 2008. Generally, half of this money is spent on information technology (data processing and data communication equipment, software, and related services) and the other half on communication technology (telecommunication equipment and related services).[8]

ICT has become a major factor for quality and efficiency of health care worldwide. ICT in health care also emerged to a leading industry branch. The percentage of health care ICT on the worldwide ICT market is difficult to estimate. The following numbers may indicate the significance of ICT in health care: In the U.S. the estimated total expenditures of ICT equipment and software in health care were about $21 billion in 2007, which is 8.1% of the total US ICT expenditures.[9] Reports from the European Union (EU)

[7]European Information Technology Observatory (EITO). ICT Market Overview. http://www.eito.com/reposi/FreeDataSheets/ICT-MarketOverview-world

[8]Bitkom. http://www.bitkom.de

[9]US Census Bureau. Information & Communication Technology Survey. http://www.census.gov/csd/ict

state that the eHealth industry in the EU (defined as comprising clinical information systems, telemedicine and homecare, and regional networks) was estimated "to be worth close to €21 billion in 2006" and that the global eHealth industry "has the potential to be the third largest industry in the health sector with a global turnover of €50–60 billion."[10] Many countries established programs to force information and communication technology especially in the eHealth segment with investment volumes between $50 million and $11.5 billion.[11]

One might have doubts about the validity of these rather rough numbers. However, they all exemplify the following: There is a significant and increasing economic relevance not only for information and communication technology in general but also in health care.

2.3.3 Changing Health Care

Now once more, what changes in health care do we expect through information and communication technology?

The developments mentioned will probably continue into the next decade at least at the same rate as given today. The development of information and communication technology will continue to have a considerable effect on our societies in general and on our health care systems in particular.[12]

The use of computer-based tools in health care is dramatically increasing, and new technologies such as mobile devices and multifunctional bedside terminals will proliferate. Those mobile information processing tools offer both communication and information processing features. Wireless networks are standard in many hospitals. Computer-based training systems strongly support efficient learning for health care professionals. Documentation efforts are continuously rising and lead to more sophisticated computer-based documentation tools (see Fig. 2.7). Decision support tools, for example, in the context of drug prescription, support high-quality care. Communication is increasingly supported by electronic means. The globalization of providing health care and the cooperation of health care professionals is increasing, and patients and health care professionals seek reliable health information on the Internet. Large health databases are available for everyone at his or her work place and global companies offer personal health records worldwide for everyone. Providing high-quality and efficient health care will continue to be strongly correlated with high-quality information and communication technology and a

---

[10]European Communities. Accelerating the Development of the eHealth Market in Europe. 2007. Luxembourg: Office for Official Publications of the European Communities; 2007. http://ec.europa.eu/information_society/activities/health/downloads/index_en.htm, last accessed May 20, 2009.

[11]G. F. Anderson, B. K. Frogner, R. A. Johns, U. E. Reinhardt, Healthcare Spending and Use of Information Technology in OECD Countries, Health Affairs, May/June 2006 25(3):819–31.

[12]President's Information Technology Advisory Committee (PITAC). Transforming Healthcare Through Information Technology – PITAC report to the president. Arlington: Nation Coordination Office for Computing; 2001.

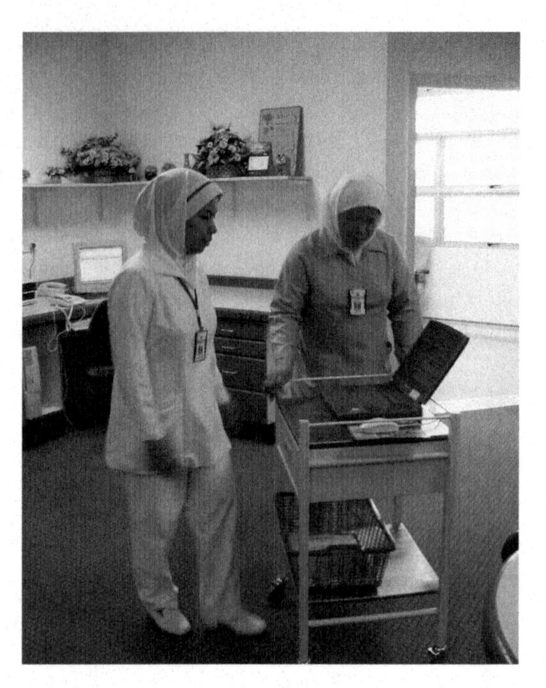

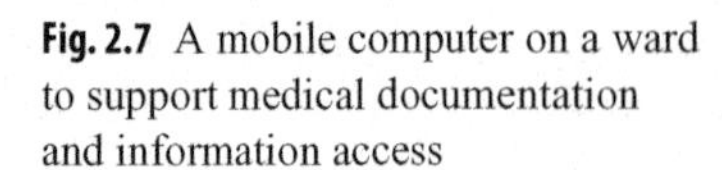

Fig. 2.7 A mobile computer on a ward to support medical documentation and information access

sound methodology for systematically processing information. However, the newest information and communication technologies do not guarantee high-quality information processing. Both information processing technologies and methodologies must adequately and responsibly be applied and, as will be pointed out later on, systematically managed.

2.4 Importance of Systematic Information Management

2.4.1 Affected People and Areas

Nearly all people and all areas of a hospital are affected by the quality of the information system, as most of them need various types of information (e.g., about the patient) in their daily work. The patient can certainly profit most from high-quality information processing since it contributes to the quality of patient care and to reducing costs.

The professional groups working in a hospital, especially physicians, nurses, and administrative personnel, and others are also directly affected by the quality of the information system. As they spend 25% or even more of their time on information handling, they directly profit from good and efficient information processing. However, they will also feel the consequences if information processing is poor.

2.4.2 Amount of Information Processing

The amount of information processing in hospitals, especially in larger ones, should not be underestimated. Let us look at a typical German university medical center. It is an enterprise encompassing staff of approximately 4,500 people, an annual budget of approximately €250 million, and, as a maximum care facility, numerous tasks in research, education, and patient care. It consists of up to 60 departments and up to 100 wards with up to 1,500 beds and about 100 outpatient units. Annually, approximately, 50,000 inpatients and 250,000 outpatients are treated, and 20,000 operation reports, 250,000 discharge letters, 20,000 pathology reports, 100,000 microbiology reports, 200,000 radiology reports, and 800,000 clinical chemistry reports are written.

Each year, approximately 300,000–400,000 new patient records, summing up to approximately eight million pieces of paper, are created (Fig. 2.8). When stored in a paper-based way, an annual record volume of approximately 1,500 m is generated. In Germany, for example, they should be archived over a period of 30 years. When stored digitally, the annual data volume needed is expected to be around 10–15 terabytes, including digital images and digital signals.

The computer-based tools of a university medical center encompass more than hundred of the computer-based application components, thousands of workstations and other

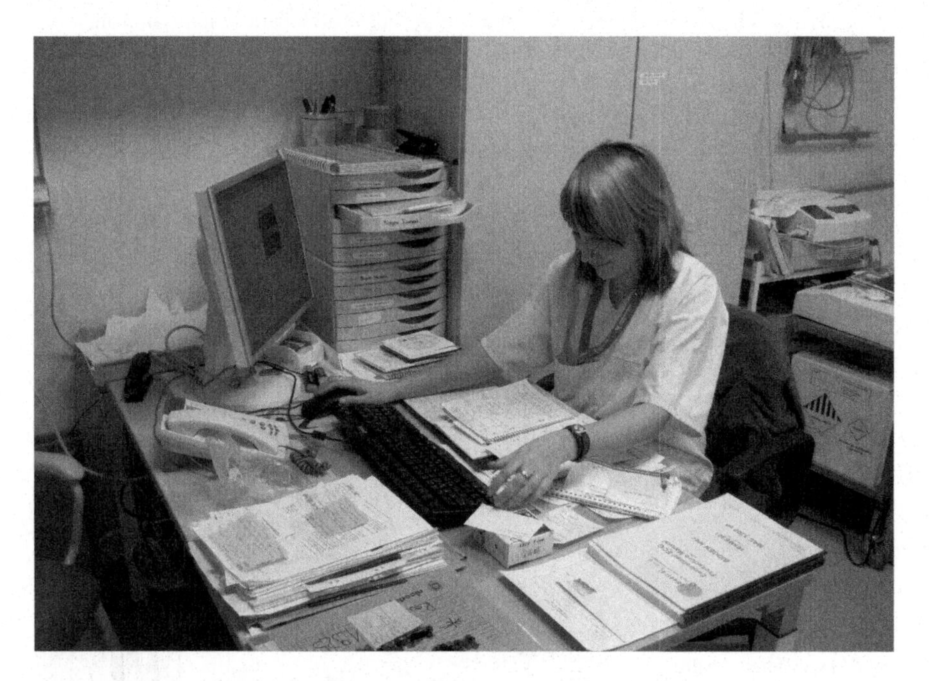

Fig. 2.8 A study nurse in an outpatient unit dealing with a multitude of paper-based forms

terminals, and more than hundred servers (larger computer systems that offer services and features to other computer systems), and the respective network.

The numbers in the majority of hospitals are much smaller. In larger ones we will find, for example, about ten departments with 600 beds and about 20,000 inpatients every year. In industrialized countries 1,500 staff members would work there, and the annual budget of the hospital would be about €80 million. Especially in rural areas, we can also find hospitals with only one department and fewer than 50 beds.

2.4.3 Sharing the Same Data

There are different reasons for pursuing holistic and integrated information processing. The most important reason is that various groups of health care professionals within and outside health care institutions need the same data (Fig. 2.9).

For example, a surgeon in a hospital documents the diagnoses and therapies of an operated patient in an operation report. This report serves as basis for the discharge letter. The discharge letter is also an important document to communicate with the admitting institution, normally a general practitioner. Diagnosis and therapy are also important for statistics about patient care and for quality management. Equally, they contain important information for the systematic nursing care of a patient. Diagnostic and therapeutic data are also relevant for billing.

In Germany, for example, some basic administrative data must be communicated to the respective health insurance company online within 3 days after patient admission and after discharge. In a coded form, they are the basis for accounting. Additionally, managing and controlling a hospital is possible only if the cost (such as consumption of materials or drugs) of the treatment can be compared to the characteristics and severity of the illness, characterized by diagnosis and therapy.

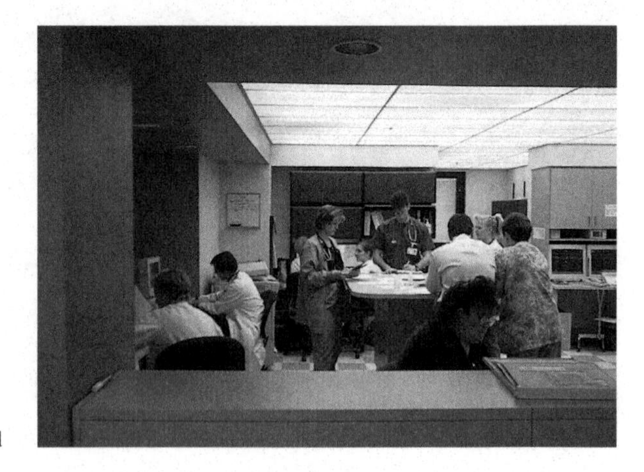

Fig. 2.9 Regular clinical round by different health care professionals on a ward

2.4.4 Integrated Information Processing to Satisfy Information Needs

Information processing has to integrate the partly overlapping information needs of the different groups and areas of a hospital (see Fig. 2.10).

Systematic, integrated information processing in a hospital has advantages not only for the patient, but also for the health care professionals, the health insurance companies, and the hospital owners. If information processing is not conducted globally across institutions, but locally, for example, in professional groups (physicians, nurses, and administrative staff) or areas (clinical departments, institutes, and administration), this corresponds to traditional separation politics and leads to isolated information processing groups, such as "the administration" or "the clinic." In this case, the quality of the hospital information system clearly decreases while the costs for information processing increase due to the necessity for multiple data collection and analysis. Finally, this has disadvantages for the patient and, when seen from a national economical point of view, for the whole population.

However, integration of information processing should consider not only information processing in one health care organization, but also information processing among different institutions (such as integrated health care delivery systems). The achievements of modern medicine, particularly in the field of acute diseases, have led to the paradoxical result that chronic diseases and multimorbidity increasingly gain in relevance. Among other reasons, this is due to more people being able to live to old age. Moreover, in many

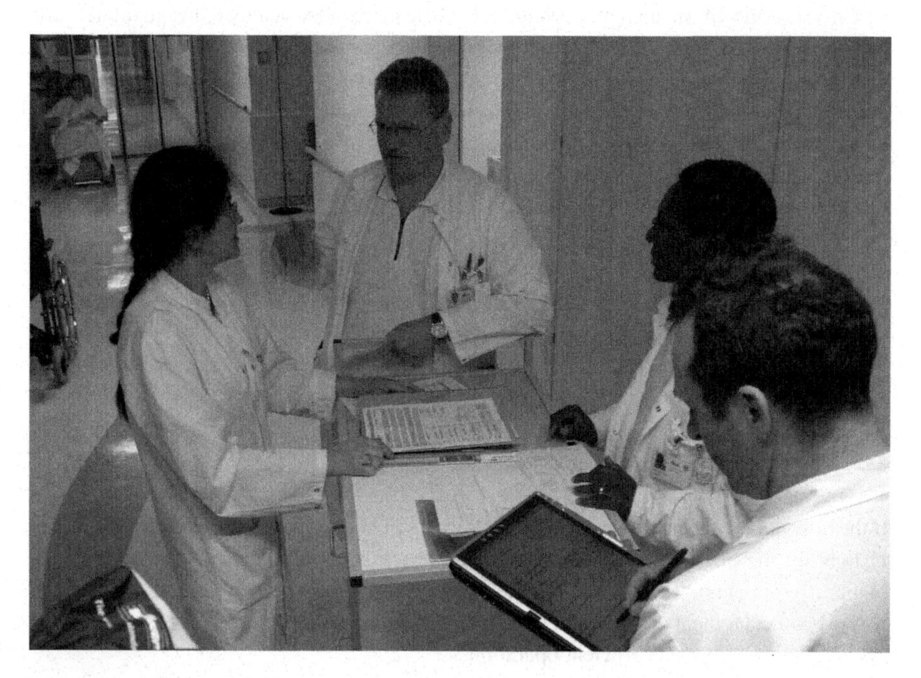

Fig. 2.10 During a ward round: Health care professionals jointly using information processing tools

countries, an increasing willingness to switch doctors and a higher regional mobility exist among patients. The degree of highly specialized and distributed patient care creates a great demand for integrated information processing among health care professionals and among health care institutions such as hospitals, general practices, laboratories, etc. In turn, this raises the need for more comprehensive documentation and efficient, comprehensive information systems.

2.4.5 Raising the Quality of Patient Care and Reducing Costs

Systematic information processing is the key factor for raising quality and reducing costs. What does "systematic" mean in this context? "Unsystematic" can, in a positive sense, mean creative, spontaneous, or flexible. However, "unsystematic" can also mean chaotic, purposeless, and ineffective, and also entail high costs compared to the benefits gained.

"Systematic" in this context means purposeful and effective, and with great benefit regarding the costs. Bearing this in mind, it is obvious that information processing in a health care institution should be managed systematically. Due to the importance of information processing as a quality and cost factor, an institution has to invest systematically in its health information system. These investments deal with both staff and tools for information processing. They aim at increasing quality of patient care and at reducing costs.

Unsystematic information processing normally leads to a low quality of health information systems, and the information needs of the staff and departments cannot be adequately satisfied. When health information systems are not systematically managed, they tend to develop in a chaotic way. This has severe consequences: decreased data quality, and higher costs, especially for tools and information processing staff, not to mention aspects such as data protection and data security violation. Even worse, insufficiently managed information systems can contribute to breakdowns in established clinical workflows, to a reduced efficiency of care, to user boycott, to decreased quality of care and – in the end – even endanger patient safety.

To adequately process information and apply information and communication technology, knowledge and skills for these tasks are required.

2.4.6 Basis of Systematic Information Processing

If the hospital management decides to invest in systematic information processing (and not in fighting the effects of chaotic information processing, which normally means much higher investments), it decides to manage the hospital information system in a systematic way. The management of a hospital information system forms and controls the information system, and it ensures its efficient operation.

2.5 Examples

2.5.1 Knowledge Access to Improve Patient Care

Imagine the following situation: Ursula B. was pregnant with quintuplets. She had already spent more than 5 months in a University Medical Center. She had to spend most of this time lying in bed. During the course of her pregnancy, her physical problems increased. From the 28th week on, she suffered severe respiratory distress.

Professor L., the pediatrician, who was also involved in her treatment, had the following question: What are the chances of the infants being born healthy at this gestational age?

He went to a computer, which is connected to the computer network of the University Medical Center. The physician called up a function "knowledge access" and, as application component, a literature database (MEDLINE[13]), which contains the current state of the art of medical knowledge worldwide (Fig. 2.11).

The following information resulted from this knowledge access: Several publications stated that only slim chances exist for all infants to survive in good health. If they are born during the 28th week of pregnancy, the chance for survival is about 15%. In case of birth during the 30th week, their chances would improve to about 75%. Also, according to the literature, further delay of the delivery does not improve the prognosis of the quintuplets.

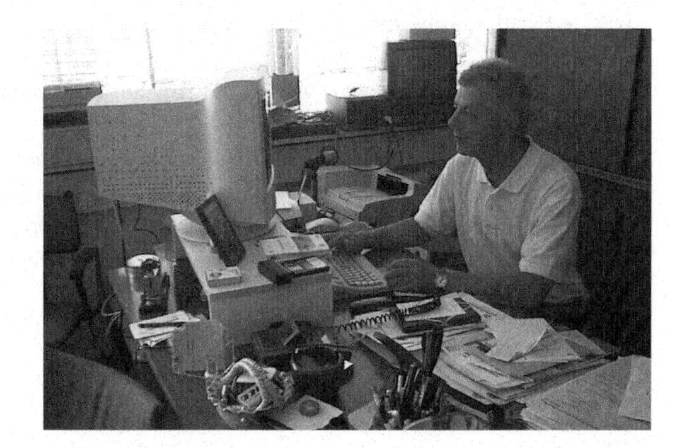

Fig. 2.11 Prof. L., Head of the Department of Pediatrics, working with a literature server

[13]Offered for free by the National Library of Medicine (NLM), Bethesda, USA, http://www.ncbi.nlm.nih.gov/entrez/query.fcgi

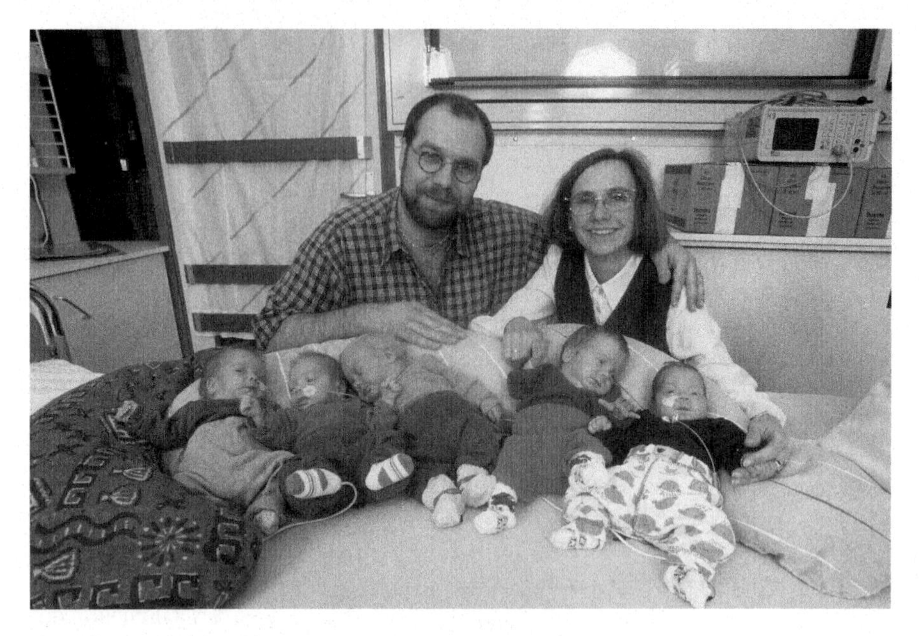

Fig. 2.12 The Heidelberg quintuplets

The physician discussed the results with the expectant mother. Despite her respiratory problems, she had the strength to endure 2 more weeks.

On January 21st of the respective year, the quintuplets were born well and healthy at the University Medical Center (Fig. 2.12). A team of 25 physicians, nurses, and midwives assisted during the delivery. Appropriate knowledge access was of crucial importance.

Today, knowledge access at a ward is in many hospitals an integrated part of a hospital information system.

You may wonder, in which year and in which medical center the quintuplets were born. It was in 1999 at the Heidelberg University Medical Center. Although this real example dates back more than 10 years we found it still worth to report on because it shows clearly how important it is to have information and knowledge available, and in this respect is pioneering for the future trends.

By the way, all quintuples are well and Prof. L., the attending physician, became their godfather.

2.5.2 Nonsystematic Information Processing in Clinical Registers

The following example shows what can happen when information processing is done in a nonsystematic (or, better, chaotic?) manner from yet another point of view.[14] Let us

[14]The example is based on a similar one in: Green SB, Byar DP. Using Observational Data from Registries to Compare Treatments: The Fallacy of Omnimetrics. Statistics in Medicine 1984;3:361–70.

Table 2.1 Example of Simpson's paradox – Success rates of Novum and Verum treatments for patients with diagnosis Δ, treated during the years δ at the Plötzberg Medical Center and Medical School (PMC)

	Success Yes	Success No	Σ	Success Rate
All patients				
Novum	333	1,143	1,476	(23%)
Verum	243	1,113	1,356	(18%)
Σ	576	2,256	2,832	
Male patients				
Novum	24	264	288	(8%)
Verum	147	906	1,053	(14%)
Σ	171	1,170	1,341	
Female patients				
Novum	309	879	1,188	(26%)
Verum	96	207	303	(32%)
Σ	405	1,086	1,491	

analyze a (fictitious) clinical register from the (fictitious) Plötzberg Medical Center and Medical School (PMC). PMC will be used in examples and exercises in this book.

Table 2.1 shows statistics with patients having diagnosis Δ, for example, rheumatism, and treated during the years δ, for example, 1991–2001, at PMC. The patients have either received standard therapy, Verum, or a new therapy, Novum.

Comparing the success rates of Novum and Verum, one might conclude that the new therapy is better than the standard therapy. Applying an appropriate statistical test would lead to a low p value and a significant result. The success rate was also analyzed by sex. This resulted in Verum leading in female patients as well as in male patients.

Is one of our conclusions erroneous? Or maybe both? What would a systematic design and analysis of such a register be? After looking at the data, one can identify a fairly simple reason for this so-called Simpson's paradox. The methodology for processing information systematically ought to prevent such errors; however, it is far more complex.

2.5.3 The WHO eHealth Resolution[15]

Nowadays computer-based information processing in health institutions and moreover health networks is referred to as eHealth. In its eHealth resolution, the World Health

[15]World Health Organization. eHealth Resolution. 58th World Health Assembly, Resolution 28. May 25, 2005. Geneva: WHO; 2005. 58th World Health Assembly's home page: http://www.emro.who.int/HIS/ehealth/PDF/EB115_R20-en.pdf

Organization (WHO) strongly recommends to systematically introduce, improve, and manage eHealth worldwide, which should lead to "eHealth for all by 2015."[16]

"The Fifty-Eighth World Health Assembly …

1. URGES Member States:
   1. to consider drawing up a long-term strategic plan for developing and implementing eHealth services that includes an appropriate legal framework and infrastructure and encourages public and private partnerships;
   2. to develop the infrastructure for information and communication technologies for health as deemed appropriate to promote equitable, affordable, and universal access to their benefits, and to continue to work with information telecommunication agencies and other partners to strive to reduce costs to make eHealth successful;
   3. to build on closer collaboration with the private and not-for-profit sectors in information and communication technologies, to further public services for health;
   4. to endeavor to reach communities, including vulnerable groups, with eHealth services appropriate to their needs;
   5. to mobilize multisectoral collaboration for determining evidence-based eHealth standards and norms, to evaluate eHealth activities, and to share the knowledge of cost effective models, thus ensuring quality, safety and ethical standards;
   6. to establish national centers and networks of excellence for eHealth best practice, policy coordination, and technical support for healthcare delivery, service improvement, information to citizens, capacity building, and surveillance;
   7. to consider establishing and implementing national public-health information systems and to improve, by means of information, the capacity for the surveillance of, and rapid response to, disease and public health emergencies.

2. REQUESTS the Director-General:
   1. to promote international, multisectoral collaboration with a view to improving compatibility of administrative and technical solutions in the area of eHealth;
   2. to document and analyze developments and trends, inform policy and practice in countries, and report regularly on use of eHealth worldwide;
   3. to provide technical support to Member States in relation to eHealth products and services by disseminating widely experiences and best practices, in particular on telemedicine technology; devising assessment methodologies; promoting research and development; and furthering standards through diffusion of guidelines;
   4. to facilitate the integration of eHealth in health systems and services, including in the training of health-care professionals and in capacity building, in order to improve access to, and quality and safety of, care;

[16]Healy JC. The WHO eHealth Resolution – eHealth for all by 2015? Methods Inf Med 2007; 46(1):2–4.

5. to continue the expansion to Member States of mechanisms such as the Health Academy which promote health awareness and healthy lifestyles through eLearning[17];
6. to provide support to Member States to promote the development, application and management of national standards of health information; and to collect and collate available information on standards with a view to establishing national standardized health information systems in order to facilitate easy and effective exchange of information among Member States;
7. to support regional and interregional initiatives in the area of eHealth among groups of countries that speak a common language."

2.5.4 Estimated Impact of eHealth to Improve Quality and Efficiency of Patient Care

This example is taken from a study report presented by Gartner on behalf of the Swedish Ministry of Health and Social Affairs.[18]

This study analyzed the potential benefits of an increased usage of eHealth in six EU member states:

"...There is a significant healthcare improvement potential using eHealth as a catalyst.... Examples of quantified potentials include:

- Five million yearly outpatient prescription errors could be avoided through the use of Electronic Transfer of Prescriptions.
- 100,000 yearly inpatient adverse drug events could be avoided through Computerized Physician Order Entry and Clinical Decision Support. This would in turn free up 700,000 bed-days yearly, an opportunity for increasing throughput and decreasing waiting times, corresponding to a value of almost €300 million.
- 49,000 cases of inpatient Hospital Acquired Infections could be avoided every year collectively through the use of Business Intelligence and Data Mining for real time detection of in-hospital infections. This could increase availability by over 270,000 bed-days, resulting in opportunity savings of over €131 million.
- 11,000 deaths caused by complications related to diabetes could collectively be reduced through Electronic Medical Records with Chronic Disease Management capabilities.
- 5.6 million admissions to hospitals for chronically ill patients could be avoided collectively through the use of Telemedicine and Home Health Monitoring.
- Nine million bed-days yearly could be freed up through the use of Computer-Based Patient Records, an opportunity for either increasing throughput or decreasing waiting times, corresponding to a value of nearly €3.7 billion.

[17] eLearning is understood in this context to mean use of any electronic technology and media in support of learning.

[18] http://www.sweden.gov.se/content/1/c6/12/98/15/5b63bacb.pdf

- Patients can become more involved and accountable for the management of their chronic conditions through access to knowledge based best practices via an EMR with Chronic Disease Management capabilities and communication with their physicians through a Patient Portal.
- Patients can have more control on how and when to engage with their physicians through technologies such as Patient Portals and Personal Health Records that enable alternative ways of communication and consultation such as e-mail and e-visits."

2.6 Exercises

2.6.1 Amount of Information Processing in Typical Hospitals

Estimate the following figures for a typical university medical center and for a typical rural hospital. To solve this exercise, look at the strategic information management plan for information processing of a hospital, or proceed with your own local investigations.

- Number of (inpatient) clinical departments and institutes
- Number of wards and outpatient units
- Number of employees
- Annual budget
- Number of beds, inpatients, and outpatients per year
- Number of new patient records per year
- Number of discharge letters per year
- Number of computer servers, workstations, and terminals
- Number of operation reports, clinical chemistry reports, and radiology reports per year

2.6.2 Information Processing in Different Areas

Find three examples of information processing for each of the following areas in a hospital, taking into account the different health care professional groups working there. Which information is processed during which activities, and which tools are used? Take non-computer-based and computer-based information processing into consideration in your examples.

- Information processing on a ward
- Information processing in an outpatient unit
- Information processing in an operating room
- Information processing in a radiology department
- Information processing in the hospital administration

2.6.3 Good Information Processing Practice

Have a look at the following typical areas of hospitals. Try to find two examples of "good" information processing practices in these areas, and two examples of "poor" information processing practices. Which positive or negative consequences for the patients could they have?

- Patient administration
- Cardiologic ward
- Laboratory

2.7 Summary

Information processing is an important quality factor, but an enormous cost factor as well. It is also becoming a productivity factor. Information processing should offer a holistic view of the patient and of the hospital. A hospital information system can be regarded as the memory and nervous system of a hospital.

Information and communication technology has become economically important and decisive for the quality of health care. It will continue to change health care.

The integrated processing of information is important, because

- all groups of people and all areas of a hospital depend on its quality,
- the amount of information processing in hospitals is considerable, and
- health care professionals frequently work with the same data.

The systematic processing of information

- contributes to high-quality patient care , and
- reduces costs.

Information processing in hospitals is complex. Therefore,

- the systematic management and operation of hospital information systems, and
- medical informatics specialists responsible for the management, and operation of hospital information systems are needed.

3 Information System Basics

3.1 Introduction

Every domain usually has its own terminology, which often differs from the ordinary understanding of concepts and terms. This chapter presents the terminology for information systems and their management, as used in this book. It is, therefore, essential to read this chapter carefully. All relevant concepts can also be found in the Thesaurus at the end of the book.

After reading this chapter, you should be able to answer the following questions:

- What is the difference between data, information, and knowledge?
- What are information systems, and what are their components?
- What is information management?

3.2 Data, Information, and Knowledge

Data constitute reinterpretable representations of information, or knowledge, in a formalized manner suitable for communication, interpretation, or processing by humans or machines. Formalization may take the form of discrete characters or of continuous signals (e.g., sound signals). To be reinterpretable, there has to be an agreement on how data represent information. For example, "Peter Smith" or "001001110" are data. A set of data that is put together for the purpose of transmission and that is considered to be one entity for this purpose is called a message.

There is no unique definition of information. Depending on the point of view, the definition may deal with a syntactic aspect (the structure), a semantic aspect (the meaning), or a pragmatic aspect (the intention or goal of information). We will simply define information as specific determination about entities such as facts, events, things, persons, processes, ideas, or concepts. For example, when a physician determines the diagnosis (facts) of a patient (person), then he or she has information.

A. Winter et al., *Health Information Systems*,
DOI: 10.1007/978-1-84996-441-8_3, © Springer-Verlag London Limited 2011

Knowledge is general information about concepts in a certain (scientific or professional) domain (e.g., about diseases, therapeutic methods). Knowledge contrasts with specific information about particular individuals of the domain (e.g., patients). The knowledge of a nurse, for example, comprises how to typically deal with patients suffering from decubitus.

For the sake of simplicity, we will often use the term information processing when we mean processing of data together with its related information and knowledge.

3.3 Information Systems and Their Components

3.3.1 Systems and Subsystems

Before talking about information systems, let us first define the concept system. As defined here, a system is a set of persons, things, events, and their relationships that forms an integrated whole. We distinguish between natural systems and artificial (man-made) systems. For example, the nervous system is a typical natural system, consisting of neurons and their relationships. A man-made system is, for example, a hospital, consisting of staff, patients, and relatives, and their interactions. If a (man-made) system consists of both human and technical components, it can be called a socio-technical system.

A system can, in principle, be divided into subsystems that comprise a subset of the components and the relationships between them. For example, a possible subsystem of the nervous system is the sympathetic nervous system. A subsystem of a hospital is, for example, a ward with its staff and patients.

Subsystems themselves are again systems.

3.3.2 Information Systems

An information system is that part of an institution that processes and stores data, information, and knowledge. It can be defined as that socio-technical subsystem of an institution, which comprises all information processing as well as the associated human or technical actors in their respective information processing roles. This means that, for example, the computers, printers, telephones, as well as the staff using them to manage information are part of the information system of an institution.

"Socio-" refers to the people involved in information processing (e.g., health care professionals, administrative staff, and computer scientists), whereas "technical" refers to information processing tools (e.g., computers, telephones, and patient records). The people and machines in an institution are considered only in their role as information processors, carrying out specific actions following established rules.

An information system that comprises computer-based information processing and communication tools is called a computer-based information system. An information system can be divided into subsystems, which are called sub-information systems. For example, the information system of an institution can be split into two sub-information systems: the part where computer-based tools are used is called the computer-based part; the rest is called the non-computer-based part of an information system.

3.3.3 Components of Information Systems

When describing an information system, it can help to look at the following typical components of information systems: enterprise functions, business processes, application components, and physical data processing systems.[1]

An enterprise function describes what acting human or machines have to do in a certain enterprise to contribute to its mission and goals. For example, *patient admission*, *medical and nursing care planning*, or *financial accounting* describe typical enterprise functions. Enterprise functions are ongoing and continuous. They describe what is to be done, not how it is done. Enterprise functions can be structured into a hierarchy of enterprise functions, where an enterprise function can be described in more detail by refined sub-functions. Enterprise functions are usually denoted by nouns or gerunds (i.e., words ending with -ing). The actions summarized by an enterprise function are in most cases significantly dealing with information processing. Later on we will focus more strictly on this aspect and therefore restrict to information processing enterprise functions (see Sect. 5.3.2.1).

For the sake of simplicity, we will refer to enterprise functions as hospital functions, if the respective enterprise is a hospital.

An activity is an instantiation of an enterprise function. For example, "the physician admits the patient Smith" is an activity of the enterprise function *patient admission*. In contrast to enterprise functions, activities have a definite beginning and end.

To describe how an enterprise function is performed, not only may information about its refined sub-functions be needed, but information about their chronological and logical sequence may also be needed. With business processes, the sequence of (sub-)functions together with the conditions under which they are performed can be described. Business processes are usually denoted by verbs, which can be followed by a noun (e.g., "admitting a patient," "planning care" or "writing a discharge letter"). Process instances are composed of the individual activities; hence they also have a definite beginning and end. While enterprise functions concentrate on the "what," business processes focus on the "how" of activities. Enterprise functions can be considered as representatives of business processes.

Whereas enterprise functions describe what is done, we now want to consider tools for processing data, in particular application components and physical data processing systems. Both are usually referred to as information processing tools. They describe the means used for information processing.

Application components support enterprise functions. We distinguish computer-based from non-computer-based application components. Computer-based application components are controlled by software products. A software product is an acquired or self-developed

[1] We will give little bit more formal definition of these terms later on in Sect. 5.3.2.

piece of software that can be installed on a computer system. For example, the computer-based application component *patient administration system* stands for the installation of a software product to support enterprise functions such as *patient admission* and *administrative discharge and billing*.

Non-computer-based application components are controlled by working plans that describe how people use certain physical data processing systems. For example, a non-computer-based application component called nursing management and documentation system is controlled by rules regarding how, by whom, and in which context given forms for nursing documentation have to be used. In this example, the paper-based forms that are used represent physical data processing systems (see Fig. 3.1).

Communication and cooperation among application components must be organized in such a way that the enterprise functions are adequately supported.

Physical data processing systems, finally, describe the information processing tools that are used to implement computer-based as well as non-computer-based application components. Physical data processing systems can be human actors (such as the person delivering mail), non-computer-based physical tools such as forms for nursing documentation, paper-based patient records or telephones, or computer systems (such as terminals, servers, and personal computers). Computer systems can be physically connected via data wires, leading to physical networks. Figure 3.2 shows some typical physical data processing

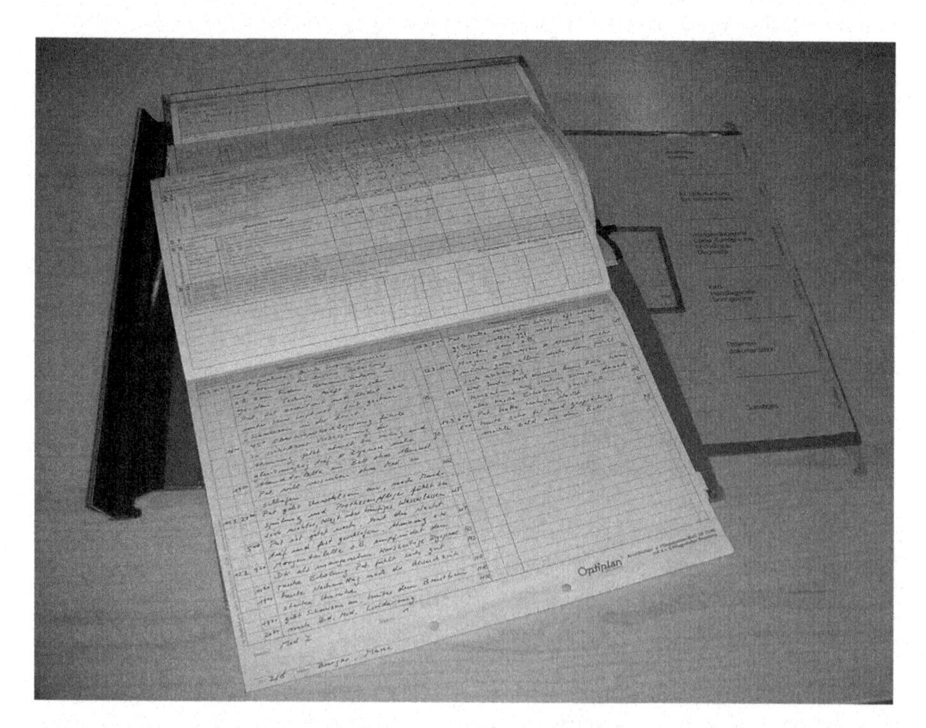

Fig. 3.1 An example for forms and folders for nursing documentation, representing a physical data processing system. The rules that describe who may use these forms, and how they should be used, make up the application component

systems. The printer, for example, could contribute in the implementation of the application component *medical documentation system* by printing documentation forms.

Details on the most relevant information processing tools in hospitals can be found in Sects. 6.4 and 6.6.

3.3.4 Architecture and Infrastructure of Information Systems

The architecture of an information system describes its fundamental organization, represented by its components, their relationships to each other and to the environment, and by the principles guiding its design and evolution.[2] The architecture of an information system can be described by the enterprise functions, the business processes, the information processing tools, and their relationships.

There may be several architectural views of an information system, for example, a functional view looking primarily at the enterprise functions, a process view looking primarily at the business processes, etc. Architectures that are equivalent with regard to certain characteristics can be summarized in a certain architectural style.

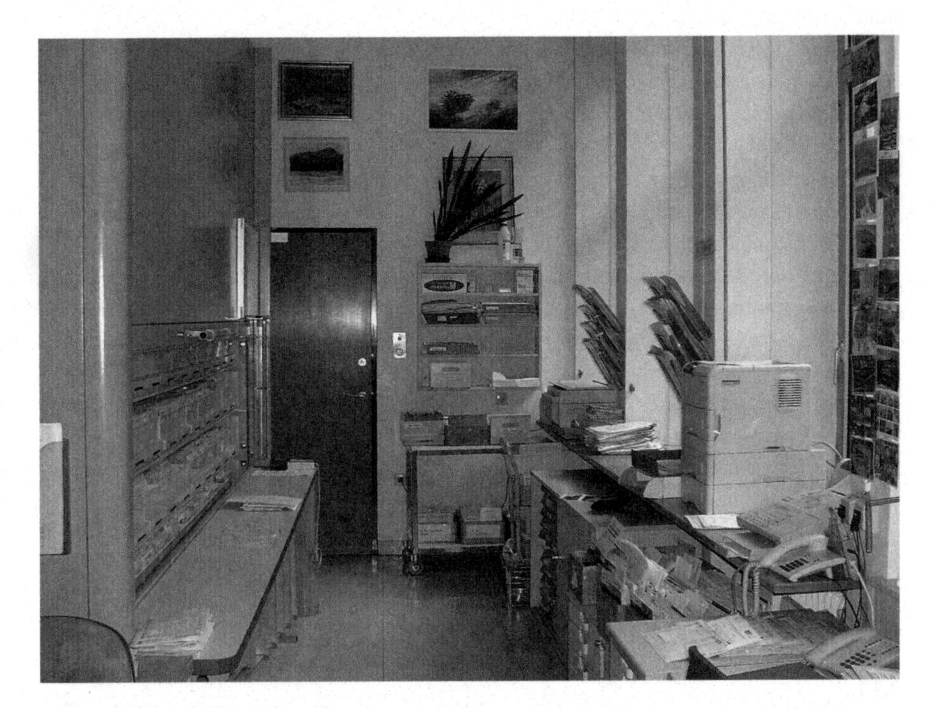

Fig. 3.2 Typical physical data processing systems in an outpatient unit (e.g., printer, telephone, and non-computer-based patient record)

---

[2]Institute of Electrical and Electronics Engineers (IEEE). Std 1471-2000: Recommended Practice for Architectural Description of Software-Intensive Systems. September 2000. http://standards.ieee.org

When the focus is put onto the types, number, and availability of information processing tools used in a given enterprise, this is also called the infrastructure of an information system.

3.4 Information Management

In general, management comprises all leadership activities that determine the institution's goals, structures, and behaviors. Accordingly, information management (or management of information systems) comprises those management activities that deal with the management of information processing in an institution, for example, a hospital. The goal of information management is systematic information processing that contributes to the institution's strategic goals (such as efficient patient care and high satisfaction of patients and staff in a hospital). Information management therefore directly contributes to the institution's success and ability to compete.
The general tasks of information management are planning, directing, and monitoring. In other words, this means

- planning the information system and its architecture,
- directing its establishment and its operation , and
- monitoring its development and operation with respect to the planned objectives .

Information management encompasses the management of all components of an information system – the management of enterprise functions and business processes, of application components, and of physical data processing systems.

Information management can be differentiated into *strategic, tactical*, and *operational information management*. *Strategic information management* deals with information processing as a whole. *Tactical information management* deals with particular enterprise functions or with application components that are introduced, removed, or changed. *Operational information management*, finally, is responsible for operating the components of the information system. It cares for its smooth operation, for example, by planning necessary personal resources, by failure management, or by network monitoring. Information management in hospitals is discussed in detail in Sect. 9.2.

3.5 Exercises

3.5.1 On the Term Information System

Try to describe in your own words, what the term information system, as introduced in Sect. 3.3, means.

3.5.2 On Enterprise Functions

Choose two different types of enterprises, for example, a bank and a theatre. Try to list five major enterprise functions for these enterprises.

3.5.3 On Application Components

Please look at Fig. 3.1. It shows a physical data processing system. Please try to formulate some rules as to how the different parts are to be used, and by whom, to implement a non-computer-based nursing documentation system as application component. Do you need any other physical data processing systems to implement this application component?

3.5.4 On Architectures and Infrastructures

Let us for this exercise focus on the architecture of houses (not on the architecture of information systems). Describe two different architectural styles for houses. Identify five items, which are important to describe the infrastructure of a certain house.

3.5.5 On Information Management

What does information management mean? Describe three information management tasks in your everyday life.

3.6 Summary

When working on information systems, we must distinguish between data, information, and knowledge:

- Data can be defined as a representation of information, or knowledge in a formalized manner, suitable for communicating, interpreting, or processing.
- Information can be defined as specific determination about entities, such as facts, events, things, persons, processes, ideas, or concepts.
- Knowledge can be defined as general information about concepts in a certain domain.

A system is a set of persons, things, events, and their relationships that form an integrated whole. Systems can be divided into subsystems.

An information system can be defined as the socio-technical subsystem of an institution, which comprises all information processing as well as the associated human or technical actors in their respective information processing roles. Typical components of information systems are:

- the enterprise functions supported;
- the business processes that take place;
- the application components that support the enterprise functions;
- the physical data processing systems the application components are executed on.

The subsystem of an information system where computer-based tools are used is called the computer-based part of the information system. The architecture of an information system describes its fundamental organization, represented by its components, their relationships to each other and to the environment, and by the principles guiding its design and evolution.

Information management comprises those management activities in an institution that deal with the management of information processing and therefore with the management of the institution's information system.

4 Health Information Systems

4.1 Introduction

An information system was previously defined as the socio-technical subsystem of an institution, which comprises all information processing as well as the associated human or technical actors in their respective information processing roles. Health information systems (HIS) are dealing with processing data, information, and knowledge in health care environments. Especially with regard to chronic diseases, it becomes more and more important to organize health care in a patient-centric way, such that all participating in- or outpatient care institutions cooperate very closely. This is also denoted as integrated care. In integrated care it is necessary to provide relevant information not only within a single institution, but wherever and whenever it is needed. This includes medical practices, rehabilitation centers, nursing centers, and even the home of the patient. We therefore differentiate institutional and transinstitutional health information systems. In the following, we will introduce hospital information systems, which are the most complex instances of institutional information systems, and transinstitutional information systems. Throughout the book we will use the term health information system and the abbreviation HIS if we discuss aspects concerning both hospital information systems and transinstitutional information systems. If we deal with properties being unique for one of these, we will use the terms hospital information system and transinstitutional information system, respectively. After reading this chapter, you should be able to answer the following questions:

- What are hospital information systems?
- What are transinstitutional health information systems?
- What are the challenges for health information systems?
- What are electronic health records?

4.2 Hospital Information Systems

With the definition of information systems in mind, a hospital information system can be easily defined. A hospital information system is the socio-technical subsystem of a hospital, which comprises all information processing as well as the associated human or technical

A. Winter et al., *Health Information Systems*,
DOI: 10.1007/978-1-84996-441-8_4, © Springer-Verlag London Limited 2011

actors in their respective information processing roles. Typical components of hospital information systems are enterprise functions, business processes, application components, and physical data processing systems (see Sect. 3.3.3). For the sake of simplicity, we will refer to enterprise functions of a hospital as hospital functions.

As a consequence of this definition, a hospital has a hospital information system from the beginning of its existence. Therefore, the question is not whether a hospital should be equipped with a hospital information system, but rather how its performance can be enhanced, for example, by using state-of-the-art information processing tools, or by systematically managing it.

All groups of people and all areas of a hospital must be considered when looking at information processing. The sensible integration of the different information processing tools in a hospital information system is important.

Hospital staff can be seen as part of the hospital information system. For example, when working in the department of patient records or as an operator in a department for information and communication technology, staff members directly contribute to information processing. However, in their role as user of the hospital information system, they use information processing tools (e.g., a nurse may use a telephone or a computer). Each employee may continuously switch between these two roles.

The goal of a hospital information system is to sufficiently enable the adequate execution of hospital functions for *patient care*, including *patient administration*, taking into account economic *hospital management* as well as legal and other requirements. Legal requirements concern, for example, data protection or reimbursement aspects. Other requirements can be, for example, the decision of a hospital executive board on how to store patient records.

To support *patient care* and the associated administration, the tasks of hospital information systems are:

- To make information, primarily about patients, available: current information should be provided on time, at the right location, to authorized staff, in an appropriate and usable form. For this purpose, data must be correctly collected, stored, processed, and systematically documented to ensure that correct, pertinent, and up-to-date patient information can be supplied, for instance, to the physician or a nurse (Fig. 4.1).
- To make knowledge, for example, about diseases, side effects, and interactions of medications available to support diagnostics and therapy.
- To make information about the quality of *patient care* and the performance and cost situation within the hospital available.

In addition to *patient care*, university medical centers undertake research and education to gain medical knowledge and to teach students.

When hospital information systems make available

- the right information and knowledge
- at the right time
- at the right place
- to the right people
- in the right form,

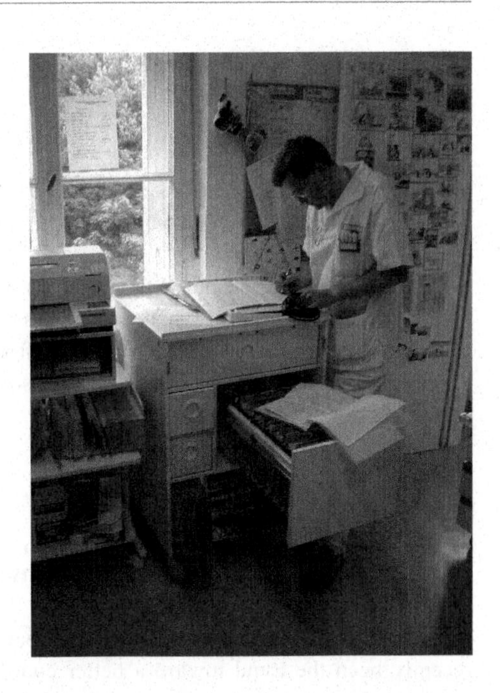

Fig. 4.1 A health care professional accessing patient information

so that these people can make the right decisions, this is also described as information and knowledge logistics.

Hospital information systems have to consider various areas of a hospital, such as

- wards,
- outpatient units,
- service units: diagnostic (e.g., laboratory department, radiology department), therapeutic (e.g., operation room), and others (e.g., pharmacy, patient records archive, library, blood bank),
- hospital administration areas (e.g., patient administration department, patient record archive, department of quality management, financial and controlling department, department of facility management, information management department, general administration department, human resources department),
- offices and writing services for (clinical) report writing.

In addition, there are the management areas, such as *hospital management*, management of clinical and non-clinical departments, administration management, and nursing management.

These areas are related to *patient care*. They could be broken down further. For university medical centers, additional areas, needed for research and education, must be added to the above list.

Obviously, the most important people in a hospital are the

- patients and, in certain respects, their
- visitors.

The most important groups of people working in a hospital are
- physicians,
- nurses,
- administrative staff,
- technical staff and
- medical informaticians and other health information management staff.

Within each group of people, different needs and demands on the hospital information system may exist, depending on the role, tasks, and responsibilities. Ward physicians, for example, require information that is different from that required by physicians working in service units or by senior physicians. Patients sometimes need similar information as physicians but in a different form.

4.3 Transinstitutional Health Information Systems

In many countries, the driving force for health care and for ICT in health care has recently been the trend toward a better coordination of care, combined with rising cost pressure. One consequence is the shift toward better integrated and shared care. This means that the focus changes from isolated procedures in one health care institution (e.g., one hospital or one general practice) to the patient-oriented care process, encompassing diagnosis and therapy, spreading over institutional boundaries (Fig. 4.2).

A group of two or more legally separated health care institutions that have temporarily and voluntarily joined together to achieve a common purpose are defined as a health care network. The information system of a health care network is called a transinstitutional health information system. Typical examples are regional health information systems, comprising the health care environment in a certain region, including, for example, hospitals, offices of general practitioners, pharmacies, rehabilitation centers, home care organizations, and even health insurances and governmental authorities.

In the United States, for example, health care institutions are merging into large integrated health care delivery systems. These are systems of health care institutions that join together to consolidate their roles, resources, and operations to deliver a coordinated range of services and to enhance effectiveness and efficiency of patient care. The situation in Europe is also changing from hospitals as centers of care delivery to decentralized networks of health care delivery institutions that are called regional networks or health care networks. Enterprise boundaries are blurring. Hospital information systems will increasingly be linked with information systems of other health care institutions.

For example, the Hannover Medical School, a large hospital with 75 departments and more than 1,400 patient beds, provides a web portal for its partners, where patient data can be shared and mutually updated by all institutions participating in patient care. Among others, a rehabilitation clinic in Fallingbostel, 50 km north of Hannover, has

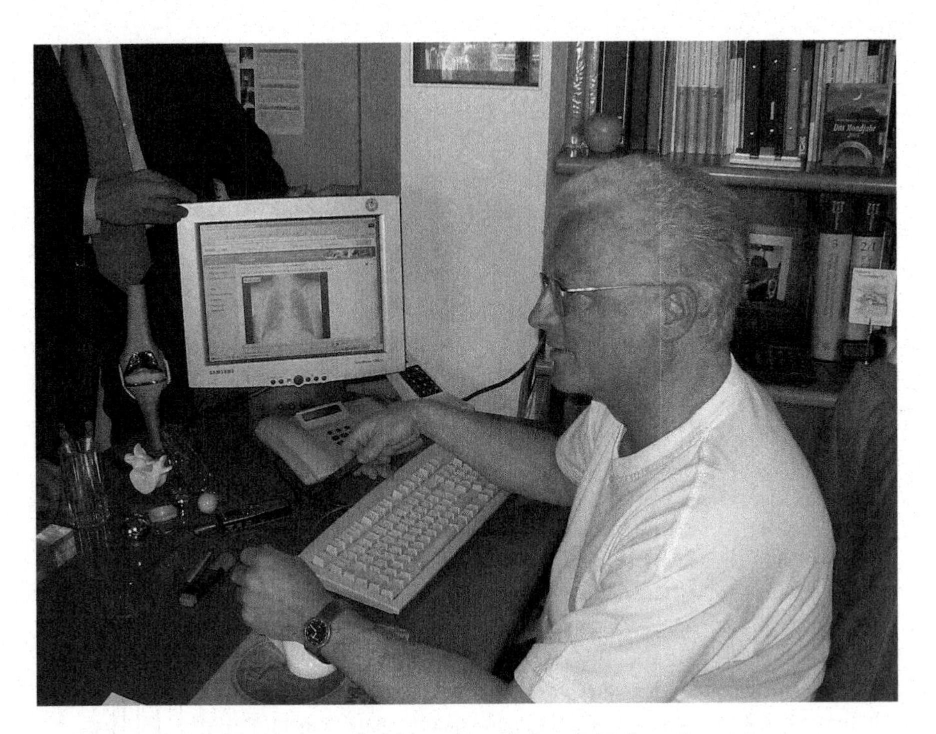

Fig. 4.2 A general practitioner accessing documents of a hospital information system

access to the data of transplant patients, who need time to recover after their operation has taken place, without the need for expensive intensive care treatment. By electronically linking both facilities, the most cost-effective treatment process and optimal time of transfer to the rehabilitation facility can be chosen without loss of quality due to information lags.

The architecture of hospital information systems must take these developments into account. They must be able to provide access or to exchange patient-related and general data (e.g., about the services offered in the hospital) across its institutional boundaries.

A lot of technical and legal issues have to be solved before computer-based transinstitutional health information systems will adequately support transinstitutional patient care. For example, a general willingness to cooperate with other health care providers must exist; optimal care processes must be defined, and recent business processes be redesigned; accounting and financing issues must be regulated; questions of data security and data confidentiality must be answered, together with questions on data ownership (patient or institution) and on responsibilities for distributed patient care; issues on long-term patient records (centralized or decentralized) must be discussed; and technical means for integrated, transinstitutional information processing must be offered (telemedicine, eHealth), including general communication standards.

4.4 Electronic Health Records as a Part of Health Information Systems

The most important enterprise functions in health care are related to diagnostics and therapy. Obviously, data that are relevant to medical decision making need to be collected and presented in a patient record.

A patient record in general is composed of all data and documents generated or received during the care of a patient at a health care institution. Nowadays, many documents in the paper-based patient record are computer printouts, such as laboratory results, or discharge summaries typed into a text processing system. The portion of documents created in computer-based form will further increase. Thus, it seems natural to strive for a patient record that is partly or completely stored on electronic document carriers: the electronic health record (EHR).

The electronic health record (EHR) is the collection of medical data relating to one subject of care, i.e., the patient, that is stored in the computer-based part of a health information system. "The EHR for a subject of care might be scattered physically across multiple (discrete or interconnected) clinical systems and repositories, each of which will hold and manage a partial EHR for each of its data subjects, scoped according to the service or community settings, clinical domains and time periods of use of that system in the life of each person."[1]

Primarily, EHRs are used to support patient care by providing relevant information about a patient whenever and wherever it is needed. Furthermore, they are needed for administrative functions, such as billing and quality management.

In the past, EHR used to be provider-centric, i.e., they only contained patient information that was recorded in one institution, for example, in a hospital or in a physician's office. Those EHR are usually called electronic patient records (EPR). Hence, potentially relevant information about the medical history of a patient that was recorded in other institutions was missing or had to be recorded again. This led to quality and efficiency problems.

Although this situation can still be found in many institutions, efforts are being made today to organize EHRs patient-centric, i.e. independent of institutional boundaries. To achieve the vision of a complete and lifetime-spanning EHR which supports health care on the one hand, but respects legal and ethical issues on the other hand, different strategies can be found. These are described in Sect. 7.3.2.

4.5 Challenges for Health Information Systems

In spite of the positive general development of health information systems, challenges can be identified that have to be resolved. Evolutionary grown information systems (remember that hospitals have an information system from the beginning of their existence) consist of a variety of components and tend to be very heterogeneous. As a consequence, major challenges exist. In anticipation of concepts that are introduced later in this book, we want to sensibilize you for the following challenges:

[1]Standard ISO/Draft International Standard 18308

- **The challenge of user acceptance**. Health care professionals or hospital managers as users of heterogeneous health information systems may have the need to overview a broad variety of data. They will have difficulties or will at least have the problem of having to use a set of application components, often with different user interfaces, overlapping features, and separate user identification procedures. This is time-consuming and potentially dangerous for the patient, as important data may not be available when needed, leading to wrong diagnostic or therapeutic decisions.
- **The challenge of data redundancy**. As different health care professionals often need the same data (see Sect. 2.3), heterogeneous information systems typically lead to data duplication: Relevant data may be documented several times at different sites and or by different providers. This double-documentation is time-consuming for staff and patients and error-prone, as documented data may be inconsistent or incomplete. In addition, uncontrolled redundancy causes considerable additional maintenance costs for updating duplicated data in (redundant) databases.
- **The challenge of transcription**. In heterogeneous architectures there is a considerable amount of transcription, i.e., the transfer of data from one storage device to another (e.g., the transfer of a patient's diagnoses from the patient record to an order entry form). Media cracks, i.e. the change of the storage media during the transcription of data, are often the cause of errors. Both may decrease the quality of data and both do increase costs as well as the health care professional's time needed for recording and accessing patient data.
- **The challenge of maintaining referential integrity**. For redundant data, either as replicates or even as duplicates, it is difficult to obtain and later maintain referential integrity, i.e., the correct assignment of entities, for example the assignment of data to a certain patient (see Sect. 6.5.2.2).
- **The challenge of costs**. Too high, in particular uncontrolled redundancy causes considerable additional maintenance costs for updating replicate data in (redundant) databases.
- **The challenge of privacy and security.** Patients' health data belong to the most sensitive data about humans. For this reason, individual patient data must only be accessible to those persons previously authorized by the patient. A health information system must guarantee this claim which is called privacy of patient data. Likewise, the information system has to ensure data security which comprises availability, confidentiality and integrity of patient data.

In transinstitutional health information systems, the problem of heterogeneity can be estimated even higher. Since these systems involve many originally autonomous information systems, some additional challenges can be identified:

- **The challenge of terminology**. Having data stored in different databases (and without a unique and comprehensive data model or data dictionary) at different sites, there is no immediate need for a unified terminology and semantics. When starting to communicate between these applications systems, this can, however, cause severe problems, and an agreement on terminology for communicating information on diagnoses and procedures is needed.

- **The challenge of stability**. Down times of one or more computer-based application systems with the consequence of significantly restricting care processes may be seldom, but they exist. The same holds for problems in accessing the non-computer-based record. But in a transinstitutional or even regional context, risk of instability is comparatively high.
- **The challenge of transinstitutional information management**. Nowadays, in many hospitals, the *operational, tactical*, and *strategic information management* is organized professionally (see Sect. 9.3). Dedicated, specialized staff is taking care of the information system. For information processing and storing within health care networks, there is often no specific person or group being responsible and having authority to decide and act.

4.6 Example

4.6.1 Architecture of a Hospital Information System

Here is an extract of the description of the architecture of the hospital information system of the Plötzberg Medical Center and Medical School (PMC). As mentioned, PMC is a fictitious institution, which will be used in examples and exercises in this book.

The hospital information system of PMC enables the hospital functions of *patient care* with *patient admission, decision making and patient information, medical and nursing care planning order entry, execution of diagnostic, therapeutic, and nursing procedures, coding of diagnoses and procedures, patient discharge and transfer to other institutions*. In addition, *supply and disposal management, scheduling and resource allocation, hospital administration,* and *hospital management* are supported.

Those hospital functions are supported by some bigger and over a hundred smaller application components (partly computer based, partly non-computer based). The most important application component is the patient administration system, the computer-based application component that supports *patient admission* and *patient discharge and transfer to other institutions*. In addition, several computer-based departmental application components are used for work organization and resource planning (e.g., in the radiology department, in the laboratory department, and in outpatient units). Nearly all computer-based application components are interconnected, using a communication server. Some computer-based application components are isolated systems without interfaces.

Non-computer-based application components are used for special documentation purposes (e.g., documentation in operation rooms), and for *order entry*.

The application components are installed on physical data processing systems. As computer-based physical data processing systems, approximately 40 application and database servers are operated, and over 4,000 personal computers are used. Over 1,000 printers of different types are installed. Most computer-based physical data processing systems are interconnected by a high-speed communication network.

As non-computer-based physical data processing systems, over 2,000 telephones and 800 pagers are used. About 1,500 different types of paper-based forms are used to support different tasks. More than 400,000 patient records are created and used each year, and a dozen local archives are responsible for patient record *archiving*. A paper-based mailing system allows for non-computer-based communication between departments.

4.7 Exercises

4.7.1 Hospital Information System as a System

As introduced, a system can be defined as a set of people, things, and/or events together with their relationships that forms an integrated whole. Which people, things, or events can you find when looking at a hospital information system? In what relationship do they stand to one another? To solve this exercise, take into account the components of hospital information systems as defined in Sect. 3.3.3.

4.7.2 Buying a Hospital Information System

Look at the definition of hospital information systems in Sect. 4.2. Based on this definition, is it possible to buy a hospital information system? Explain your answer. What do vendors of hospital information systems thus really sell?

4.7.3 Transinstitutional Health Information Systems

Patient-centered (not just institution-centered) care is obviously playing a major role. Mention the challenges, which transinstitutional health information systems are facing. Try to argue from your point of view, why these challenges are greater than the same ones within one hospital.

4.8 Summary

Information systems that are dealing with processing data, information, and knowledge in health care environments are called health information systems.

Health information system can be differentiated as institutional health information system, for example, hospital information systems, and transinstitutional health information systems that span the borders of two or more legally separated institutions. Transinstitutional health information systems play a vital role in supporting integrated care.

Important challenges of health information systems are:

- the challenge of user acceptance,
- the challenge of data redundancy,
- the challenge of transcription,
- the challenge of maintaining referential integrity,
- the challenge of costs,
- the challenge of privacy and security.

In transinstitutional health information systems, some additional challenges can be identified:

- the challenge of terminology,
- the challenge of stability,
- the challenge of transinstitutional information management.

The electronic health record (EHR) is the collection of medical data relating to one *patient* that is stored in the computer-based part of a health information system. EHRs are needed to support functions of *patient care* as well as for administrative functions.

Modeling Health Information Systems 5

5.1 Introduction

Modeling HIS is an important precondition for their management: What we cannot describe, we usually cannot manage adequately.

After defining the concepts necessary for dealing with this chapter, we will present some types of information system models describing different aspects of HIS. We will then focus on the so-called "three-layer graph-based metamodel" ($3LGM^2$), which has been developed for describing, evaluating and planning health information systems. $3LGM^2$ models and their application for information management will play an important role throughout this book. Finally, we introduce reference models and a specific reference model that facilitates modeling information systems in hospitals.

After reading this section, you should be able to answer the following questions:

- What are models, metamodels and reference models?
- What are typical metamodels for modeling various aspects of HIS?
- What is $3LGM^2$?
- What are typical reference models for HIS?

5.2 On Models and Metamodels

When dealing with systems in general and with HIS in particular, we need models of systems.

5.2.1 Definitions

Definition 5-1: Model
A model is a description of what the modeler thinks to be relevant of a system.

A. Winter et al., *Health Information Systems*,
DOI: 10.1007/978-1-84996-441-8_5, © Springer-Verlag London Limited 2011

In the sciences, models commonly represent simplified depictions of reality or excerpts of it. Models are adapted to answer certain questions or to solve certain tasks. Models should be appropriate for the respective questions or tasks. This means that a model is only "good" when it is able to answer such a question or solve such a task. For example, a model that only comprises the patients (and not the nurses) of a ward cannot be used for nurse staffing and shift planning. Since we are dealing with information management, this means that models should present a simplified but appropriate view of a HIS in order to support information management. Examples of respective questions to be answered could be:

- Which hospital functions are supported by a HIS?
- Which information processing tools are used?
- What information is needed, if a patient shall be admitted to the hospital? What information can be provided afterwards?
- What will happen if a specific server breaks down?
- How can the quality of information processing be judged?

The better a model assists its users, the better the model is. Thus, the selection of a model depends on the problems or questions to be answered or solved.

A large number of different classes of models exists. Each class of models is determined by a certain metamodel. A metamodel can be understood as a language for constructing models of a certain class and a guideline for using the language.

Definition 5-2: Metamodel
A metamodel is a modeling framework, which consists of

- modeling syntax and semantics (the available modeling concepts together with their meaning), i.e. the modeling language,
- the representation of the concepts (how the concepts are represented in a concrete model, e.g., in a graphical way),
- and (sometimes) the modeling rules (e.g., the modeling steps), i.e. the guideline for applying the language.

Just as different views on HIS exist, there also exist various metamodels. Typical types of metamodels for HIS are:

- functional metamodels, focusing on hospital functions that are supported by the information system;
- technical metamodels, which are used to build models describing the information processing tools used;
- organizational metamodels, which are used to create models of the organizational structure of HIS;
- data metamodels, which are used for building models of the structure of data processed and stored inside a HIS;

- business process metamodels, which focus on the description of what is done in which chronological and logical order;
- information system metamodels, which combine different metamodels into an integrated, enterprise-wide view on information processing in an institution.

The art of HIS modeling is based on the right selection of a metamodel. Thus, for HIS modeling, you should consider the following steps:

1. Define the questions or tasks to be solved by the HIS model.
2. Select an adequate metamodel.
3. Gather the information needed for modeling.
4. Create the model.
5. Analyze and interpret the model (answer your questions).
6. Evaluate if the right metamodel was chosen, that is, if the model was adequate to answer the questions. If not, return to step 2.

5.2.2 Types of Models

Depending on the type of metamodel used, models can be arranged according to different types.

5.2.2.1 Functional Models

Functional models represent the enterprise functions of an institution (what is to be done). In a hospital, their elements are the hospital functions that are supported by the application components of the hospital information system. The relationships of the hospital functions can, for example, represent the information exchanged between them. In addition, enterprise functions are often described in a hierarchical way, comprising more global enterprise functions (such as *patient administration*) and more specific (refined) enterprise functions (such as *administrative discharge and billing*).

Typical questions to be answered with functional models are:

- Which enterprise functions are relevant in a given institution?
- Which specific enterprise functions are part of which global enterprise functions?
- Which enterprise functions share the same data?

Typical representations of functional models are (hierarchical) lists of enterprise functions, as well as graphical presentations. Table 5.1 presents an extract from a three-level hierarchy of hospital functions:

Table 5.1 An extract from the functional HIS model, describing hospital functions relevant for patient care and hospital administration at the Plötzberg Medical Center and Medical School (PMC)

Patient care	Order entry	Preparation of an order
		Appointment scheduling
	Patient discharge and transfer to other institutions	Administrative discharge and billing
		Medical discharge and medical report writing
		Nursing discharge and nursing report writing
Hospital administration	Patient administration	Patient identification and checking for recurrent
		Administrative admission
		Visitor and information service
	Information Management	Strategic information management
		Tactical information management
		Operational information management

5.2.2.2 Technical Models

Technical models describe the information processing tools used. As concepts, they typically provide physical data processing systems (e.g., computer systems, telephones, forms, pagers, records) and application components. As relationships, they provide the data transmission between physical data processing systems (e.g., network diagrams), or the communication between application components.

Typical questions that can be answered with technical models are:

- Which information processing tools are used?
- Which application components communicate with each other?
- What are the data transmission connections between the physical data processing systems?
- What does the network technology look like?
- What technical solutions are used to guarantee the security and reliability of information processing tools?

Technical models are typically presented as lists (e.g., lists of information processing tools used) or as graphs (e.g., graph of the network architecture of computer systems). Examples of graphical models are presented in Figs. 5.1 and 5.2.

5.2.2.3 Organizational Models

Organizational models describe the organization of a unit or area. For example, they may be used to describe the organizational structure of a hospital (e.g., consisting of

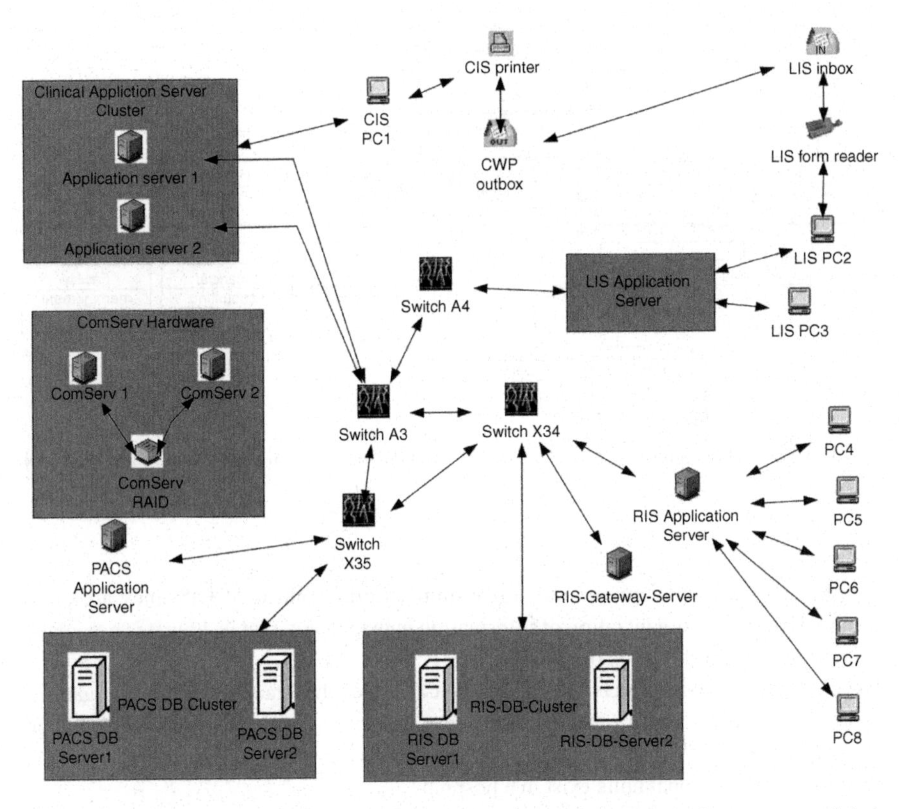

Fig. 5.1 An extract of a technical HIS model with some physical data processing systems and their data transmission links of the hospital information system of the Plötzberg Medical Center and Medical School (PMC)

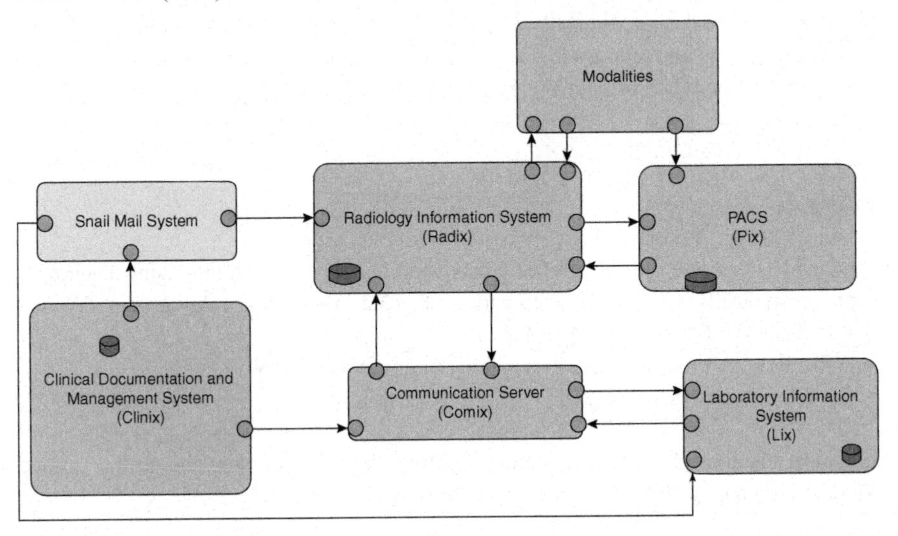

Fig. 5.2 An extract of a technical HIS model with some application components and their communication links of the hospital information system of the Plötzberg Medical Center and Medical School (PMC)

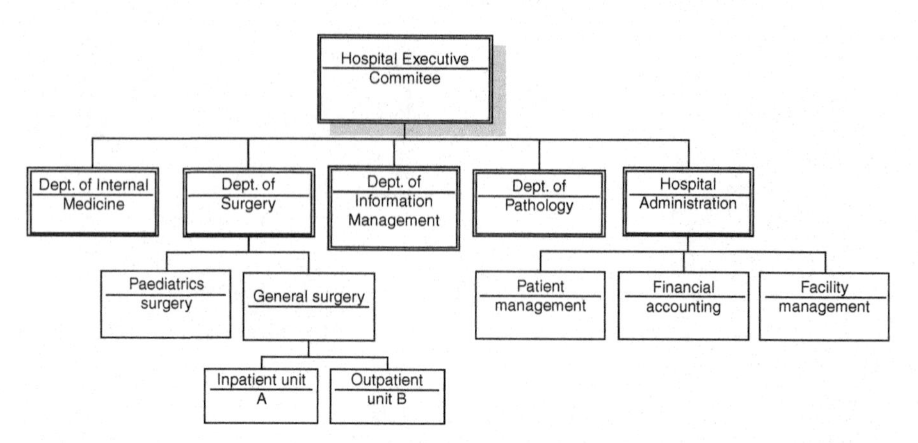

Fig. 5.3 An extract from the organizational model of Plötzberg Medical Center and Medical School (PMC)

departments with inpatient and outpatient units). In the context of HIS, they are often used to describe the organization of information management, that is, how it is organized in order to support the goals of the hospital.
The concepts of those models are usually units or roles that stand in a certain organizational relationship to each other. Typical questions to be answered with organizational models are:

- Which organizational units exist in a hospital?
- Which institutions are responsible for information management?
- Who is responsible for information management of a given area or unit?

Organizational models are typically represented as a list of organizational units (e.g., list of the departments and sections in a hospital), or as a graph (e.g., graphical description of the organizational relationships). An example is presented in Fig. 5.3.

5.2.2.4 Data Models

Data models describe the data processed and stored in an information system. Their concepts are typically entity types (compare sect. 5.3.2.1) and their relationships. Typical questions to be answered with data models are:

- What data are processed and stored in the information system?
- How are data elements related?

A typical metamodel for data modeling is offered by the class diagrams in the Unified Modeling Language (UML).[1] An example is presented in Fig. 5.4.

[1]Object Management Group (OMG): Unified Modeling Language – UML. http://www.uml.org

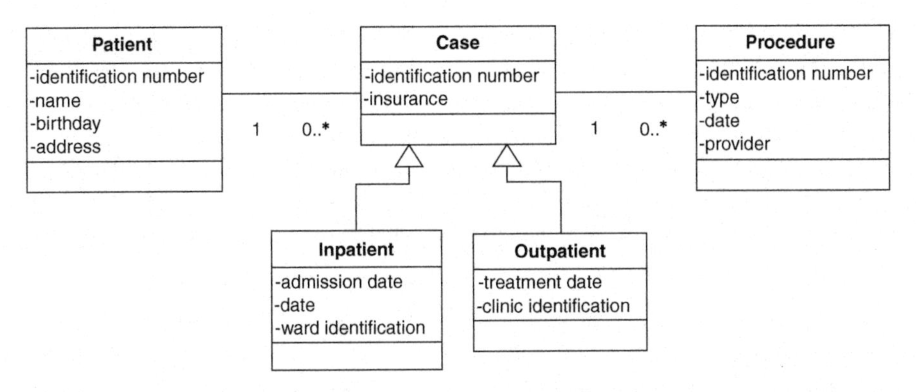

Fig. 5.4 A simplified data model (UML class diagram), describing the relationships between the entity types patient, case, and procedure, as extract from the data model of the HIS of the Plötzberg Medical Center and Medical School (PMC)

5.2.2.5 Business Process Models

Business process models focus on a dynamic view of information processing. The concepts used are activities and their chronological and logical order. Often, other concepts are added, such as the role or unit that performs an activity, or the information processing tools that are used. The following perspectives usually can be distinguished:

- Functional perspective: What activities are performed, and which data flows are needed to link these activities?
- Behavioral perspective: When are activities performed, how are they performed, and where are they performed? Do they use mechanisms such as loops and triggers? What mechanisms trigger the start of the overall process?
- Organizational perspective: Where and by whom are activities being performed? Which different roles participate in the activities?
- Informational perspective: Which entity types or entities (documents, data, products) are being produced or manipulated? Which tools are used for this?

Typical questions to be answered with business process models are:

- Which activities are executed with regard to a given enterprise function?
- Who is responsible and which tools are used in a given process?
- Which activity is the pre- or postcondition for a given activity?
- What are the weak points of the given process and how can they be improved?

Due to the number of different perspectives, various business process metamodels exist. Examples are metamodels for simple process chains, event-driven process chains, activity diagrams, and Petri nets.

Simple process chains describe the (linear) sequence of process steps. They describe the specific activities that form a process, in addition to the responsible role (e.g., a physician).

Event-driven process chains add dynamic properties of process steps: events and logical operators (and, or, xor) are added to the enterprise functions, allowing the more complex modeling of branching and alternatives. In addition, some instances of event-driven process chains allow the addition of entity types (e.g., a chart).[2]

Activity diagrams (as part of the modeling technique of the Unified Modeling Language, UML) also describe the sequence of process steps, using activities, branching, conditions, and entity types (Fig. 5.5). In addition, the method allows for splitting and synchronization of parallel subprocesses.[3]

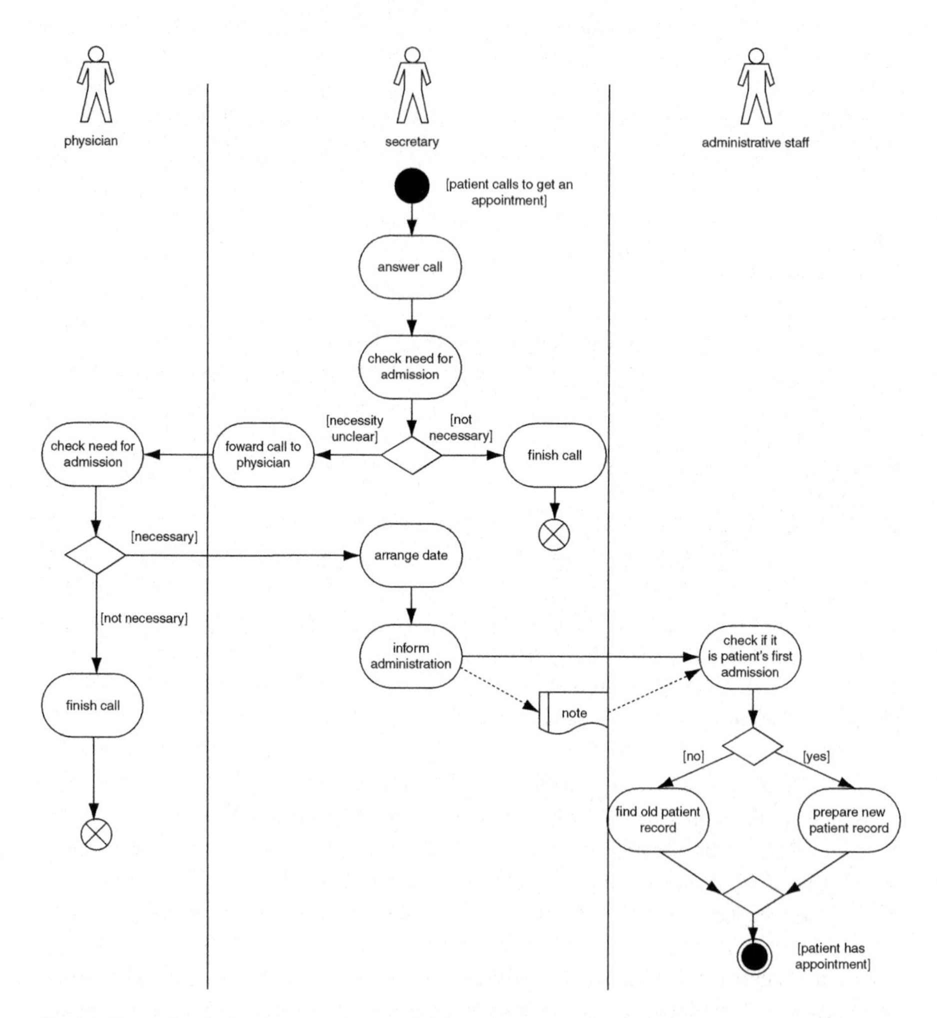

Fig. 5.5 Example of a business process model, based on a UML activity diagram, describing a part of the *admission* process in the Department of Child and Juvenile Psychiatry at Plötzberg Medical Center and Medical School (PMC)

[2]Scheer AW. ARIS – Business Process Modeling. Berlin: Springer; 2000.

[3]Object Management Group (OMG): Unified Modeling Language – UML. http://www.uml.org

Finally, Petri nets describe the dynamic properties of processes in a more formal way than the other methods.[4]

5.2.2.6
Information System Models

Information system models comprise all modeling aspects discussed so far, that is, functional modeling, technical modeling, organizational modeling, data modeling, and process modeling. But beyond this, information system models consider the dependencies of these models and, therefore, offer a more holistic view.
Typical questions to be answered with enterprise modeling are:

- Which hospital functions are supported by which information processing tools?
- Are the information processing tools sufficient to support the hospital functions?
- Is the communication among the application components sufficient to fulfill the information needs?
- Which aims of the enterprise will be affected by a certain application component?
- In which area of the institution are specific data on specific objects used?

5.3
A Metamodel for Modeling Health Information Systems on Three Layers: 3LGM²

Let us now introduce a specific information system metamodel for modeling health information systems. This metamodel is called the three-layer graph-based metamodel (3LGM²). It aims to support the systematic management of HIS and especially the structural quality assessment of information processing in health care institutions. We will use this metamodel further on in this book.
Typical questions to be answered with models derived from the 3LGM² metamodel are:

- Which hospital functions are supported?
- Which information is needed or updated when performing a hospital function?
- Which application components are used, and how do they communicate?
- Which physical data processing systems are used?
- Which hospital functions are supported by which application component?
- Which application components are installed on which physical data processing systems?
- What is the overall architecture of the hospital information system?

3LGM² combines functional, technical, organizational, and some aspects of business process metamodels. It is represented in UML notation. As the name indicates, the 3LGM² distinguishes three layers of information systems:

- domain layer;
- logical tool layer;
- physical tool layer.

[4] Mortensen KH, Christensen S, editors. Petri Nets World. http://www.daimi.au.dk/PetriNets

There are three variants of the $3LGM^2$: $3LGM^2$-B, $3LGM^2$-M and $3LGM^2$-S. The main difference between the variants is the provision of different concepts for describing the communication between application components in an information system. $3LGM^2$-B, which is the basis for $3LGM^2$-M and $3LGM^2$-S, consists of concepts describing basic elements of a HIS architecture. $3LGM^2$-M extends $3LGM^2$-B by concepts for modeling message-based communication. For architectures in which computer-based application components provide services to be used by other computer-based application components (so-called service-oriented architectures), the concepts of $3LGM^2$-S are useful for modeling.

The following sections provide the theoretical background for the further use of $3LGM^2$ in this book. Section 5.3.1 introduces those UML concepts needed for understanding the description of $3LGM^2$ in UML notation. Section 5.3.2 explains $3LGM^2$-B with its basic concepts of the three layers of $3LGM^2$. Sections 5.3.3 and 5.3.4 introduce the additional concepts of $3LGM^2$-M and $3LGM^2$-S.

5.3.1 UML Class Diagrams for the Description of $3LGM^2$

The metamodel $3LGM^2$ is formalized with the help of class diagrams according to the Unified Modeling Language (UML). For a more thorough understanding of UML, you may refer to a respective textbook, but the necessary basics are explained in this section.

$3LGM^2$ class diagrams consist of classes, abstract classes and associations between classes.

Every $3LGM^2$ concept is described by a class. Classes contain the attributes and methods of a set of similar entities. Every class is given an unambiguous class name. For example, computer-based application component is a class of the $3LGM^2$ metamodel. In a concrete $3LGM^2$ model, we use instances of classes for modeling. A *patient administration system* could be an instance of the class computer-based application component.

As introduced in Sect. 3.3.3, both computer-based application components and non-computer-based application components are application components. In $3LGM^2$, we therefore refer to application component as an abstract class, because we can build no instances of application component in a concrete model. Instead, we have to use its $3LGM^2$ subclasses computer-based application component or non-computer-based application components for building instances. The names of abstract classes are written in italics in UML class diagrams; arrows relate the subclasses to the abstract class (see Fig. 5.6).

Associations link classes. For example, application component is linked with component interface by the association "has" in $3LGM^2$ (see Sect. 5.3.2.2). Associations are represented by lines between classes and are often named. At the two ends of an association line, the multiplicity specifies how many instances of a class can be linked with how many instances of the opposite class (see Fig. 5.7).

If it is necessary to specify an association by attributes or by associations to other classes, an association class is used (see Fig. 5.8). In $3LGM^2$, we use for example the association class 'support' to further specify the relationships between enterprise functions and application components (see Sect. 5.3.2.4).

In the 3LGM² metamodel, we often use associations between one class and itself in order to be able to sub- or superordinate certain instances of this class. For example, both

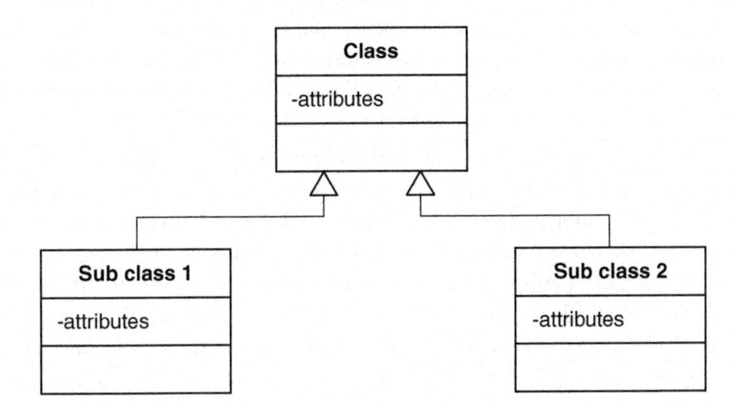

Fig. 5.6 Abstract classes and subclasses in a UML class diagram

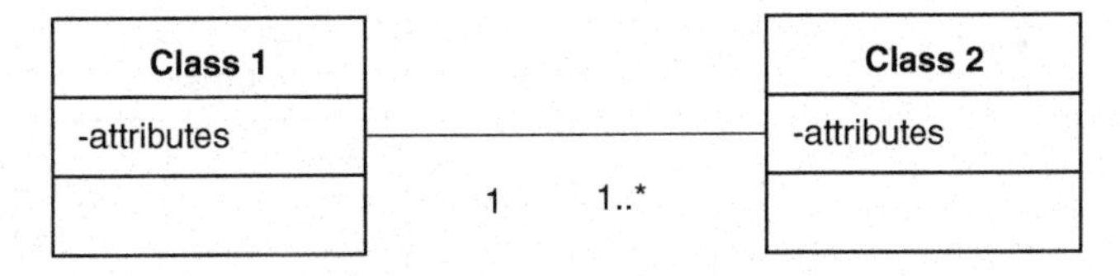

Fig. 5.7 Associations between classes in a UML class diagram

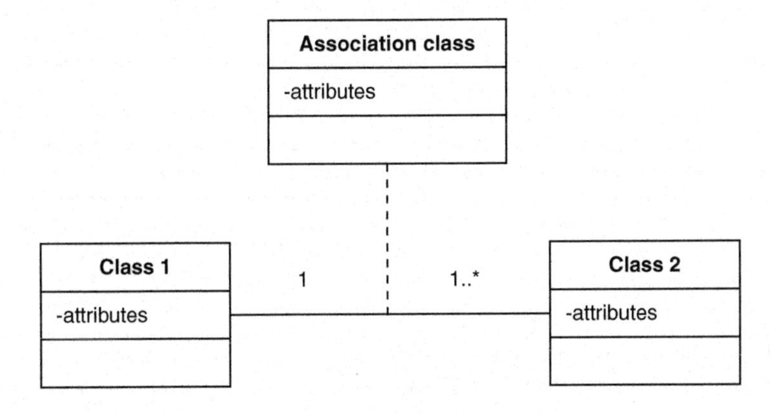

Fig. 5.8 Association classes in a UML class diagram

the operation theatre with room number OP1 and the building B123 are instances of the same class of locations in a certain hospital. But since room OP1 is located in B123 it can be subordinated to that building. In a similar but not identical way the enterprise function 'execution of radiological procedures' can be subordinated to *execution of diagnostic and therapeutic procedures*.

As these examples show, it is helpful to distinguish between two different meanings of subordination in $3LGM^2$ models: decomposition and specialization.

Decompositions describe part-of relationships as with OP1 and B123. The respective superordination is called a composition. See Fig. 5.9 for its description in a UML class diagram.

Specializations describe refinement relationships as with 'execution of radiological procedures' in comparison to *execution of diagnostic and therapeutic procedures*. The respective superordination is called generalization. See Fig. 5.10 to understand how this is described in a UML class diagram. In specializations, attribute values of the superordinated instance are inherited to the subordinated instance. For example, if *execution of diagnostic and therapeutic procedures* is supported by a certain computer-based application component X, then 'execution of radiological procedures' is also considered to be supported by X since it is actually just one special way of *execution of diagnostic and therapeutic procedures*.

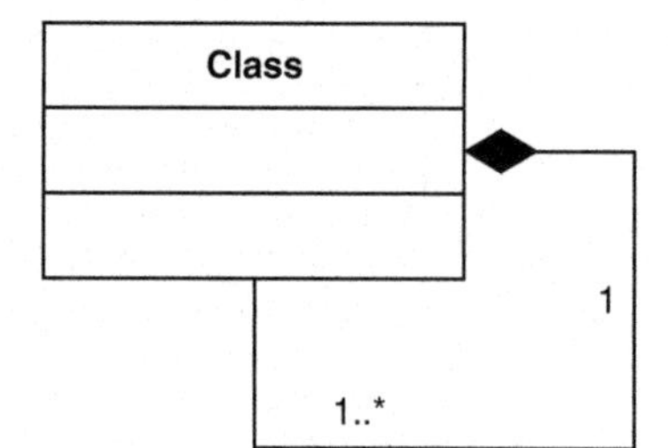

Fig. 5.9 Decomposition as one type of association between one class and itself in a UML class diagram

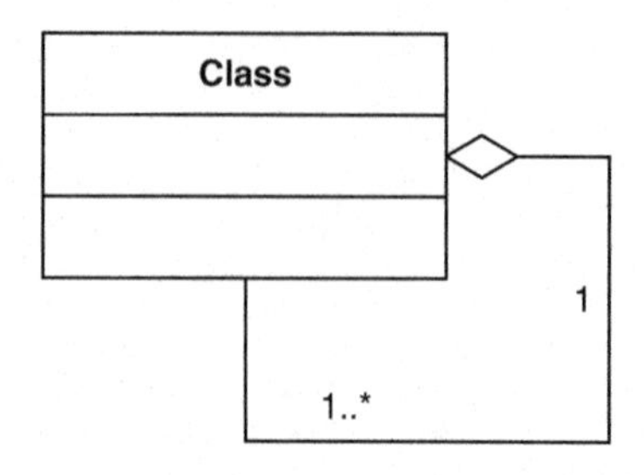

Fig. 5.10 Specialization as another type of association between one class and itself in a UML class diagram

5.3.2 3LGM²-B

5.3.2.1 Domain Layer

The domain layer of 3LGM² describes what kinds of activities in a health care institution are enabled by its information system and what kind of data should be stored and processed. This layer is independent of the implemented information processing tools.

There are myriads of physical or virtual objects in a health care institution (e.g., patient John Doe, or epicrisis of patient Jane Smith dated from 2010-06-10). Data represent information about those objects and are the values of attributes of the objects. Objects being similar with respect to their attribute categories are summarized as object classes (e.g., class patient as set of all objects which are human beings and receive care in a health care institution).

> Definition 5-3: Entity type
> An entity type is a representation of
> 1. an object class and of
> 2. the data representing information concerning the objects of this object class, if these data are stored or could or should be stored in the information system.

We use the label of an object class as term for the respective entity type. For the sake of simplicity we say "data about an entity type" if we think about the data being represented by the entity type.

For example an entity type patient represents

- the class of all patients in a certain hospital and
- the data describing these patients like their name, birthday, home address, social security number, height, weight etc. as it is stored in a certain information system.

Note, that we must not confuse the entity type with the respective object class and the data describing its objects. The entity type is only their representation or surrogate in an information system's model.

Information processing activities at a certain time and place in an information system use certain data in order to update or delete other data. Using the concept entity type we can say, that an activity interprets data about certain entity types and updates data of certain entity types. Again simplifying we say that the activity interprets entity types and updates entity types.

If we look at enterprise functions as introduced in Sect. 3.3.3 and focus on their information processing aspects, we can then define them formally as follows:

> Definition 5-4: Enterprise function
> The class of all activities interpreting the same set of entity types and updating the same set of entity types is called an information processing enterprise function (short: enterprise function). An enterprise function is a directive in an institution on how to interpret data

about entity types and then update data about entity types as a consequence of this interpretation. The goal of data interpretation and updates is part of or contributes to (sub) goals of the institution. A function has no definitive beginning or end.

Similar to an activity, an enterprise function is said to interpret entity types and update entity types.

For example, if Dr. Doe plans clinical care for her patient Smith this morning (i.e. an activity), this will result in interpreting data about Smith's diagnoses and the hospital's clinical pathways and then updating data about concrete plans for medical or nursing procedures. The class of all similar activities of all doctors and nurses may be called *medical and nursing care planning* and is an enterprise function of a hospital. The enterprise function contributes significantly to the hospital's goal of treating patients and updates the entity types medical procedure and nursing procedure depending on the interpreted entity types diagnosis and clinical pathway.

Enterprise functions and entity types can be structured hierarchically by specialization and decomposition. When an enterprise function or an entity type is specialized, all its subelements are a further refinement of the enterprise function or the entity type and independent of the respective superelement. For an enterprise function it means that the activities regarding this enterprise function are executed differently in different contexts. The enterprise function *execution of diagnostic procedures*, for example, has different specializations in different diagnostic departments. Similarly, an entity type can have different forms for slightly different purposes: A finding from a radiology department is different from a finding from a laboratory; but both are specializations of findings, which is the generalized term. By contrast, when an enterprise function or an entity type is decomposed, all its subelements form a proper subset of the enterprise function or the entity type. An activity regarding an enterprise function is only completed if all activities regarding all its decomposed subfunctions are completed. For example, the activities regarding *patient admission* are only completed if among others *administrative admission*, *medical admission* and *nursing admission* have been performed. A decomposed entity type is only complete when all its subordinate entity types are available. A patient history, for example, must contain all clinical data about a patient, including medical and nursing anamnesis, findings, discharge summary etc.

Interpreting and updating relationships between enterprise functions and entity types are inherited to their subelements, no matter whether the enterprise functions or entity types were decomposed or specialized.

Enterprise functions are performed in certain organizational units of health care institutions. Organizational units like a radiology department can be decomposed, but not specialized.

Definition 5-5: Organizational unit

An organizational unit is a part of an institution which can be defined by responsibilities.

Note that enterprise functions, entity types, and organizational units are just part of a static view of a hospital. However, so-called information processes can be modeled by bringing enterprise functions, which interpret and update entity types, into a logical and chronological order.

Definition 5-6: Information process

An information process is a logical and chronological sequence of enterprise functions which interpret or update data about entities.

In contrast to most business process models (see Sect. 5.2.2.5), information processes do not contain a behavioral perspective.

The concepts introduced here and their mutual associations are illustrated in Fig. 5.11 by using UML as explained in Sect. 5.3.1.

A graphical representation of enterprise functions and entity types on the domain layer is shown in Fig. 5.12 where enterprise functions are represented as rectangles and entity types are represented as ovals. An arrow from an entity type to an enterprise function represents an interpreting access, from an enterprise function to an entity type an updating access. Dashed arrows point from decomposed elements towards their composition. This may also be illustrated by positioning decomposed elements on or into their composition. Arrows with empty heads point from specialized elements to their generalization.

Which entity types and which enterprise functions of an information system are modeled, depends on the health care institution and on the modeling purpose. Reference models may offer recommendations about important entity types and enterprise functions for certain kinds of hospitals (see Sects. 5.4 and 5.5).

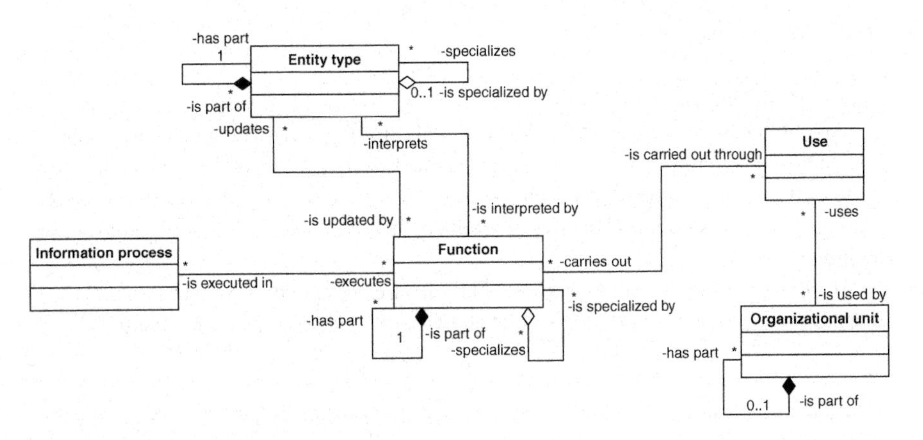

Fig. 5.11 Concepts of the 3LGM² Domain Layer

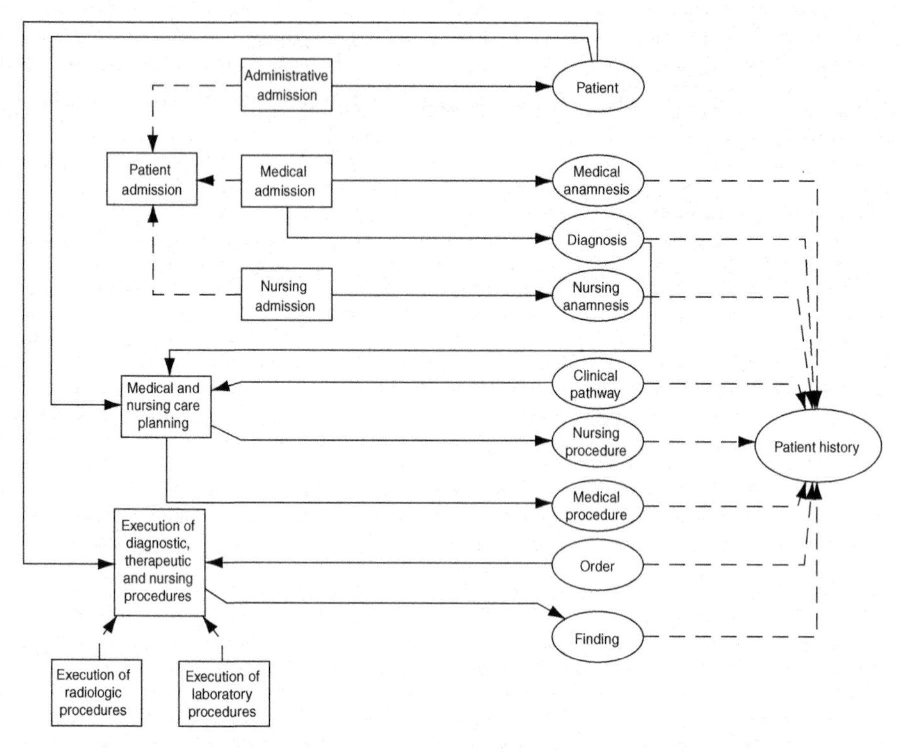

Fig. 5.12 Example of a 3LGM² Domain Layer

5.3.2.2 Logical Tool Layer

At the logical tool layer (UML metamodel, Fig. 5.13), application components (see Sect. 3.3.3.) are the center of interest.

Definition 5-7: Application component

An application component is a set of actually usable rules, which control data processing of certain physical data processing systems. Rules are considered to be actually usable, if they are implemented such that they are ready to support certain enterprise functions in a certain enterprise or support communication between application components.

If the rules are implemented as executable software, the application component is called computer-based application component. Otherwise it is called non-computer-based.

Application components, either computer-based or non-computer-based, support enterprise functions. A software product is a set of rules, represented by software being stored at a certain medium but not implemented and actually executable yet. This is what we can buy. A computer-based application component cannot be bought in a shop anyway but has

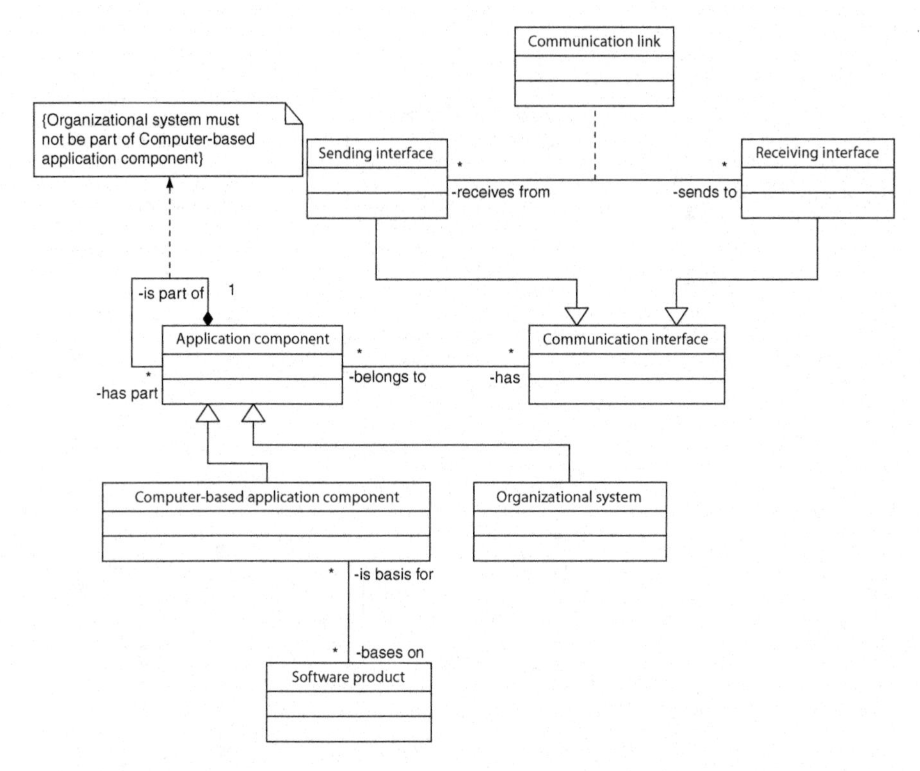

Fig. 5.13 Concepts of the 3LGM² logical tool layer. Lines denote interlayer relationships between logical tool layer and domain layer

to be constructed by customizing a buyable software product onsite. Non-computer-based application components (synonym: organizational systems) are controlled by conventional rules, which can be summarized as working plans describing how people use non-computer-based data processing systems (see Sect. 3.3.3.).

Application components are responsible for the storage and for the communication of data about certain entity types. Application components use communication interfaces for the communication among each other. A communication interface can either send or receive data about entity types. For communication among application components, communication links can be defined. A communication link connects a communication interface of one application component with a communication interface of another application component and communicates data about a certain entity type. Application components have to communicate by respective use of their interfaces to ensure that enterprise functions can interpret and update entity types as described at the domain layer. Application components may be decomposed.

Application components of an information system are objects, which actually can be experienced by staff members in an institution. But nevertheless, they are not tangible. Therefore, we refer to application components also as logical tools. Consequently, we call the layer describing the application components the logical tool layer. This is in contrast to the tangible tools, which we refer to as physical (see Sect. 5.3.2.3).

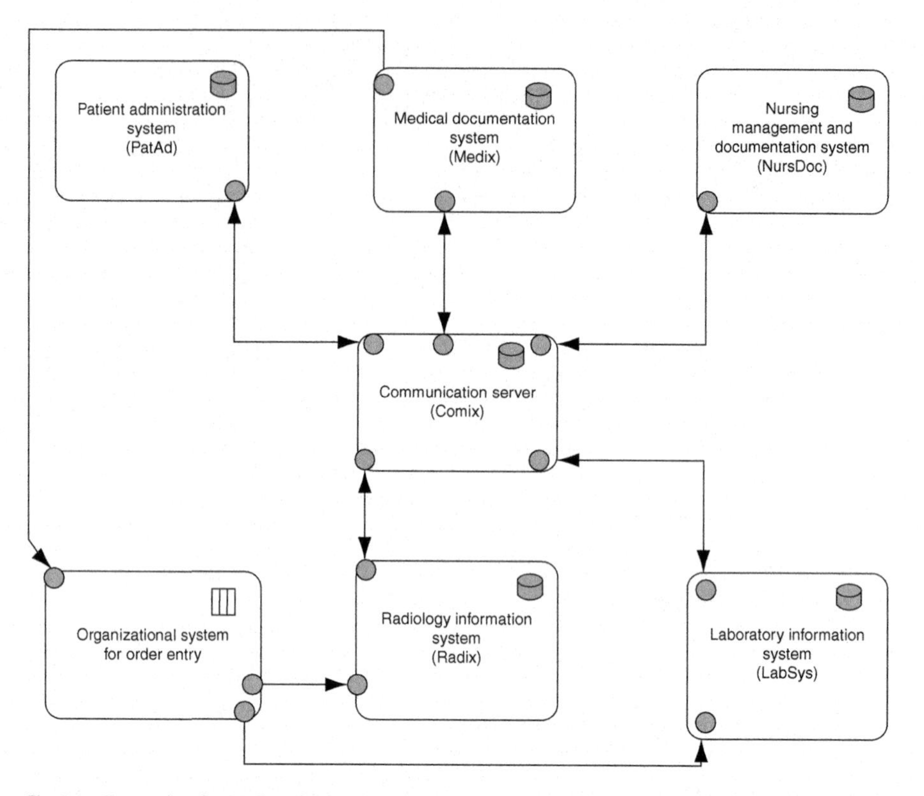

Fig. 5.14 Example of a 3LGM² logical tool layer

Figure 5.14 shows an example of a logical tool layer. In this example, the application components are depicted as large rounded rectangles, and the relationships between them via communication interfaces (small circles) are depicted as arrows. The direction of the arrows represents the direction of the communication. Names of software products being used for a computer-based application component are put in parentheses.

5.3.2.3 Physical Tool Layer

The physical tool layer (UML metamodel, Fig. 5.15) is a set of physical data processing systems.

> Definition 5-8: Physical data processing system
>
> A physical data processing system is a physically touchable object or a simulated physically touchable object being able to receive, store, forward, or purposefully manipulate data. We denote receiving, storing, forwarding and purposeful manipulation of data as data processing. This data processing is controlled by rules.

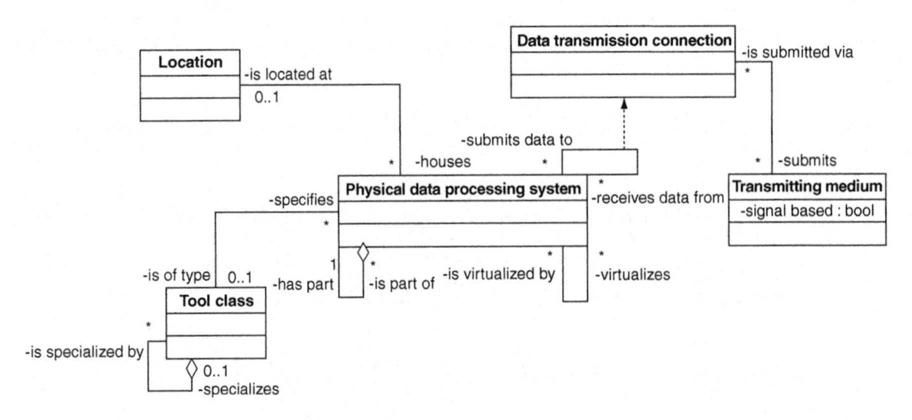

Fig. 5.15 Concepts of the 3LGM² physical tool layer. Dotted lines denote interlayer relationships between logical tool layer and physical tool layer

The rules mentioned here are identical to those mentioned in the definition of an application component.

Physical data processing systems can even be human actors (such as persons delivering mail), non-computer-based physical tools (such as printed forms, telephones, books, paper-based patient records, administrative stickers), or computer systems (such as terminals, servers, personal computers, switches, routers).

Physical data processing systems like a specific server or a specific personal computer can be assigned to a tool class (e.g., server, personal computer) and a location. Physical data processing systems are physically connected via so-called data transmission connections (e.g., communication network, courier service) which can use different transmitting media. A transmitting medium is either signal-based (e.g., copper cable, optical fiber) or non-signal-based (e.g., sheet of paper, CD-ROM, memory stick).

Physical data processing systems can be refined by decomposition (see Sect. 5.3.1). A physical data processing system can be part of exactly one physical data processing system.

Additionally, physical data processing systems can be virtualized. We speak of virtualization when, either, one or more physical data processing systems simulate one physical data processing system, or one physical data processing simulates one or more physical data processing systems. In the first case, we call the simulated physical data processing system a cluster. In the latter case, we call the simulated physical data processing systems virtual machines. In a cluster, for example, different servers could, depending on their capacity, alternatively run a certain computer-based application component. However, the cluster can be administrated as one (virtual) server. By contrast, with the help of virtual machines, different operating systems or different instances of one operating system can be run on one physical server, for example. Both virtual machines and clusters are called virtual physical data processing systems, since they can be used as physical data processing systems for example to implement application components, but are not physical in the sense of being touchable physically. See Fig. 5.16 for the representation of virtualization in 3LGM² models.

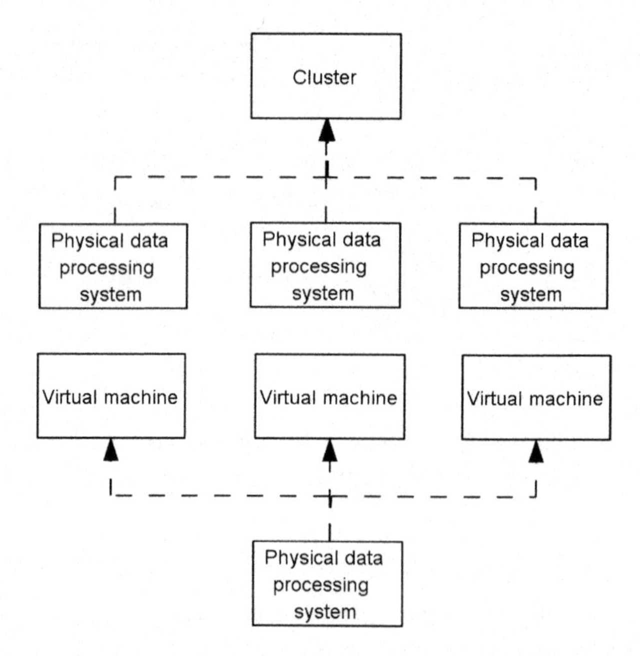

Fig. 5.16 On the top, the concept of a cluster virtualizing several physical data processing systems is illustrated. At the bottom, there is one physical data processing system which is virtualized into several virtual machines

Figure 5.17 shows an example of a physical tool layer. Data transmission connections between physical data processing systems are depicted as lines. The figure also shows decompositions, virtual machines and clusters. Information about locations and tool classes is not represented graphically.

5.3.2.4 Interlayer Relationships

A variety of dependencies, called interlayer relationships, exist among components of different layers. Relationships exist between concepts of the domain layer and the logical tool layer and between concepts of the logical tool layer and the physical tool layer (see Fig. 5.18).

Considering the domain layer and the logical tool layer, the most important relationships are between enterprise functions and application components. These relationships are handled by the class use and the association class support in 3LGM². If a computer-based application component is used for a certain enterprise function there are two possibilities. Either the computer-based application component is immediately used for supporting the activities regarding an enterprise function (class use), or the computer-based application component only mediates the use of another computer-based application component which supports the enterprise function (class support). The answers to the

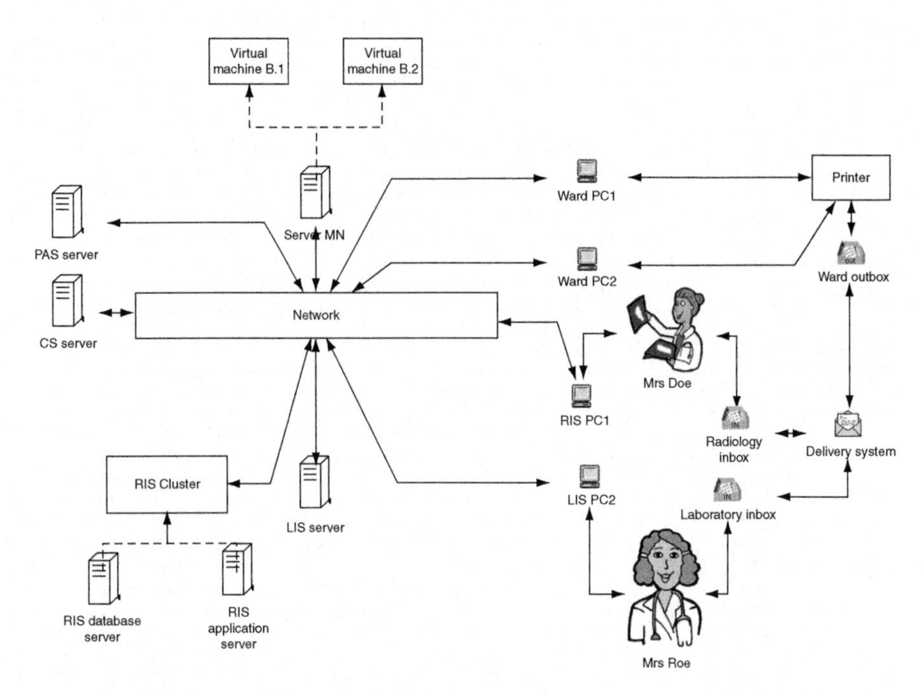

Fig. 5.17 Example of a 3LGM² physical tool layer

following two questions help to understand how to assign enterprise functions to application components.

- Which application components are necessary to support an enterprise function completely?

  In a 3LGM² model, we specialize or decompose enterprise functions to that level of detail needed to describe the support of the enterprise functions by single application components. That means, if we think of the hierarchy of enterprise functions in a 3LGM² model as a tree in graph theory, then each of the tree's "leaf functions" must completely be supported by one application component of the information system. We only assign application components to the "leaf functions" of the tree. For example, if we find that the enterprise function *medical and nursing care planning* needs joint support of two application components X and Y, we have to specialize or decompose the enterprise function in a way, that the resulting subfunctions are supported by X and Y respectively. If X is used by clinicians and Y is used by nurses it could be a solution to decompose the enterprise function into 'medical care planning' and 'nursing care planning'. If X is used in department D1 and Y in department D2, a specialization into 'medical and nursing care planning in D1' and 'medical and nursing care planning in D2' could be a solution. The next paragraph will help to identify the example's latter case as a functional redundancy which might not be expressed by specializing *clinical and nursing care planning* but by assigning D1 and D2 as alternative/redundant application components supporting the enterprise function.

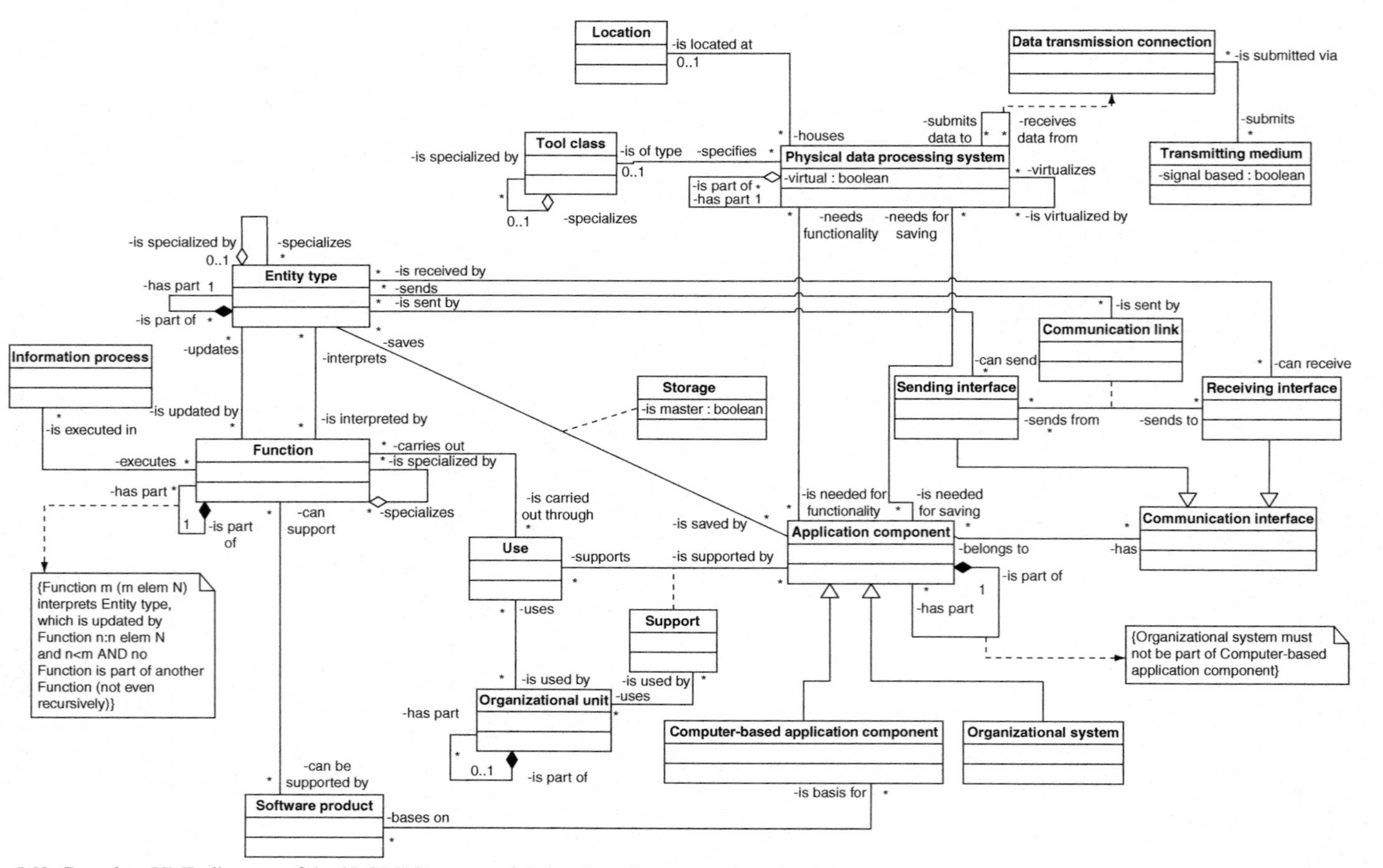

Fig. 5.18 Complete UML diagram of the 3LGM²-B metamodel showing all concepts, intra- and interlayer relationships

- Which possible alternatives are there to support an enterprise function?
  An enterprise function F is sometimes supported alternatively by more than one application component. That means, no matter if one of these application components fails, enterprise function F can still be performed. In this case, we have a functional redundancy which may be an indication for superfluous application components. However, as one application component often supports a variety of enterprise functions which in turn can also be supported by a variety of application components, it is quite complicated to determine an information system's set of redundant application components which could be shut down without losing the support of any enterprise function. Section 8.7.4. provides a deeper understanding of functional redundancy, its calculation and its effects on health information systems.

Further relationships between classes of the domain layer and classes of the logical tool layer regard entity types (compare Fig. 5.13):

- At the logical tool layer, application components, both computer-based and non-computer-based, can store data about entity types. If an entity type E is updated by an enterprise function and this entity type's data are stored in an application component, we call this combination the 'documentation of entity type E'.
- For every entity type E can be stated whether an application component storing data about E is master for E and, therefore, in case of redundant data storage, contains the 'original' data about that entity type. 'Original' means that data about E stored in other application components have to be considered as copies of the 'original' data. Consequently, only data in master application components can be updated directly by users; data integrity in the other application components has to be maintained by sending new copies of the original data to these non-master application components (for details see Sect. 6.5.5.2).
- Additionally, entity types can be related to communication links and interfaces in order to express their ability to send or receive data about these entity types.

Between the logical tool layer and the physical tool layer, there exist two relationships which link application components and physical data processing systems. One of these relationships states that an application component needs physical data processing systems to be able to provide its features. For example, a certain computer-based application component has to be installed on a certain server to make its features available. Furthermore, if application components store entity types, they need physical data processing systems that can store data. Thus, the second relationship between application components and physical data processing systems expresses that an application component needs physical data processing systems for storage.

Figure 5.19 combines Figs. 5.12, 5.14 and 5.17 in order to illustrate the different interlayer relations mentioned before. Note that relationships between entity types and application components or communication links and interfaces are not represented graphically.

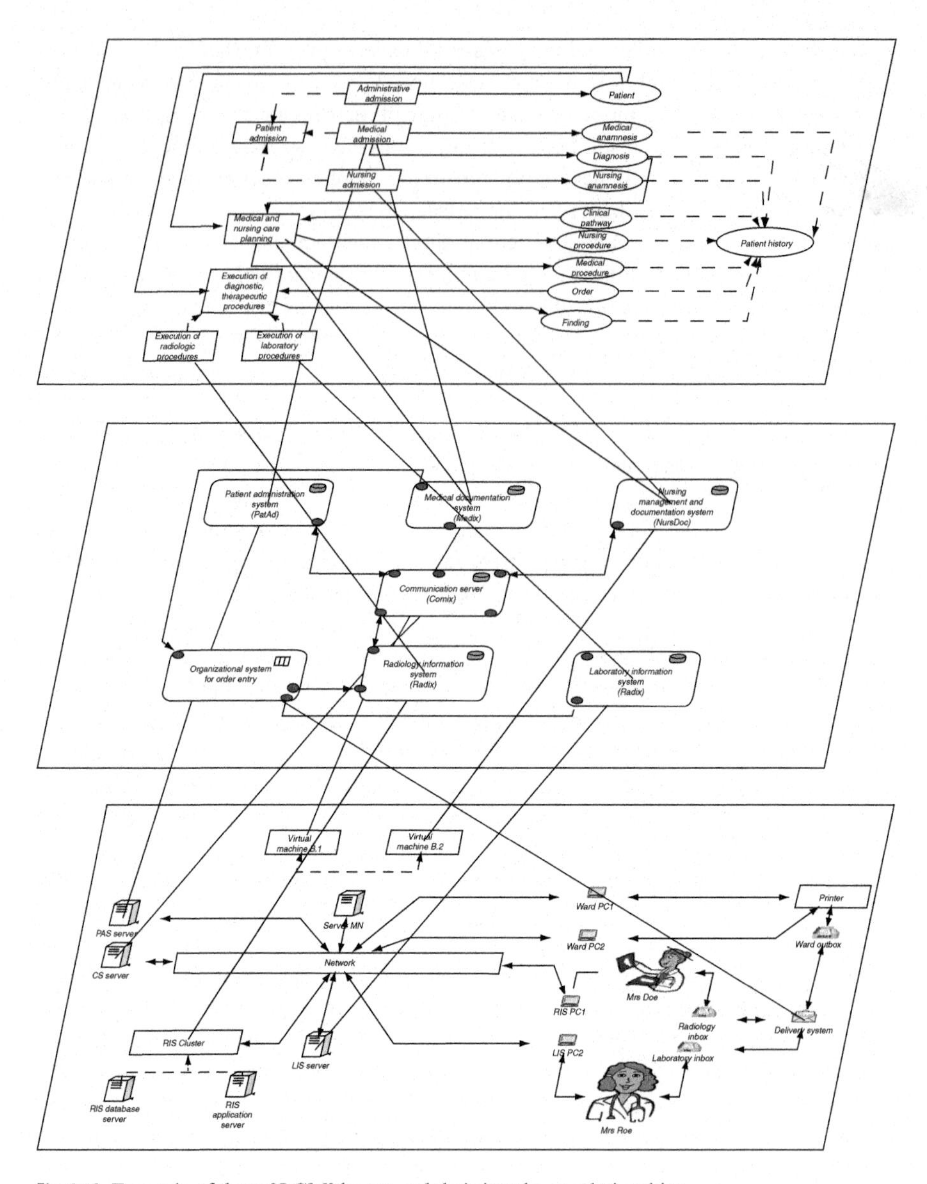

Fig. 5.19 Example of three 3LGM² layers and their interlayer relationships

5.3.3 3LGM²-M

In addition to the concepts of 3LGM²-B, the variant 3LGM²-M provides the new concepts message type and communication standard for modeling message-based communication at the logical tool layer (compare Fig. 5.20).

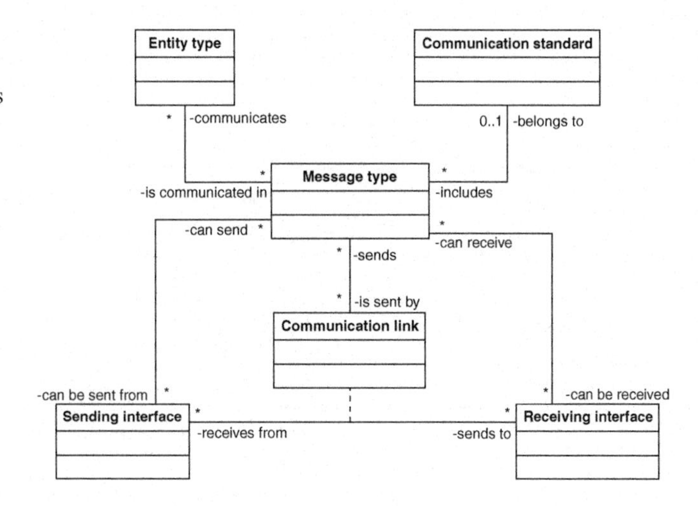

Fig. 5.20 Concepts of 3LGM²-M. The diagram only contains the new concepts message type and communication standard and their relationships with other concepts

A message is a set of data that are arranged as a unit in order to be communicated between application components. A message type describes a class of uniform messages and determines which data about which entity types is communicated by a message belonging to this message type. That means, in the 3LGM²-M metamodel there is a connection between message types and entity types expressing that messages of this type communicate data about these entity types. In contrast to 3LGM²-B, message types, but not the entity types themselves, are used to describe, what data are communicated over sending interfaces, communication links and receiving interfaces.

A message type can belong to a communication standard and a communication standard is used to group message types. In general, communication standards describe how messages of a certain data format are communicated when a certain event occurs. In medical informatics, HL7 and DICOM are well-known examples for communication standards (see Sect. 6.5.4 for details). In 3LGM²-M, we do not model events.

5.3.4 3LGM²-S

3LGM²-S is suitable for modeling service-oriented architectures (see Sect. 6.5.5.3). It extends 3LGM²-B by the new concepts 'service' and 'service class', and replaces the concepts 'sending interface' and 'receiving interface' by 'providing interface' and 'invoking interface' at the logical tool layer (compare Fig. 5.21).

As in 3LGM²-B and 3LGM²-M, we proceed on the assumption that an application component implements certain features which are functionalities directly contributing to the fulfillment of one or more enterprise functions. Thus, we define service the following way.

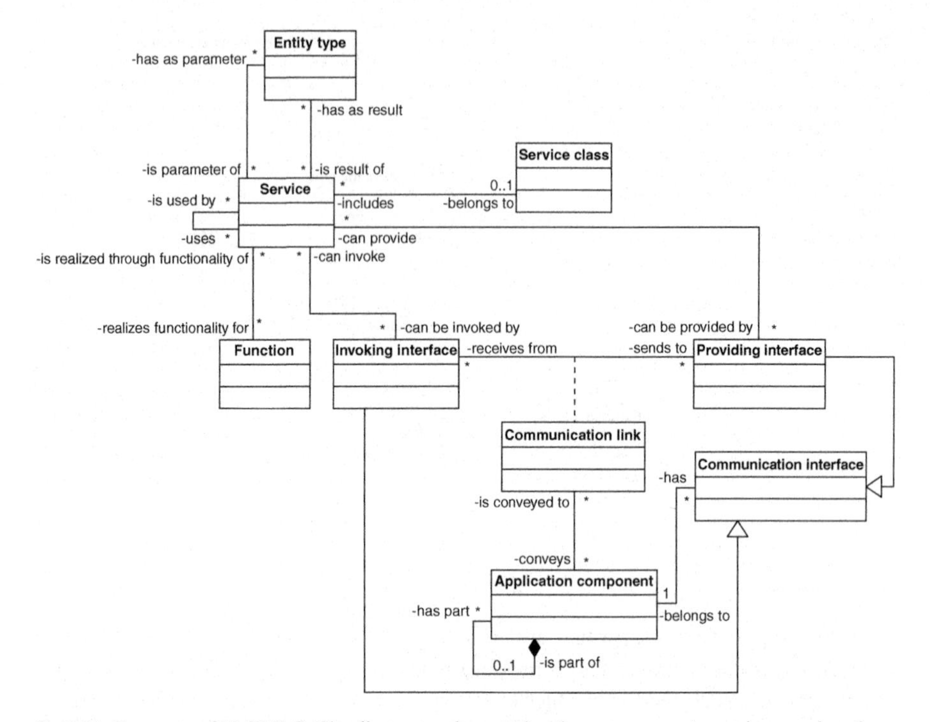

Fig. 5.21 Concepts of 3LGM²-S. The diagram only contains the new concepts service, service class, invoking interface and providing interface and their relationships with other concepts

> Definition 5-9: Service
>
> A service is a feature provided by an application component in order to be used by other application components.

If we want to express that some services are of similar type, we can summarize them in a service class.

As their names imply, providing interfaces and invoking interfaces, each belonging to only one application component, are able to provide or to invoke services.

5.4 On Reference Models

Until now we talked about HIS metamodels, that is, about languages to describe health information systems from various views. To support HIS modeling, modelers often ask for examples of models of typical HIS realized by one of the typical metamodels mentioned in Sect. 5.2.1 They would like to use them as a pattern which can be customized to the specific situation he or she has to model. We call this kind of models reference models.

According to the type of metamodel used, a reference model supports the construction of models of a certain class of systems and helps to deal with a certain class of questions or tasks concerning these systems.

Definition 5-10: Reference Model

A model is called a reference model for a certain class of systems and a certain class of questions or tasks dealing with these systems, if it provides model patterns supporting

- the derivation of more specific models through modifications, limitations, or completions (generic reference models) or
- direct comparison of different models with the reference model concerning certain quality aspects of the modeled systems (e.g., completeness, styles of system's architecture) (nongeneric reference models).

A specific model may be considered a variant of a generic reference model developed through specialization (modifications, limitations, or completions). This variant is an instance of the metamodel that also underlies the corresponding reference model. For example, a model of the processes in a hospital information system of a specific hospital may be derived from a general reference model on HIS processes. Both the specific model and the used reference model are instances of the same business process metamodel.

A reference model should be followed by a description of its usage, for example, how specific models can be derived from the reference model, or how it can be used for the purpose of comparison.

Specific models can be compared with a reference model, and consequently models can also be compared with each other, judging their similarity or difference when describing certain aspects.

For example, business reference models describe models of processes, data, and organization of a certain class of institutions (e.g., hospitals). They deal with information processing in these institutions.

If such a reference model focuses on the processes in the institution, it will be based on a business process metamodel (see Sect. 5.2.2.5) and can be called a business process reference model. If it focuses on the data and their types and relationships it will be based on a data metamodel (see Sect. 5.2.2.4) and can be called a data reference model. The exemplary data model outlined in Fig. 5.4 can be used as a data reference model.

Reference models can be normative in the sense that they are broadly accepted and have practical relevance. Reference models are more likely to be accepted if they are not only reliable and well-tested, but also recommended by a respected institution. For example, the initiative Integrating the Healthcare Enterprise (IHE) (see Sect. 6.5.4.6) provides a comprehensive set of models describing how to use communication standards like HL7 and DICOM in typical health care settings. These models can be regarded as reference models. Actually many experts in the field use these reference models like norms or standards, although they are explicitly not. Obviously they became normative because they are widely used especially in commercial invitations of tenders for software supporting radiology departments.

5.5 A Reference Model for the Domain Layer of Hospital Information Systems

As the identification and modeling of adequate enterprise functions and entity types for a hospital is rather time- and consequently cost-intensive, a functional reference model for the domain layer of hospital information systems was developed[5]. It consists of hierarchically structured sets of hospital functions and entity types. The reference model focuses on the activities in *patient care*. Thus, the main enterprise function is *patient care*, and there are maintenance functions supporting *patient care* like *supply management, scheduling and resource allocation, hospital administration, hospital management* and *research and teaching* (compare Fig. 5.22).

Furthermore, in that reference model the enterprise functions bear a relation to each other by entity types which they can update or interpret. For defining entity types within the reference model of the domain layer the Health Level 7 Reference Information Model[6] (HL7-RIM) had been used.

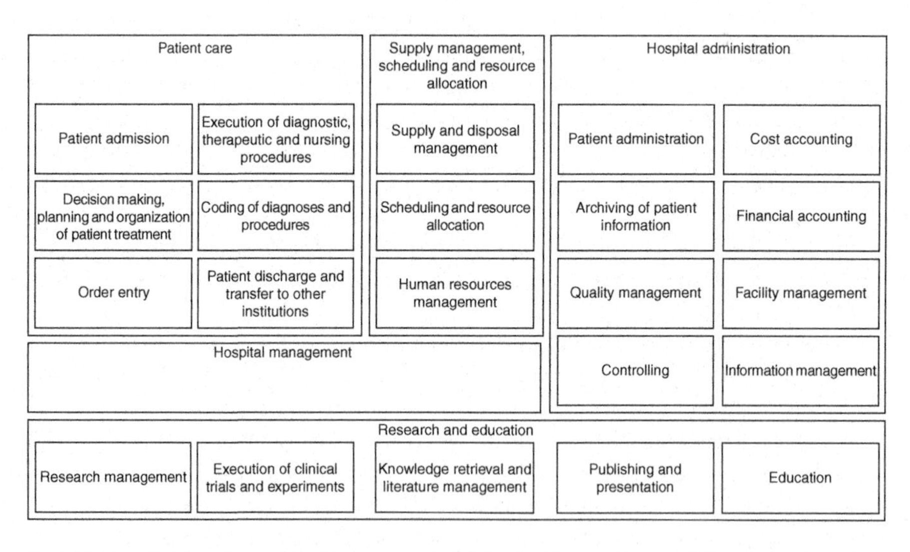

Fig. 5.22 Hospital functions of the Reference Model for the Domain Layer of Hospital Information Systems (presented until second hierarchy level)

[5]Hübner-Bloder G, Ammenwerth A, Brigl B, Winter A. Specification of a Reference Model for the Domain Layer of a Hospital Information System. In: Engelbrecht R, Geissbuhler A, Lovis C, Mihalas G (eds.): Connecting Medical Informatics and Bio-Informatics. Proceedings of Medical Informatics Europe (MIE 2005), Geneva, Aug 08–Sep 01 2005. Studies in Health Technology and Informatics, Volume 116. Amsterdam: IOS Press, 2005; pp 497–502.

[6]http://www.hl7.org/Library/data-model/RIM/modelpage_mem.htm

The Reference Model for the Domain Layer of Hospital Information Systems is available as a 3LGM² model[7] and can for this reason be immediately used for modeling hospital information systems. Following the definition of reference models in sect. 5.4 the Reference Model of the Domain Layer can be used as a model pattern for the domain layer of hospital information systems and, additionally, can help to compare hospital information systems by means of a uniform terminology used for the domain layer. That is, for each enterprise function of the Reference Model of the Domain Layer the support by application components in different information systems can be determined.

The Reference Model for the Domain Layer of Hospital Information Systems is used as a basis for describing entity types and enterprise functions throughout this book. Thus Sect. 6.3, which introduces the enterprise functions of a hospital, follows the structure of that reference model and all examples concerning entity types and enterprise functions are taken from it.

5.6 Exercises

5.6.1 Typical Implementation of Hospital Functions

Look at the hospital functions presented in Fig. 5.22 and describe how they are implemented in your hospital. Try to classify each hospital function according to how it is typically supported by application components, which are

- non-computer-based,
- computer-based,
- or a mix of computer-based and non-computer-based application components.

If in your hospital a hospital function is supported by a mix of computer-based and non-computer-based application components, find out what subfunction is supported by computer-based application components and what subfunction is supported by non-computer-based application components.

5.6.2 3LGM² as a Metamodel

3LGM² is a metamodel. Look at the definition of metamodels in Sect. 5.2.1 and find the various concepts in the 3LGM² (e.g., for modeling syntax and semantics, representation, and modeling rules).

[7]http://www.3lgm2.de//Modelle/Referenzmodelle_und_Beispielmodelle/RM_DomainLayer_version2_English.z3lgm

5.6.3 Modeling with $3LGM^2$

The following description of a sub-information system of a hospital is given:

> *Patient admission* is supported by an application component called PATADMIN, which is installed at the hospital's central server. The administration personnel work with two personal computers. The patient data are stored in the Oracle-based medical database system (MEDDB). After the *patient admission* is completed, patient data are transmitted to the computer-based application components at the laboratory department (LABSYS) and at the radiology department (RADSYS). For communication with paper-based application components, i.e., for ordering or clinical documentation, labels containing the identifying patient data as text and as barcodes are printed.

5.6.3.1 HIS Components

Identify the $3LGM^2$-relevant components of the described HIS and assign them to one of the three layers and use the correct $3LGM^2$ terms. Which necessary information to get a complete model of this sub-information system is missing?

5.6.3.2 Create the Model

Design a $3LGM^2$ model[8] with the three layers that includes the components and their relationships.

5.6.3.3 Interlayer Relationships

Describe which interlayer relationships are given and add them to the model.

5.6.3.4 New Enterprise Function

Add the enterprise function *execution of nursing procedures* to the $3LGM^2$ model of our example. In this example, nurses use paper-based forms to document their activities. The non-computer-based organization system 'Nursing Documentation System' describes how

---

[8]You can download a free test version of the $3LGM^2$ tool for creating $3LGM^2$-conform models from http://www.3lgm2.de/en/ (English) or www.3lgm2.de (German). At this website you can also find all $3LGM^2$ models used in this book.

the nurses have to document and which forms have to be used. This enterprise function mainly requires general patient data, which are printed on labels and stuck to the forms, and nursing knowledge. It results in information about executed nursing procedures. Add the necessary elements in all three layers of the graphical model.

5.7 Summary

HIS models are used to support the description, management, and operation of HIS. A good model adequately supports information managers in these tasks.

According to their different purposes, different metamodels (modeling languages) exist for HIS. This leads, for example, to functional models, technical models, organizational models, data models, business process models, and information system models.

The art of HIS modeling is based on the right selection of a metamodel with respect to the tasks to be supported and the questions to be answered.

A typical metamodel for modeling health information systems is the three-layer graph-based metamodel ($3LGM^2$). It is used to describe the static view of a HIS over three layers: the domain layer, the logical tool layer, and the physical tool layer.

The domain layer describes a hospital independent of its implementation by its enterprise functions and the interpreted and updated entity types. At the logical tool layer, application components are described that support the hospital functions. The physical tool layer comprises a set of physical data processing systems that support the application components.

There are several relationships between classes of the different layers. Enterprise functions are related to their supporting application components; entity types are related to storing application components and to communication links. Updating an entity type when performing an enterprise function and storing it afterwards in an application component is called documentation. The application components are related to the physical data processing systems on which they are implemented.

Reference models are specific models that provide model patterns. They can be used to derive concrete models or to compare models. A typical reference model for hospital functions is the Reference Model for the Domain Layer of Hospital Information Systems, which provides a thorough set of patterns for modeling entity types and enterprise functions.

Architecture of Hospital Information Systems

6

6.1 Introduction

After having introduced health information systems in general we will at first turn our attention to hospital information systems (HIS). According to our previous definition of health information systems a HIS is the socio-technical subsystem of a hospital which comprises all information processing as well as the associated human or technical actors in their respective information processing roles.

We now take a closer look at what HIS look like. We will do that rather synthetically. This means that we will first look at all the detailed components a HIS consists of and afterwards we will explain step by step how these components can be synthesized, that is, assembled in order to achieve what users nowadays experience as the HIS.

Therefore we start by discussing the kind of data that has to be processed in hospitals and then present hospital functions that interpret or update these data. We introduce typical information processing tools and typical architectures first at the logical and then at the physical tool layer of HIS. At each layer we explain how these tools can be assembled and integrated for the better support of users.

After reading this chapter, you should be able to answer the following questions:

- What kind of data has to be processed in hospitals?
- What are the main hospital functions?
- What are the typical information processing tools in hospitals?
- What are the different architectures of a HIS?
- How can integrity and integration be achieved within a HIS?

6.2 Domain Layer: Data to Be Processed in Hospitals

Since the HIS is that subsystem of the hospital dealing with processing of information – or more precisely processing of data – we first want to introduce the kind of data that are typical for hospitals. As explained in Sect. 5.3.2.1 we can express "kind of data" by entity types.

A. Winter et al., *Health Information Systems*,
DOI: 10.1007/978-1-84996-441-8_6, © Springer-Verlag London Limited 2011

After this section, you should be able to answer the following question:

- What kind of data has to be processed in hospitals?

6.2.1 Entity Types Related to Patient Care

Below typical entity types representing certain object classes and data (see definition 5.3) related to the patient and his or her histories are shortly described. The entity types are listed in alphabetical order.

Entity type	Description of an instance of the represented object class
Case	Mostly comprises a patient's stay in a hospital from patient admission to patient discharge or several ambulatory treatments related to one disease; information about a case includes the case identification number (CIN)
Clinical pathway	Is an evidence-based approach that describes which activities have to be performed for a specific group of patients when and by whom
Clinical trial	Is a research study testing a new treatment, medication, or medical device on patients. Results obtained in a trial may be used for care and data recorded during care are necessary input for trials
Diagnosis	Is the identified cause or nature of a disease or medical condition
Diagnosis class	Is an aggregation of diagnoses with similar properties
Discharge summary	Shortly summarizes diagnoses, treatment, and recommendations which are necessary for the health care institutions providing further treatment
External finding	Is a finding of a previously treating health care provider
Finding	Summarizes the results of diagnostic procedures such as lab and x-ray examinations
Informed consent	Is a patient's consent to the proposed treatment
Medical anamnesis	Comprises all information needed as a basis for medical care planning
Medical procedure	Is a procedure carried out by a doctor, e.g., radiological examination, operation
Nursing anamnesis	Comprises all information needed as a basis for nursing care planning
Nursing procedure	Is a procedure carried out by a nurse, e.g., taking blood, taking the temperature
Order	Is a request for a diagnostic, therapeutic, or drug service, e.g., a laboratory order or a radiological order
Patient	Is a person who is a subject of care; information about a patient includes the patient identification number (PIN)

(continued)

Entity type	Description of an instance of the represented object class
Patient transport	Comprises information about where a patient has been or where and how he or she is to be transported there
Procedure	Is the generalization of a medical procedure and nursing procedure
Procedure class	Is an aggregation of procedures with similar properties
Sample	Is a specimen taken from a patient, e.g., a blood sample or a urine sample
Transfer	Comprises all information about the transfer of a patient, e.g., referring doctor and reasons for referring

6.2.2 Entity Types About Resources

A hospital must guarantee that all resources needed for *patient care* are available continuously. The following resources are necessary:

Entity type	Description of an instance of the represented object class
Appointment	Determines which persons have to be at a certain place at a given time. Examples are appointment for patient admission, examination, or surgery
Bed	Must be managed according to its occupation
Health care professional	Is one who treats, according to his or her specialization (e.g., nephrology or pediatrics), patients with certain diagnoses. Examples are physicians and nurses
Drug	Is a substance administered to a patient for treatment, diagnosis, or prevention
Food	Must be provided according to different nutritional needs of patients, e.g., normal diet and light diet
Human resource	Is a person working in the hospital, i.e., a doctor, nurse, administrative staff member, IT staff member, etc.
Laundry	Is scrubs, linen, etc.
Material	Is medical strip, bandage, needle, etc.
Means of transport	Comprises information about all means of transport, e.g., stretcher, ambulance, flying ambulance
Medical and nursing knowledge	Is stored in the doctors' and nurses' heads as well as in available media
Medical device	Is a technical or mechanical device used for diagnosis and treatment
Room	Is an operating room (OR), doctor's office, or waiting room
Service	Is a non-medical service provided in the hospital

6.2.3 Entity Types Related to Administration

Besides information about resources, hospital administration needs the following entity types:

Entity type	Description of an instance of the represented object class
Patient record archive	Describes how and where the electronic or paper-based patient record can be found
Classification	Consists of a set of classes summarizing concepts not to be distinguished during analysis
Classification of diagnoses	Is, for example, the International Classification of Diseases (ICD)
Classification of procedures	Is, for example, the International Classification of Procedures in Medicine (ICPM)
Cost unit	Is information about a person or an institution responsible for bearing the costs or a part of the costs for the services to be provided
Bill	Is demanded payment
Budget	Consists of all planned costs and revenues
Information system model	Is a model describing the architecture of the hospital's information system
Facility and area	Lists and describes the facilities of the hospital
Notification	Is the obligation hospitals have to inform the local health authority if a notifiable infection or disease such as HIV, hepatitis, or anthrax occurred
Service catalog	Contains all available orders
Third-party fund	Is a fund of external institutions financing certain projects

6.2.4 Entity Types Related to Management

Management relates to the hospital as a whole and, thus, needs compressed information about the hospital's operating. The following entity types are necessary for management.

Entity type	Description of an instance of the represented object class
Business strategy	Defines the hospital's long-term strategic goals
Controlling report	Summarizes monitored key performance indicators (KPIs) and compares them to the expected future state
Strategic information management plan	Is a strategic plan which gives directives for the construction and development of a hospital's information system
Health care regulation	Is a regulation or law to be observed by health care institutions (see examples in Sect. 8.4.3)

(continued)

Entity type	Description of an instance of the represented object class
Key performance indicator	Is a quantitative measurement for monitoring the achievement of strategic goals (facility management KPI, information system KPI, human resource KPI, patient administration KPI, resource KPI)
Project	Is a unique undertaking that is characterized by management by objectives, by restrictions with regard to available time and resources, and by a specific project organization (DIN 69901)
Quality report	Is an openly published report about a hospital's performance

6.3 Domain Layer: Hospital Functions

In the previous section, we introduced different entity types which represent object types and the respective data typically processed and stored in HIS. We will now elucidate how and where data about these entity types are processed in hospitals. As explained in Sects. 3.3.3 and 5.3.2.1 we use enterprise functions to summarize classes of information-processing activities. And since we focus on hospitals, we call them hospital functions here. These hospital functions can also be considered as representatives of processes.

We will present hospital functions and their interpreted and updated entity types in greater detail, but we will not (yet) focus on how they are typically supported by various computer-based or non-computer-based information-processing tools. For the hospital functions the interpreted and updated entity types will be outlined graphically in respective figures.

After this section, you should be able to answer the following questions:

- What are the main hospital functions that have to be supported by a HIS?
- What information is interpreted or updated by hospital functions?
- Which functional aspects have to be considered when implementing information-processing tools?
- What are examples for hospital processes?

6.3.1 Patient Care

6.3.1.1 Patient Admission

Patient admission (short: *admission*) aims at recording and distributing the patient demographics and insurance data as well as medical and nursing data of the patient history (see Fig. 6.1). In addition, each patient must be correctly identified, and a unique patient and case identifier must be assigned.

This hospital function can be decomposed as follows (see Fig. 6.2):

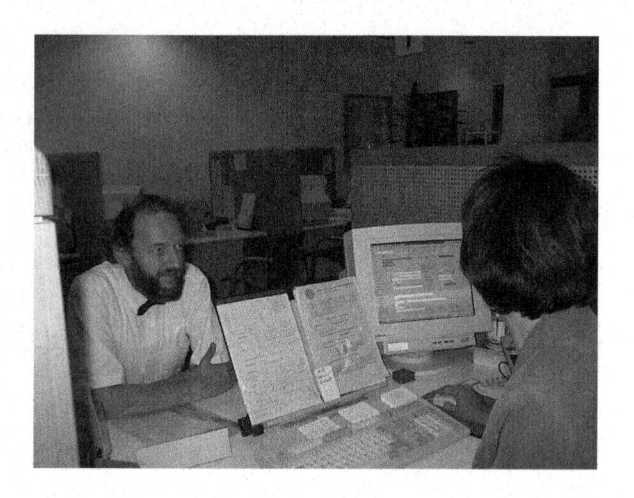

Fig. 6.1 A patient being admitted in a patient admission department

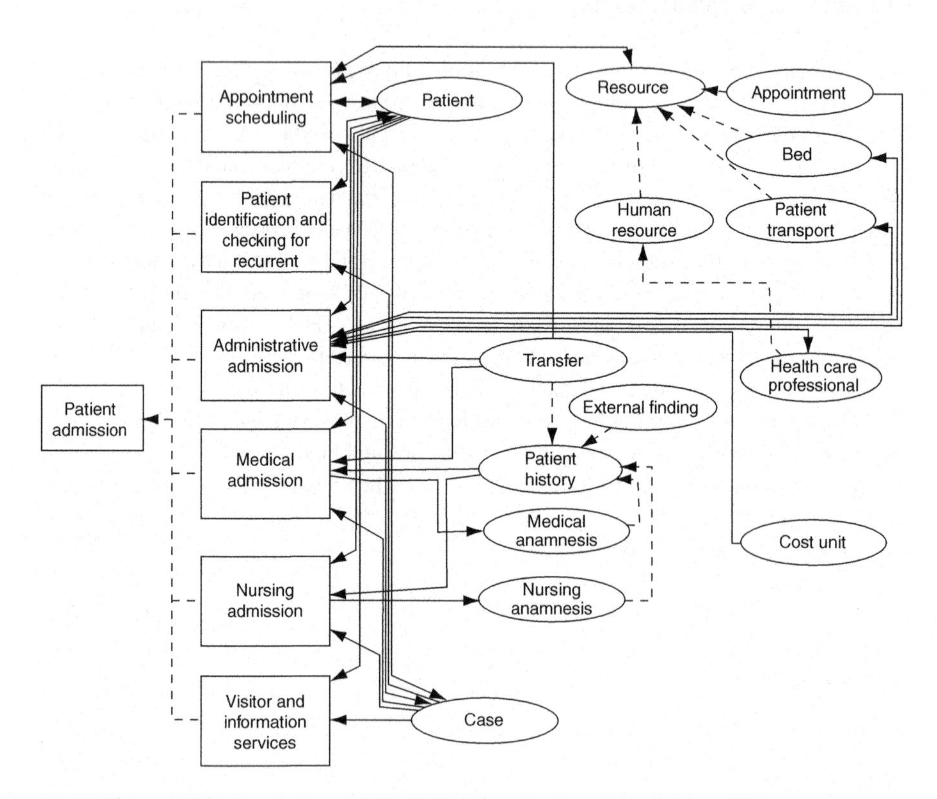

Fig. 6.2 Extract of the domain layer of the 3LGM²-based reference model describing the enterprise function *patient admission*, its subfunctions, and interpreted and updated entity types

Appointment Scheduling

The hospital must be able to schedule an appointment for a patient's visit. In addition, unplanned *patient admissions* must be possible (e.g., in case of emergencies).

Patient Identification and Checking for Recurrent

A unique patient identification number (PIN) must be assigned to each patient. This PIN should be valid and unchangeable lifelong (i.e., the PIN should not be based on changeable patient's attributes such as the name) (see also Sect. 6.5.2.1). The PIN is the main precondition for a patient-oriented combination of all information arising during previous, recent, as well as future hospitalizations. Before a PIN can be assigned, the patient must be correctly identified, usually based on a health insurance card and on available administrative patient master information (such as name and date of birth). If the patient has already been in the hospital, he or she must be identified as recurrent, and previously documented information must be made available (such as previous diagnoses and therapies). If the patient is in the hospital for the first time, a new PIN must be assigned. In addition, the hospital must be able to distinguish different cases or hospital stays of a patient. Therefore, in addition to the PIN, a case identification number (CIN) is usually assigned (see *administrative admission*).

Administrative Admission

Administrative admission starts following patient identification. It creates a so-called case, being the aggregation of several contacts, clustered according to specific clinical and/or organizational purposes of the hospital. In case of inpatient treatment, a case summarizes the hospital stay from *patient admission* until *discharge*. Each case is uniquely identified by its CIN. Important administrative data such as insurance data, details about special services, patient's relatives, admitting physician, and transfer diagnoses must be recorded. The patient is assigned to a ward and a bed. Some of the administrative data must be available to other hospital functions through the help of certain organization media (such as labels and magnetic cards; see Fig. 6.3). Administrative data form the backbone of information processing. In case of changes, patient data must be maintained and communicated. If the admitting physician has communicated relevant information (e.g., previous laboratory findings), this information must be communicated to the responsible physician in the hospital. *Administrative admission* is usually done either in a central patient admission area or directly on the ward (e.g., during emergencies or on the weekend).

Even in emergencies *patient admission* is necessary. At least *patient identification and checking for recurrent* has to be performed in order to assign a proper PIN and CIN. In these cases a short version of *administrative admission* may be applicable. If the patient is unconscious and does not bear an identity card, only a dummy name may be recorded to provide PIN and CIN. It will be no problem to replace the dummy name by the correct name later.

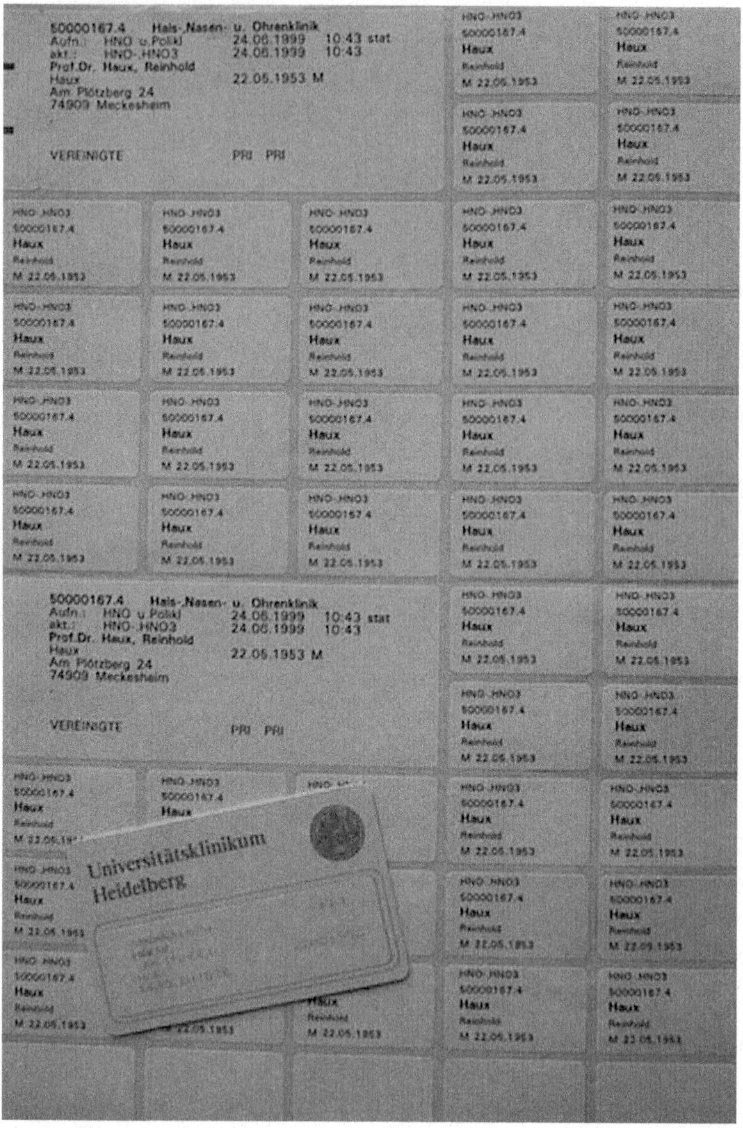

50000167.4 Hals-,Nasen- u. Ohrenklinik
Aufn.: HNO u.Polikl 24.06.1999 10:43 stat
akt.: HNO-HNO3 24.06.1999 10:43
Prof.Dr. Haux, Reinhold
Haux 22.05.1953 M
Am Plötzberg 24
74909 Meckesheim
VEREINIGTE PRI PRI

HNO-HNO3
50000167.4
Haux
Reinhold
M 22.05.1953

HNO-HNO3
50000167.4
Haux
Reinhold
M 22.05.1953

50000167.4 Hals-,Nasen- u. Ohrenklinik
Aufn.: HNO u.Polikl 24.06.1999 10:43 stat
akt.: HNO-HNO3 24.06.1999 10:43
Prof.Dr. Haux, Reinhold
Haux 22.05.1953 M
Am Plötzberg 24
74909 Meckesheim
VEREINIGTE PRI PRI

Universitätsklinikum
Heidelberg

Fig. 6.3 Typical organizational media: a magnetic card and stickers with patient identification data

Medical Admission

Subsequently, the responsible physician will carry out the *medical admission*. This typically comprises the patient history (disease history, systems review, social history, past medical history, family history, medication). Some of this information may be collected from documents of the referring physician and is taken to the hospital by the patient himself or herself.

As a result of *medical admission* the admission diagnosis has to be stated and to be coded according to ICD10 (see Sect. 6.5.3.2).

The basic patient history data have to be made available for other hospital functions. For the patient history there may also be department-specific, (semi-)standardized data entry forms available. The collected information should be available during the whole stay. *Medical admission* is usually done at the ward.

Nursing Admission

The responsible nurse will proceed with the *nursing admission*. This typically comprises the introduction of the patient to the ward and the nursing history. Administrative data and the reason of hospitalization are already at her or his disposal. For the nursing history there may be computer-based or department-specific, (semi-)standardized data entry forms available. These may contain information about the current diagnosis and therapy, orientation, communication ability, social contacts, nutrition, mobility, personal hygiene, and vital signs. The collected information should be available during the whole stay. *Nursing admission* is usually done at the ward.

Visitor and Information Service

The hospital management must always have an overview of the recent bed occupation, that is, about the patients staying at the hospital. This is, for example, important for the clerks at the information desk, who must be able to inform relatives and visitors correctly (see Fig. 6.4), and also for some general hospital management statistics.

6.3.1.2
Decision Making, Planning, and Organization of Patient Treatment

All clinical procedures of health care professionals must be discussed, agreed upon, efficiently planned, and initiated. This process is repeated each time new information is available.

This hospital function can be decomposed as follows (see Fig. 6.5):

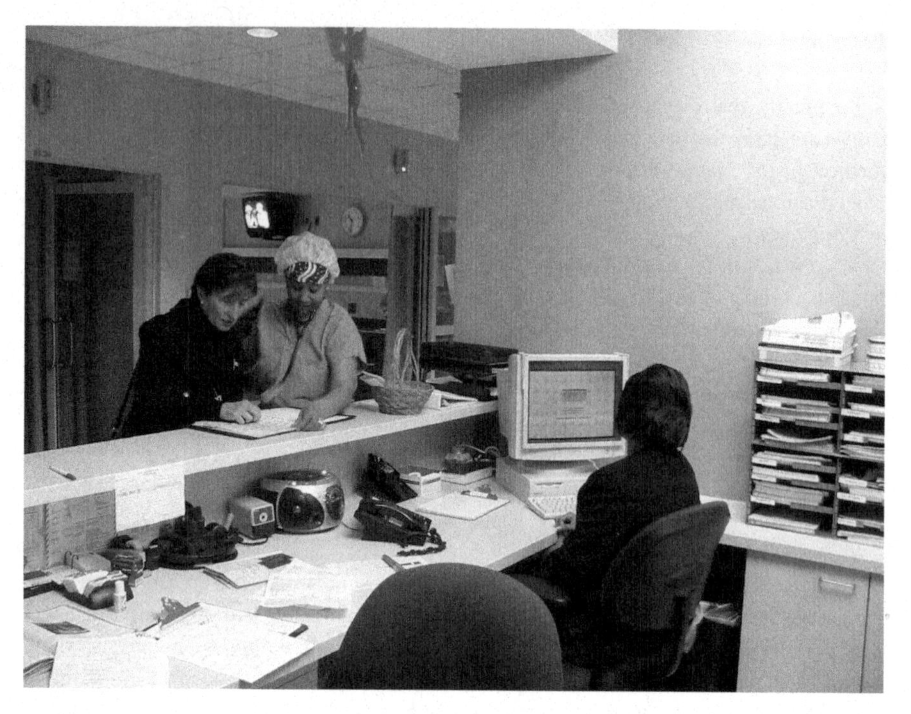

Fig. 6.4 Informing patients' relatives on a ward

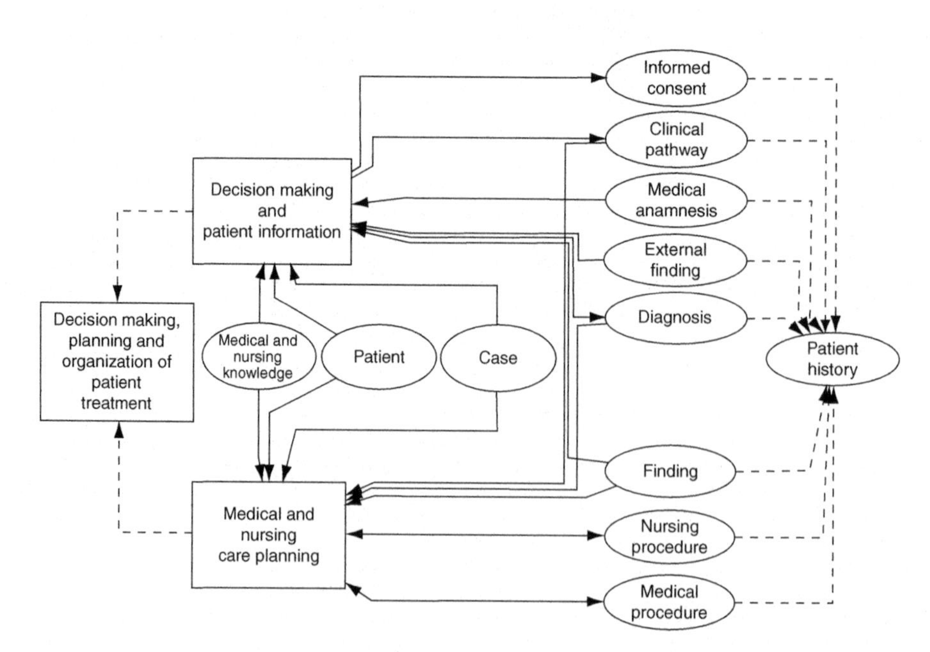

Fig. 6.5 Extract of the domain layer of the 3LGM²-based reference model describing the enterprise function *decision making, planning and organization of patient treatment*, its subfunctions, and interpreted and updated entity types

Decision Making and Patient Information

Responsible team members must decide upon the next steps such as certain diagnostic or therapeutic procedures. Depending on the complexity of a diagnostic or therapeutic decision, they should be able to consult internal or external experts (e.g., in specialized hospitals) to get a second opinion. In this context, (tele-)conferences may help. Staff members must be able to access all relevant patient data specific to a situation, in addition to general clinical knowledge (e.g., guidelines and standards) supporting patient care. Medication prescription may be supported by providing knowledge about adverse drug events. Decisions about clinical procedures must be documented. The patient should be involved in the decision-making process, the consequences of the planned diagnostic or therapeutic procedures should be explained, and his or her informed consent must be documented as well. Decision making is a permanent enterprise function which is triggered by new information about the patient.

Medical and Nursing Care Planning

The next steps now have to be planned in detail. For each medical procedure (such as a radiological examination, an operation, or a chemotherapeutic treatment) as well as for each nursing procedure, the type, extent, duration, and responsible person have to be determined. In nursing, care planning is documented in nursing care plans, containing nursing problems, nursing goals, and planned nursing procedures (Fig. 6.6). If

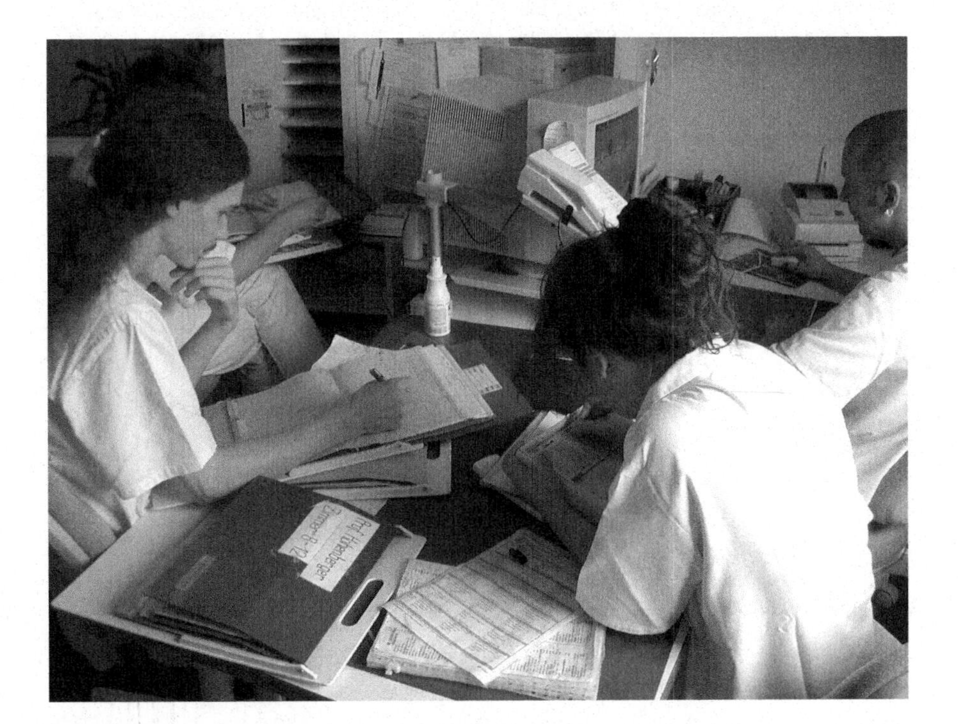

Fig. 6.6 Paper-based nursing documentation on a ward

necessary, other health care professionals are ordered to execute the planned clinical procedures (e.g., medical bandaging orders, which have to be executed by a nurse).

Care planning in cancer treatment is often performed in tumor board reviews. This means that a number of physicians who are experts in different specialties (disciplines) review and discuss the medical condition and treatment options of a patient.

6.3.1.3 Order Entry

Diagnostic and therapeutic procedures must often be ordered at specialized service units (e.g., laboratory, radiology, or pathology). These units execute the ordered procedures and communicate the findings or results back to the ordering department.

This hospital function can be decomposed as follows (see Fig. 6.7):

Preparation of an Order

Depending on the type of order, specimens that must be unambiguously assigned to a patient are submitted (e.g., blood sample). Depending on the available service spectrum offered by a service unit, which may be presented in the form of service catalogs, the health care professional selects the appropriate service on an order entry form (Fig. 6.8). Patient and case identification, together with relevant information such as recent diagnoses, relevant questions, service ordered (e.g., laboratory, radiology), and other comments (e.g., on special risks), are documented. An order should be initiated only by authorized persons.

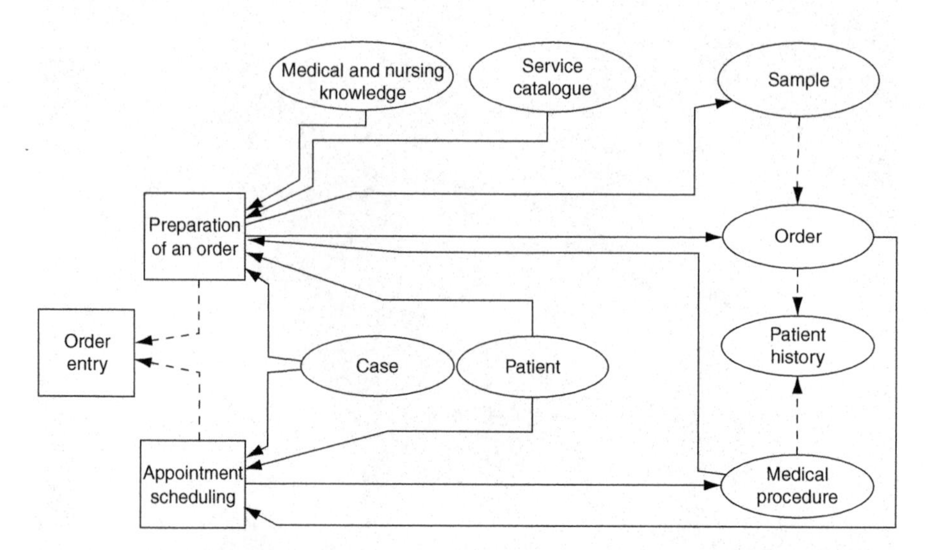

Fig. 6.7 Extract of the domain layer of the 3LGM²-based reference model describing the enterprise function order entry, its subfunctions, and interpreted and updated entity types

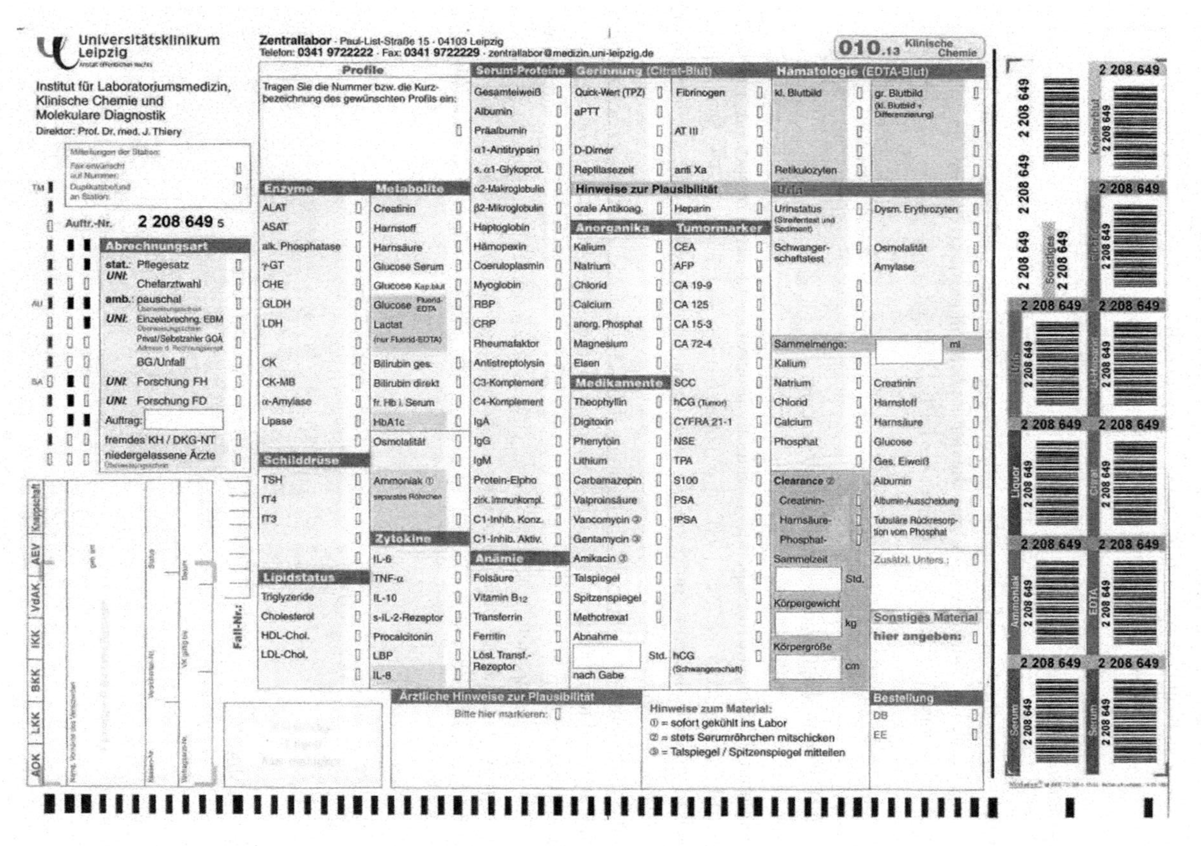

Universitätsklinikum Leipzig

Institut für Laboratoriumsmedizin, Klinische Chemie und Molekulare Diagnostik
Direktor: Prof. Dr. med. J. Thiery

Mitteilungen der Station: Fax erwünscht auf Nummer; Duplikatsbefund an Station

Zentrallabor · Paul-List-Straße 15 · 04103 Leipzig
Telefon: 0341 9722222 · Fax: 0341 9722229 · zentrallabor@medizin.uni-leipzig.de

010.13 Klinische Chemie

Auftr.-Nr. 2 208 649 5

Abrechnungsart: stat.: Pflegesatz; UNI: Chefarztwahl; amb.: pauschal; UNI: Einzelabrechng. EBM; Privat/Selbstzahler GOÄ; BG/Unfall; UNI: Forschung FH; UNI: Forschung FD; Auftrag:; fremdes KH / DKG-NT; niedergelassene Ärzte

Profile: Tragen Sie die Nummer bzw. die Kurzbezeichnung des gewünschten Profils ein:

Enzyme: ALAT, ASAT, alk. Phosphatase, γ-GT, CHE, GLDH, LDH, CK, CK-MB, α-Amylase, Lipase

Metabolite: Creatinin, Harnstoff, Harnsäure, Glucose Serum, Glucose Kap.blut, Glucose Fluorid-EDTA, Lactat (nur Fluorid-EDTA), Bilirubin ges., Bilirubin direkt, fr. Hb i. Serum, HbA1c, Osmolalität, Ammoniak ① separates Röhrchen

Schilddrüse: TSH, fT4, fT3

Lipidstatus: Triglyzeride, Cholesterol, HDL-Chol., LDL-Chol.

Zytokine: IL-6, TNF-α, IL-10, s-IL-2-Rezeptor, Procalcitonin, LBP, IL-8

Serum-Proteine: Gesamteiweiß, Albumin, Präalbumin, α1-Antitrypsin, s. α1-Glykoprot., α2-Makroglobulin, β2-Mikroglobulin, Haptoglobin, Hämopexin, Coeruloplasmin, Myoglobin, RBP, CRP, Rheumafaktor, Antistreptolysin, C3-Komplement, C4-Komplement, IgA, IgG, IgM, Protein-Elpho, zirk. Immunkompl., C1-Inhib. Konz., C1-Inhib. Aktiv.

Anämie: Folsäure, Vitamin B12, Transferrin, Ferritin, Lösl. Transf.-Rezeptor

Gerinnung (Citrat-Blut): Quick-Wert (TPZ), aPTT, D-Dimer, Reptilasezeit, Fibrinogen, AT III, anti Xa

Hinweise zur Plausibilität: orale Antikoag., Heparin

Anorganika: Kalium, Natrium, Chlorid, Calcium, anorg. Phosphat, Magnesium, Eisen

Tumormarker: CEA, AFP, CA 19-9, CA 125, CA 15-3, CA 72-4, SCC, hCG (Tumor), CYFRA 21-1, NSE, TPA, S100, PSA, fPSA, hCG (Schwangerschaft)

Medikamente: Theophyllin, Digitoxin, Phenytoin, Lithium, Carbamazepin, Valproinsäure, Vancomycin ③, Gentamycin ③, Amikacin ③, Talspiegel, Spitzenspiegel, Methotrexat, Abnahme, Std. nach Gabe

Hämatologie (EDTA-Blut): kl. Blutbild, gr. Blutbild (kl. Blutbild + Differenzierung), Retikulozyten

Urin: Urinstatus (Streifentest und Sediment), Dysm. Erythrozyten, Schwangerschaftstest, Osmolalität, Amylase, Sammelmenge: ml, Kalium, Natrium, Chlorid, Calcium, Phosphat, Creatinin, Harnstoff, Harnsäure, Glucose, Ges. Eiweiß, Albumin, Albumin-Ausscheidung, Tubuläre Rückresorption vom Phosphat

Clearance ②: Creatinin-, Harnsäure-, Phosphat-; Sammelzeit Std.; Körpergewicht kg; Körpergröße cm; Zusätzl. Unters.:

Sonstiges Material hier angeben:

Ärztliche Hinweise zur Plausibilität: Bitte hier markieren:

Hinweise zum Material:
① = sofort gekühlt ins Labor
② = stets Serumröhrchen mitschicken
③ = Talspiegel / Spitzenspiegel mitteilen

Bestellung: DB, EE

Fall-Nr.:

AOK, LKK, BKK, IKK, VdAK, AEV, Knappschaft

Kapillarblut, Sonstiges, Citrat, Urin, Li-Heparin, Liquor, Citrat, Ammoniak, EDTA, Serum, Serum — 2 208 649

Fig. 6.8 A paper-based order entry form for laboratory testing

When computer-based tools for order entry are used, computerized decision support systems could alert the physician in case of medication errors, for example, when a medication is ordered to which the patient is allergic. The order must quickly and correctly be transmitted to the service unit. If a specimen is transferred, it must be guaranteed that the order and the specimen can be linked to each other at the service unit. If necessary, modification to already transferred orders by the ordering health care professional should be possible.

Appointment Scheduling

Depending on the type of order, the patient's appointments must be scheduled (e.g., in radiological units). During scheduling, the demands of all parties (e.g., ordering physician, service unit, patient, transport unit) must be fairly balanced.

6.3.1.4 Execution of Diagnostic, Therapeutic and Nursing Procedures

The planned diagnostic, therapeutic, or nursing procedures (such as operations, radiotherapy, radiological examinations, medication) must be executed (Fig. 6.9). The hospital must offer adequate tools and resources (e.g., staff, room, equipment) for the execution of the necessary procedures.

It is important that changes in care planning that may be due to new findings are promptly communicated to all involved units and persons, enabling them to adapt to the new situation. All clinically relevant patient data (such as vital signs, orders, results, decisions) must be recorded as completely, correctly, and quickly as necessary. This supports the coordination of patient treatment among all involved persons, and also the legal justification for the actions taken. Data should be recorded in as structured a way as possible, so as to allow for

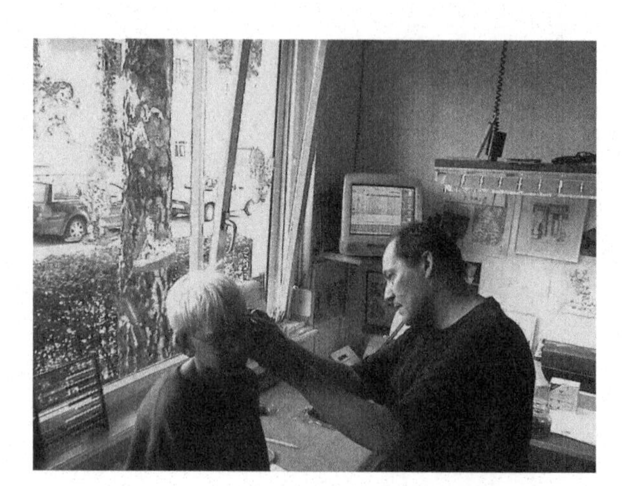

Fig. 6.9 Clinical examination conducted by a pediatrician

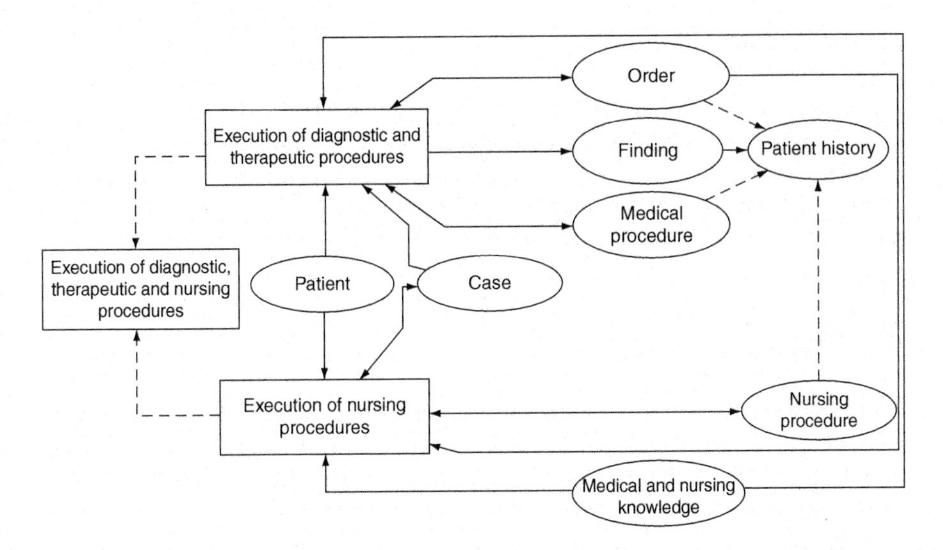

Fig. 6.10 Extract of the domain layer of the 3LGM²-based reference model describing the enterprise function *execution of diagnostic, therapeutic and nursing procedures*, its subfunctions, and interpreted and updated entity types

data aggregation and statistics, computerized decision support, or retrieval of data. It is important that data can be linked by PIN and CIN, even when data originate from different areas (such as ward, service unit, outpatient unit). Usually, the hospital has to fulfill a lot of different legal reporting (such as epidemiological registers) and documentation requirements. The items to be documented depend partly on the documenting unit and the documenting health care professional group (such as documentation by health care professionals, documentation in outpatient units or in operation rooms). Clinical information should also be available for other functions such as *financial accounting*, *controlling*, *quality management*, or *research and education*.

This hospital function can be decomposed as follows (see Fig. 6.10):

Execution of Diagnostic and Therapeutic Procedures

The planned diagnostic and therapeutic procedures must be executed. All procedures must be documented. Findings and reports must be transmitted (as quickly as necessary) back to the ordering unit and presented to the responsible health care professional. They must be unambiguously assigned to the correct patient. The responsible physician should be informed about new results, and critical findings should be highlighted.

The hospital function *execution of diagnostic and therapeutic procedures* can be specialized, for example, to execution of operations, execution of irradiation, execution of chemotherapy, execution of radiological examinations, execution of lab examinations, and execution of prophylaxis and medication.

Execution of Nursing Procedures

The planned nursing procedures (concerning excretion, decubitus, hair und nail care, skin care, wound treatment, body washing, oral and dental care, nutrition and liquid balance, thrombosis) are executed. All patient care procedures, their impact on the patient's health status, and changes to the care plan have to be documented. The responsible physician must be informed about therapy-relevant facts.

6.3.1.5 Coding of Diagnoses and Procedures

The hospital must be able to document and code all diagnoses stated and all medical procedures carried out in a correct, complete, quick, and patient-oriented way. These data are the basis for the hospital's billing. Diagnoses and medical procedures are also used for controlling. In addition, some of the data must be documented and communicated due to legal requirements.

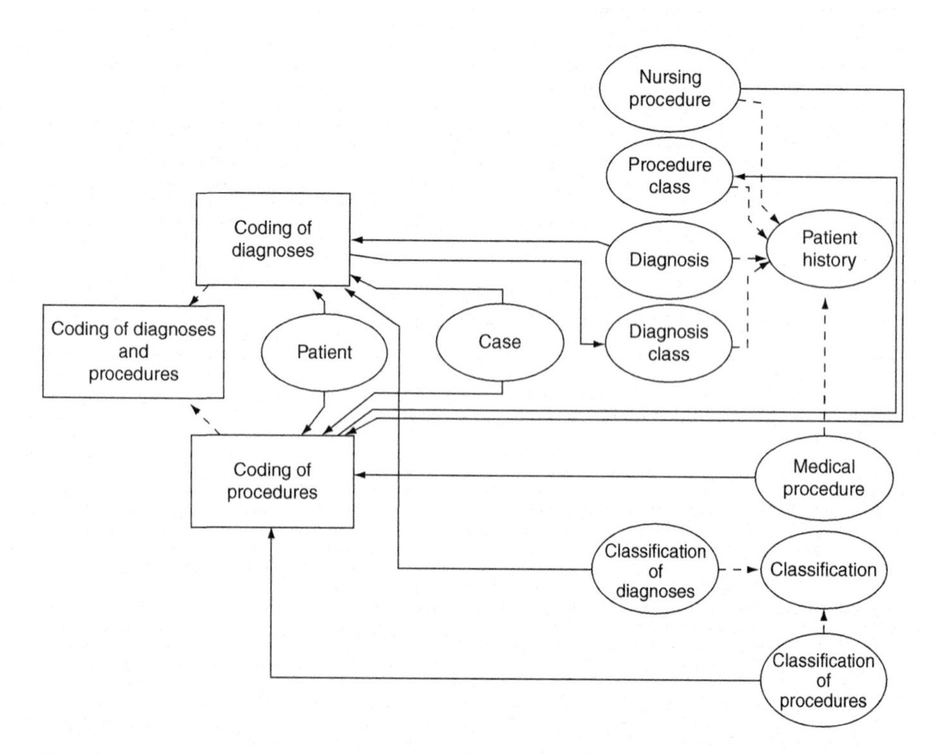

Fig. 6.11 Extract of the domain layer of the 3LGM²-based reference model describing the enterprise function *coding of diagnoses and procedures*, its subfunctions, and interpreted and updated entity types

Diagnoses and medical procedures are recorded and coded in a standardized way (e.g., using the ICD-10[1] for diagnoses codes), and then processed. Diagnoses and medical procedures should be at least partly derivable from clinical documentation. To support their documentation, adequate coding catalogs must be offered and maintained, containing lists of typical diagnoses and medical procedures relevant for a unit or a hospital.

The enterprise function *coding of diagnoses and procedures*, its decomposition in subfunctions, and the entity types to be interpreted and updated are summarized in Fig. 6.11.

6.3.1.6 Patient Discharge and Transfer to Other Institutions

When patient treatment is terminated, the patient is discharged and then sometimes transferred to other institutions (e.g., a general practitioner (GP) or a rehabilitation center) (Fig. 6.12). *Patient discharge and transfer to other institutions* (short: *discharge*) covers *administrative, medical, and nursing discharge.*

This hospital function can be decomposed as follows (see Fig. 6.13):

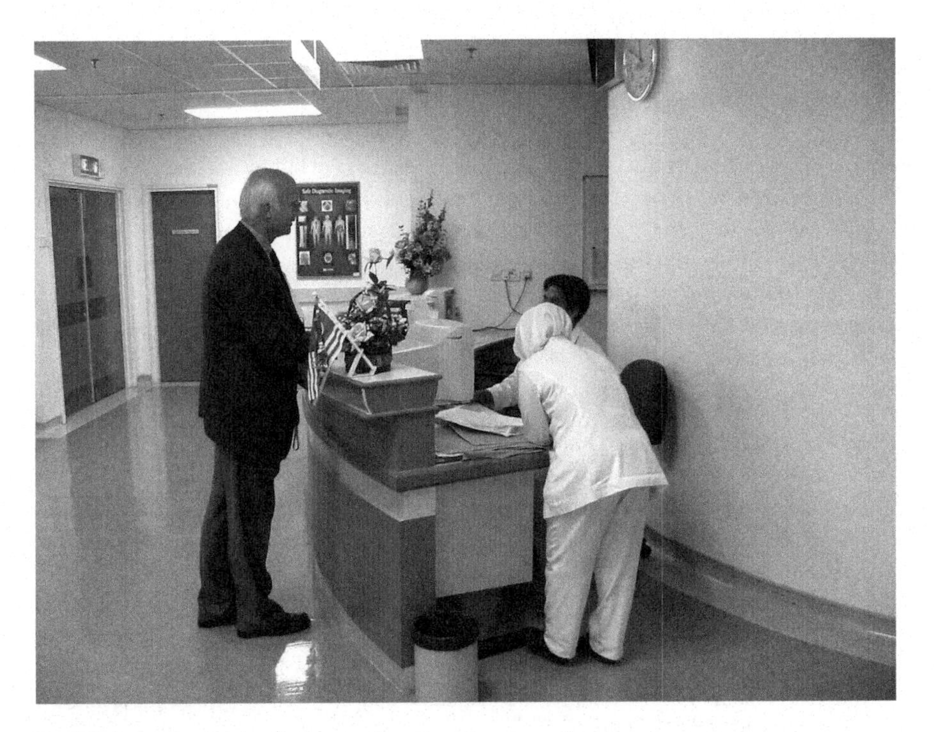

Fig. 6.12 Preparing for the *discharge* of a patient from a ward

[1]World Health Organization (WHO): Tenth Revision of the International Statistical Classification of Diseases and Related Health Problems (ICD-10). Geneva: World Health Organization. http://www.who.int/whosis/icd10

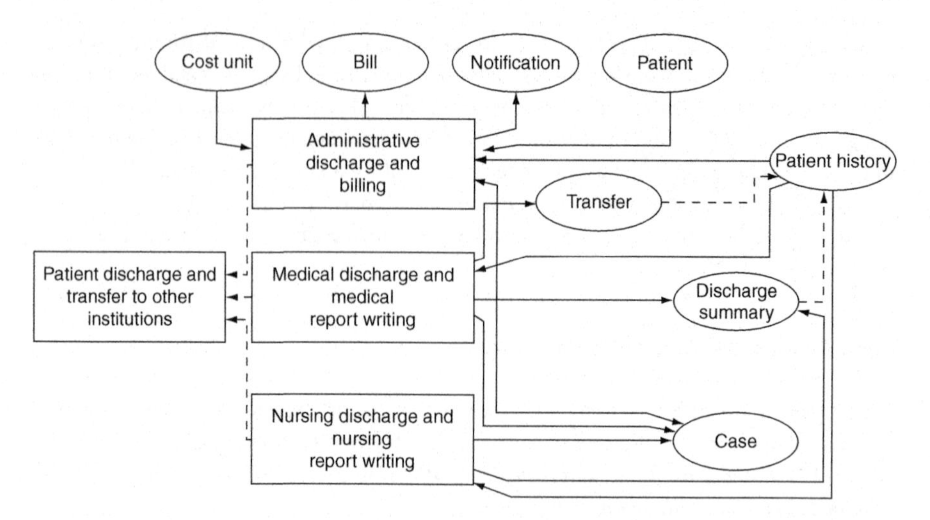

Fig. 6.13 Extract of the domain layer of the 3LGM²-based reference model describing the enterprise function *patient discharge and transfer to other institutions*, its subfunctions, and interpreted and updated entity types

Administrative Discharge and Billing

The process of administrative patient discharge initiates final billing and the fulfillment of legal reporting requirements (e.g., statistics on diagnoses and procedures). During the last years Diagnosis Related Groups (DRG [2]) systems have been introduced for patient billing in most of the industrial countries. This means that bills for patient treatment are no longer calculated based on daily rates, but on the DRG in which a patient case was classified. Diagnoses, procedures, patient's age, and some more criteria serve as an input for the calculation of a DRG.

Medical Discharge and Medical Report Writing

Medical discharge entails completing of documentation and writing of a discharge report by the attending physician. The medical report includes relevant diagnoses, important findings, therapeutic procedures, current patient state, and recommendations for further treatment. The hospital must be able to transmit this and other information (e.g., radiological images) to other institutions as quickly as possible. To speed up this process, a short report (i.e., physician's discharge letter) is often immediately communicated to the next institution, containing, for example, the diagnoses and therapeutic treatments. It is then followed by a more detailed report.

[2]http://www.fas.org/ota/reports/8306.pdf

Nursing Discharge and Nursing Report Writing

Nursing discharge entails completing of documentation and writing of a nursing report by the attending nurse. The nursing report comprises, for example, information about activity level, diet, and wound care.

6.3.2 Supply and Disposal Management, Scheduling, and Resource Allocation

The hospital must offer sufficient and well-organized resources for *patient care*. This is true for wards (ward management), outpatient units (outpatient management), and service units (department management). Efficient process organization is extremely important for hospitals, for example, in outpatient units or service units, and it can be supported, for example, by providing working lists for individual staff members, by issuing reminders about appointments, or by visualizing actual process flow. The HIS must be able to support communication between all persons involved in *patient care*. This comprises synchronous (e.g., telephone) and asynchronous (e.g., blackboards, brochures, e-mail) communication. Staff members must be able to be contacted within a prescribed period of time.

6.3.2.1 Supply and Disposal Management

Supply and disposal of materials, food, drugs, and so on must be guaranteed. All departments of the hospital should be able to order from up-to-date catalogs. The corresponding service units (stock, pharmacy, and kitchen) must be able to deliver correctly and on time.

Supply and disposal management can be decomposed as follows (see Fig. 6.14):

Catering

According to their health status, patients have different nutritional needs. It must be ensured that the patients are provided with the right dietary food at the right time.

Material and Medication Management

Nurses and doctors must be able to anticipate lack of material like medical strips, bandages, or needles to order new material from a central supplier in time (see Fig. 6.15).

Laundry Management

The hospital must permanently be supplied with linen, towels, sterile scrubs, surgical masks, etc.

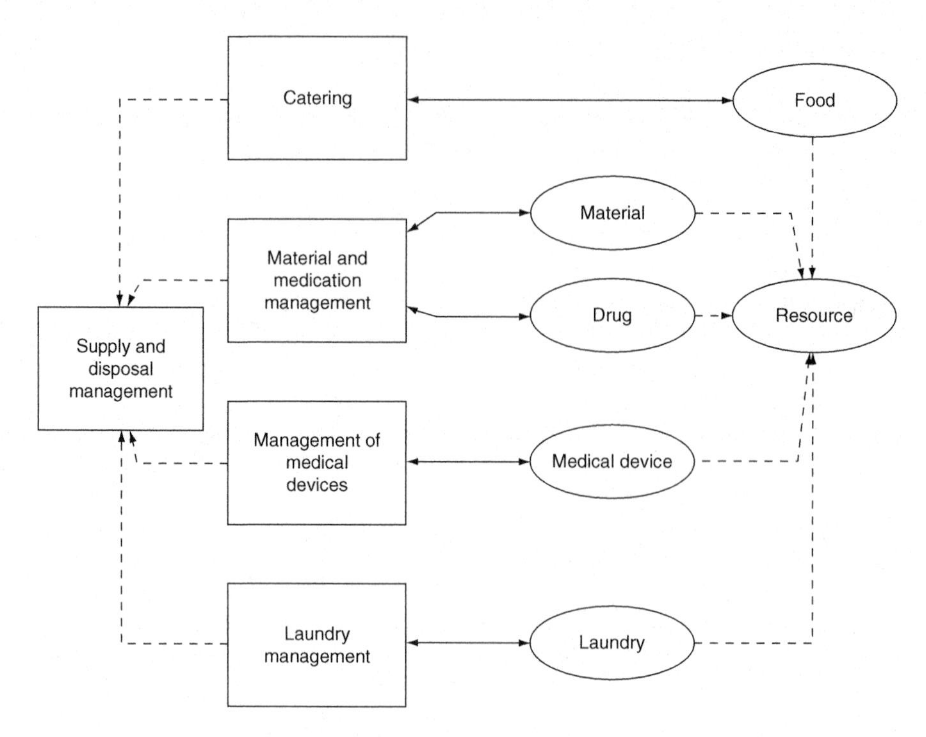

Fig. 6.14 Extract of the domain layer of the 3LGM²-based reference model describing the enterprise function *supply and disposal management*, its subfunctions, and interpreted and updated entity types

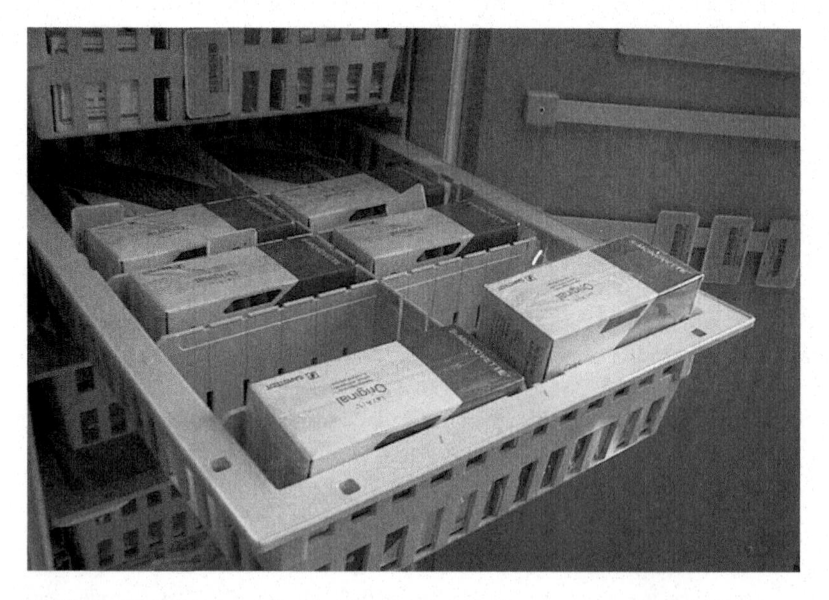

Fig. 6.15 The stock of drugs on a hospital ward

Management of Medical Devices

In addition to other resources, medical devices must be registered and maintained according to legislation. Due maintenance must be organized, documented, and completed.

6.3.2.2
Scheduling and Resource Allocation

Various resources are needed for *patient care*, and resource management comprises staff planning, bed planning, room planning, and device planning. All resource-planning activities must be coordinated. When procedures are scheduled, the demands of both the service unit and the ordering unit with regard to scheduling the appointment must be considered. Request, reservation, confirmation, notification, postponement, and cancellation must be supported. All involved staff members and patients should be informed about the appointments. Postponements and cancellations should be communicated in time to all persons involved.

This hospital function can be decomposed into *appointment scheduling*, *scheduling and resource planning with the medical service unit*, and *scheduling and resource planning with the patient transport service* (see Fig. 6.16). *Appointment scheduling* was also listed as a subfunction of *patient admission*.

6.3.2.3
Human Resources Management

This contains all tasks for the development and improvement of the productivity of staff. It comprises, for example, staff and position planning, staff register, staff scheduling, and staff payroll.

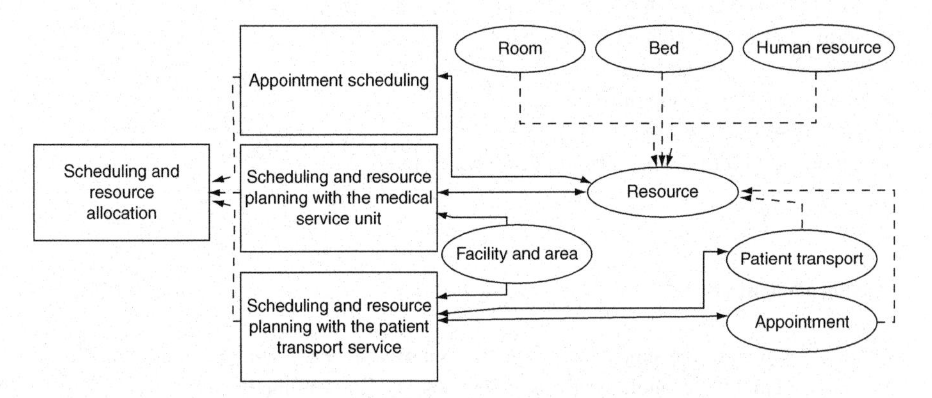

Fig. 6.16 Extract of the domain layer of the 3LGM²-based reference model describing the enterprise function *scheduling and resource allocation*, its subfunctions, and interpreted and updated entity types

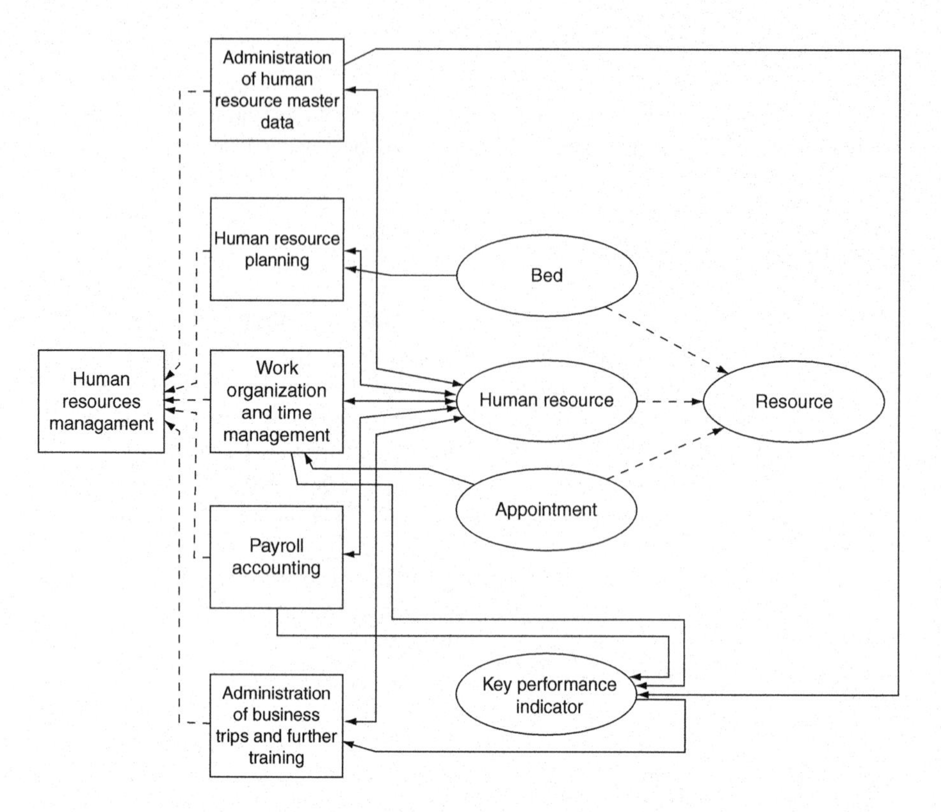

Fig. 6.17 Extract of the domain layer of the 3LGM²-based reference model describing the enterprise function *human resources management*, its subfunctions, and interpreted and updated entity types

This hospital function can be decomposed as follows (see Fig. 6.17):

- administration of human resource master data;
- human resource planning;
- work organization and time management;
- payroll accounting;
- administration of business trips and further training.

6.3.3 Hospital Administration

Hospital administration supports the organization of *patient care* and guarantees the financial survival and the economic success of the hospital. Its subfunctions are:

6.3.3.1
Patient Administration

Patient administration comprises the administrative tasks in a hospital dealing more or less immediately with patients. Thus it is an aggregation of the subfunctions of *administrative admission, patient identification and checking for recurrent, visitor and information service* (see Sect. 6.3.1.1), and *administrative discharge and billing* (see Sect. 6.3.1.6).

6.3.3.2
Archiving of Patient Information

Relevant data and documents containing patient information must be created, gathered, presented, and stored such that they are efficiently retrievable during the whole process of patient treatment. The storage of these data and documents is primarily done in patient records. Today, usually a mixture of paper-based and computer-based patient records is used. Certain legal requirements usually must be considered.

This hospital function can be decomposed as follows (see Fig. 6.18):

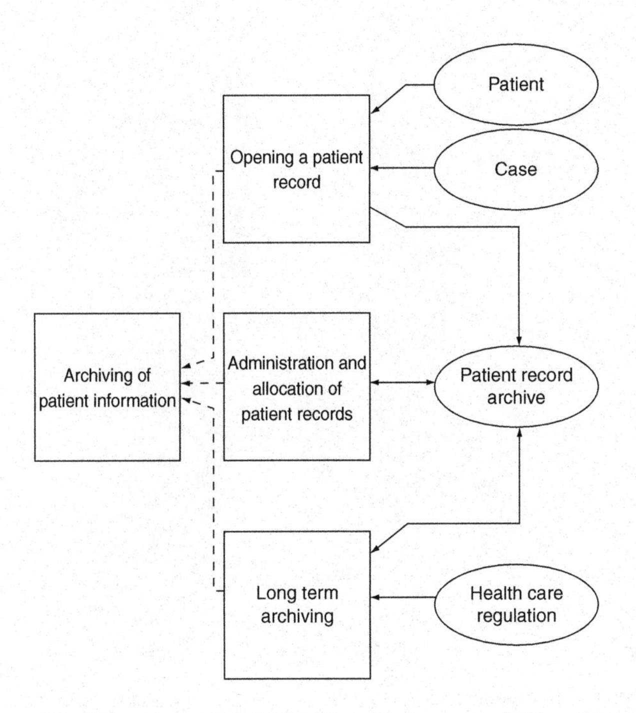

Fig. 6.18 Extract of the domain layer of the 3LGM²-based reference model describing the enterprise function *archiving of patient information*, its subfunctions, and interpreted and updated entity types

Opening of a Patient Record

Administrative admission triggers the *opening of a patient record*. The patient record may be electronic or paper-based or a mixture of both. For the filing formats of documents standards have to be established and used.

Administration and Allocation of Patient Records

A paper-based hospital archive must be able to manage patient records and make them available upon request within a defined time frame. The exact location of each record should be known (e.g., in which archive, on which shelf). Robot systems may store and gather paper-based records automatically (see Fig. 6.19). Lending and return of records (e.g., for patients coming for multiple visits) have to be organized, while respecting different access rights that depend on the role of the health care professionals in the process of *patient care*.

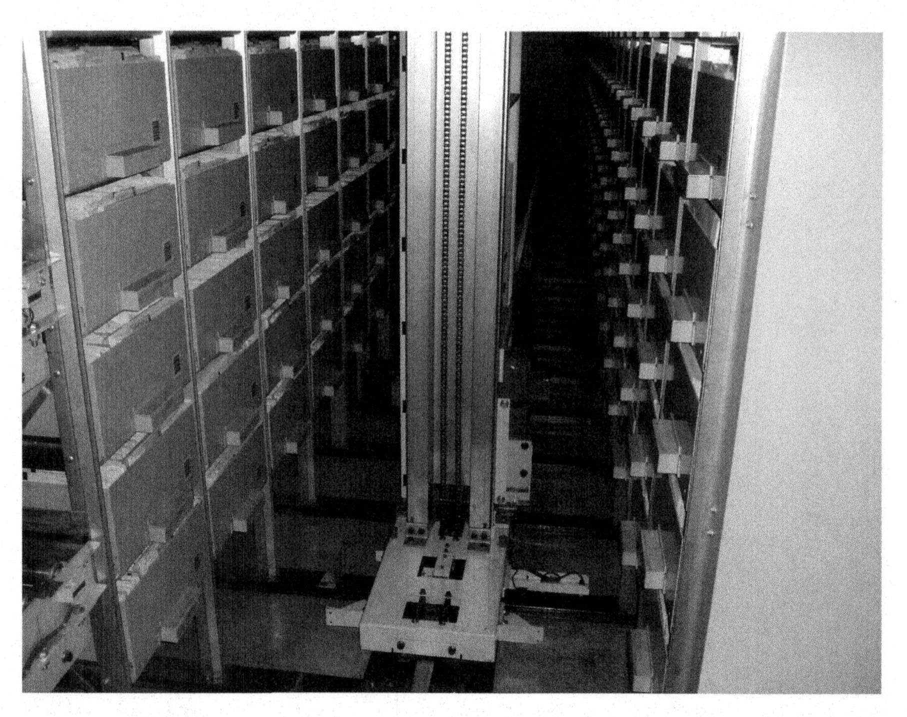

Fig. 6.19 A paper-based hospital archive with a robot system for storing and gathering boxes filled with patient records

Long-Term Archiving

After the *discharge* of the patient, patient records must be archived for a long time (e.g., for 10 or 30 years, depending on the legal regulations). The archive must offer enough space to allow the long-term storage of patient records (see Sect. 6.7.4.1). Their authenticity and correctness can be proven more easily, for example, in case of legal action, when they are archived in accordance with legal regulations.

6.3.3.3 Quality Management

Quality management comprises all activities of a health care institution's management to assure and continuously improve the quality of *patient care*. This includes setting goals, defining responsibilities, and establishing and monitoring the processes to achieve these goals. This covers, for example, internal reporting containing quality indices. *Quality management* requires information about patients and treatments as well as knowledge about diagnostic and therapeutic standards.

This hospital function can be decomposed as follows (see Fig. 6.20):

Internal Quality Management

Internal quality management assures a defined quality of all processes and outcomes of the hospital. An internal reporting system, which presents quality-related indicators, is also covered. Medical, nursing, and administrative guidelines may be defined, stored, and presented. There exists a structured complaint management.

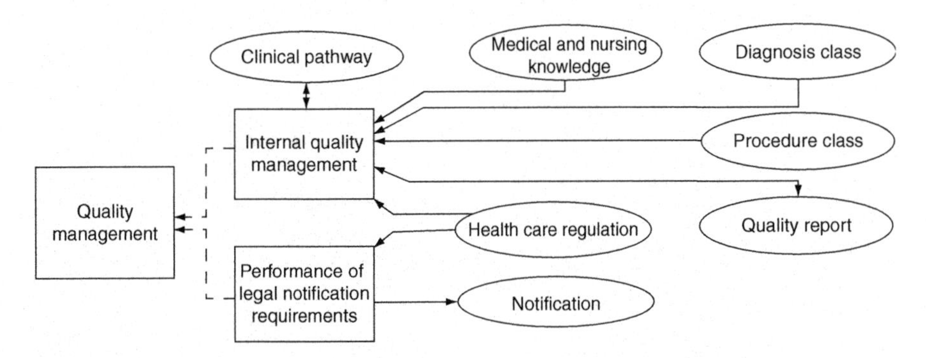

Fig. 6.20 Extract of the domain layer of the 3LGM²-based reference model describing the enterprise function *quality management*, its subfunctions, and interpreted and updated entity types

Performance of Legal Notification Requirements

Legal notification requirements for quality assurance must be completed.

6.3.3.4 Cost Accounting

For *controlling* purposes, it is necessary to keep track of services, their costs, and who has received them. *Cost accounting* usually investigates which costs incur (cost-type accounting), where costs incur (cost center accounting), and for what activities or services costs incur (cost unit accounting). According to the accounting purpose, the time period to be observed and the scope of the costs to be accounted have to be defined. The results of *cost accounting*, that is, KPIs, serve as input for controlling (see Figs. 6.21 and 6.22).

6.3.3.5 Controlling

The hospital must be able to gather and aggregate data about the hospital's operation in order to control and optimize it. This covers, for example, staff controlling, process controlling, material controlling, and financial controlling. In hospitals, for example, the number of patient cases, the length of patient stays in the hospital, and the case mix index, which is calculated from the patients' DRGs, are KPIs serving as input for controlling reports (see Figs. 6.22 and 6.23).

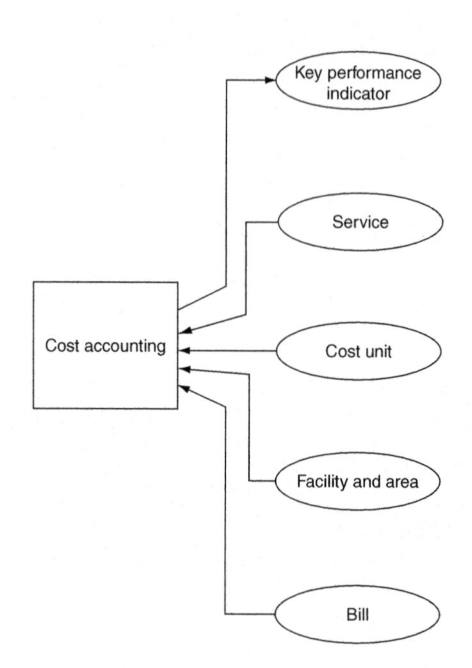

Fig. 6.21 Extract of the domain layer of the 3LGM²-based reference model describing the enterprise function *cost accounting*, its interpreted and updated entity types

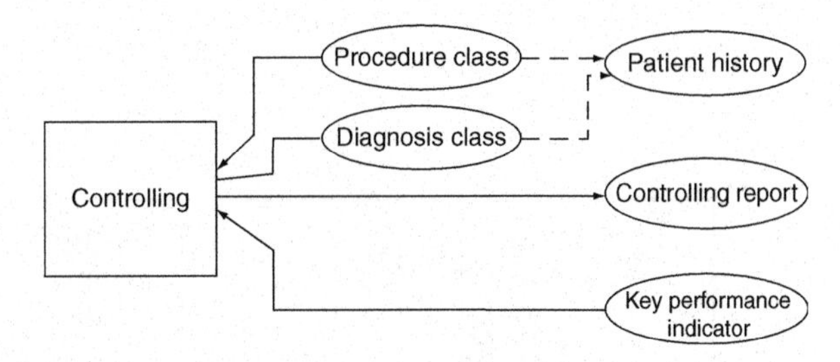

Fig. 6.22 Extract of the domain layer of the 3LGM²-based reference model describing the enterprise function *controlling* and its interpreted and updated entity types

6.3.3.6
Financial Accounting

All the hospital's financial operations have to be systematically recorded to meet legal requirements. *Financial accounting* comprises, for example, debtor accounting, credit accounting, and asset accounting. It needs information from bills and creates new values for KPIs (see Fig. 6.24). The hospital must support general statistical analysis, for example, calculation and analysis of economic data.

6.3.3.7
Facility Management

Facility management comprises the management of buildings, areas, and utilities of the hospital and also influences KPIs (see Fig. 6.25).

6.3.3.8
Information Management[3]

Information management plans the information system of an enterprise and its architecture, directs its establishment and its operation, and monitors its development and operation with respect to the planned objectives. Different management levels have different perceptions and interests.

This hospital function can be decomposed as follows (see Fig. 6.26):

Strategic Information Management

Strategic information management deals with the enterprise's information processing as a whole and establishes strategies and principles for the evolution of the information system.

[3] *Now we've come full circle. Our book deals with information management and especially strategic information management. Since information systems are subject of information management and information systems shall support all necessary functions of an enterprise, they shall support information management as well. For a more thorough explanation of strategic information management refer to Chap. 9.*

Klinische Scorecard

(Angabe gruppierter Fälle inklusive Jahreslieger, Überlieger und Fehler-DRGs sowie ausländischer Patienten und anderer außerbudgetärer Fälle)

▼ DRG-Scorecard

	Ist Monat 12.2009	Plan Monat 12.2009	Ist Monat 12.2009	Plandifferenz (normlert - in %)	Ist 01.2009 - 12.2009	Plan 01.2009 - 12.2009	Plandifferenz (normlert - in %)
Anzahl Fälle	3.928	4,351	3.792	-10	47.107	50.035	-6
CMI (effektiv)	1,573	1,433	1,583	10	1,513	1,433	6
CM (effektiv)	6.180	6,233	6.003	-1	71.255	71.684	-1
Anzahl Kurzliegerfälle	515	507	582	-2	6.772	5.829	-16
Abschlagstage Kurzlieger	596	574	683	-4	7.729	6.606	-17
Abschläge Kurzlieger (CM)	-193	-161	-195	-20	-2.331	-1,855	-26
Anzahl Langliegerfälle	296	280	257	-6	-3.217	3.222	-0
Zuschlagstage Langlieger	2.845	2.510	2.882	-13	31.023	28.861	-7
Zuschläge Langlieger (CM)	474	392	530	-21	4.802	4.513	-6
Anzahl Verlegungsfälle	65	159	71	59	779	1.829	57
Abschlagstage Verlegungen	311	693	406	55	3.969	7.965	50
Abschläge Verlegungen (CM)	-44	-77	-53	43	-557	-884	37
PCCL (Mittel)	1,306	1,285	1,300	2	1.289	1,285	0
Verweildauer (Mittel)	8,000	7,664	8,052	-4	7,847	7,498	-5
Patientenalter (Mittel)	47,7		46,0		47,5		

Fig. 6.23 Excerpt from a DRG scorecard, which is an important part of a hospital's controlling report (in German). The left column lists a set of key performance indicators (KPIs) to be controlled (e.g., "Verweildauer (Mittel)": patients' average length of stay). The next columns contain for some time periods values as recorded (e.g., "Ist Monat 12 2009": values recorded in December 2009) or as planned (e.g., "Plan Monat 12 2009": values planned for December 2009)

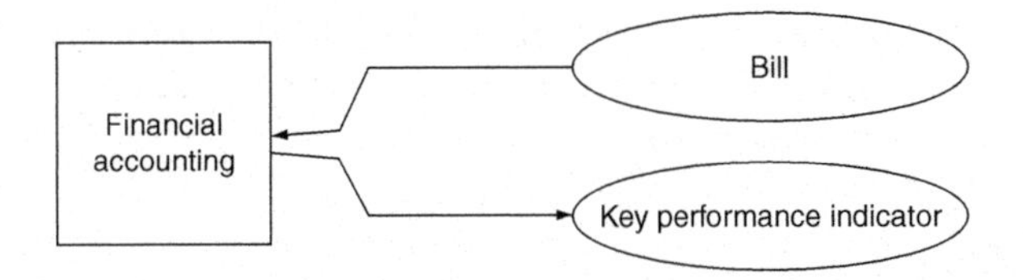

Fig. 6.24 Extract of the domain layer of the 3LGM²-based reference model describing the enterprise function *financial accounting*, its interpreted and updated entity types

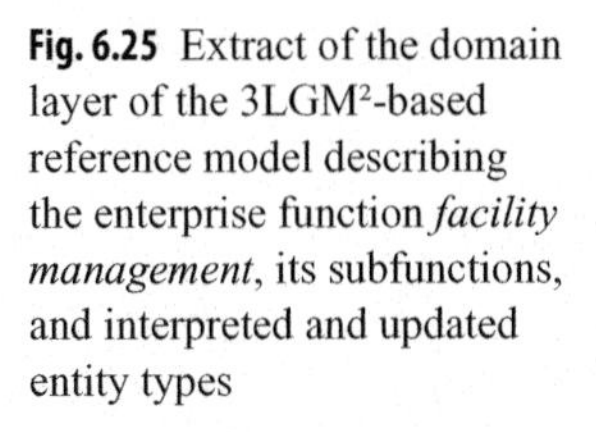

Fig. 6.25 Extract of the domain layer of the 3LGM²-based reference model describing the enterprise function *facility management*, its subfunctions, and interpreted and updated entity types

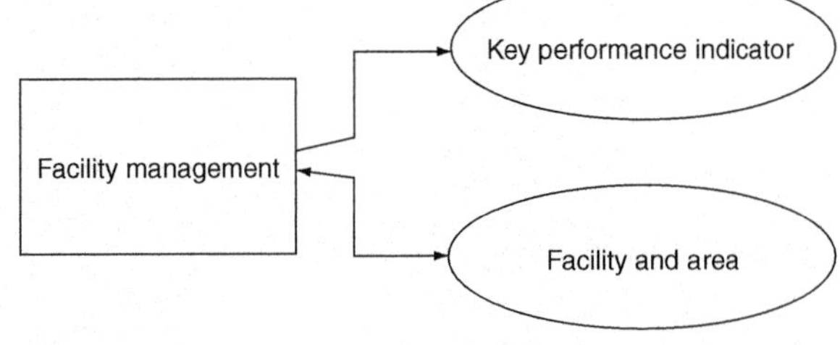

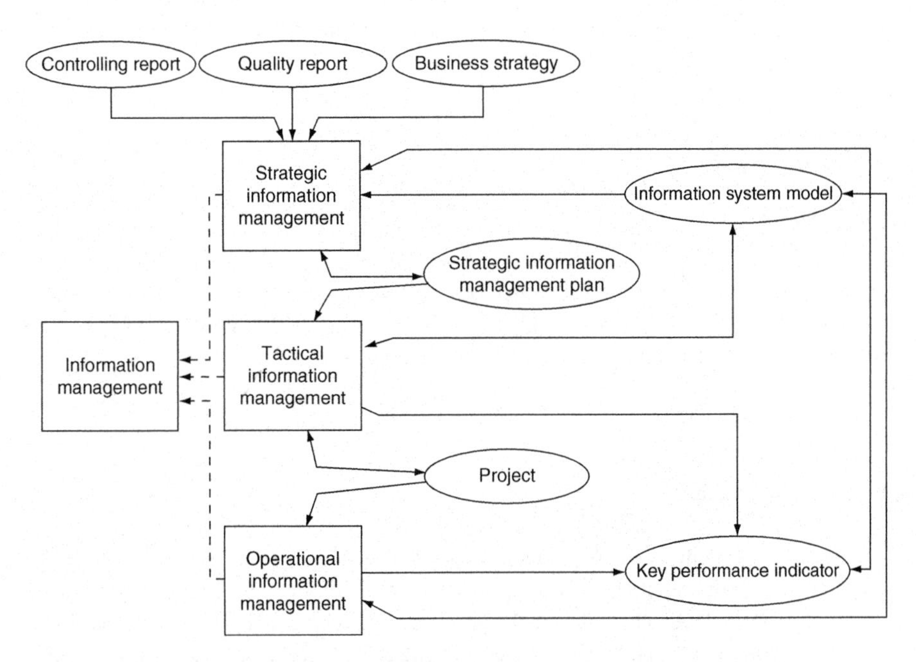

Fig. 6.26 Extract of the domain layer of the 3LGM²-based reference model describing the enterprise function *information management*, its subfunctions, and interpreted and updated entity types

An important result of strategic management activities is a strategic information management plan, which is aligned with the hospital's business strategy. It includes the direction and strategy of information management and the architecture of the enterprise information system.

Tactical Information Management

Tactical information management deals with particular enterprise functions or application components that are introduced, removed, or changed. Usually these activities are done in the form of projects. Such tactical information management projects are initiated by *strategic information management*. Thus, *strategic information management* is a vital necessity for *tactical information management*. The result of tactical information management projects is the information system.

Operational Information Management

Operational information management is responsible for operating the components of the information system. It cares for its smooth operation in accordance with the strategic information management plan. Additionally, *operational information management* plans, directs, and monitors permanent services for the users of the information system.

6.3.4 Hospital Management

Hospital management decides on questions of fundamental importance for the hospital development (hospital goals, strategic decisions, personnel decisions and decisions about budget, investments, and key treatments). *Hospital management* has to focus on high quality of *patient care* taking into account economic as well as legal and other requirements. Information needed and produced is shown in Fig. 6.27.

6.3.5 Research and Education

Especially in academic centers efficient *research and education* must be supported. The objective of clinical research is the generalization of findings and experiences to gain new knowledge. Data documented during the patient treatment process may be used for retrospective analysis, to find hints for generalization and generate hypotheses for new studies.

This hospital function can be decomposed as follows (see Fig. 6.28):

Fig. 6.27 Extract of the domain layer of the 3LGM²-based reference model describing the enterprise function *hospital management*, its interpreted and updated entity types

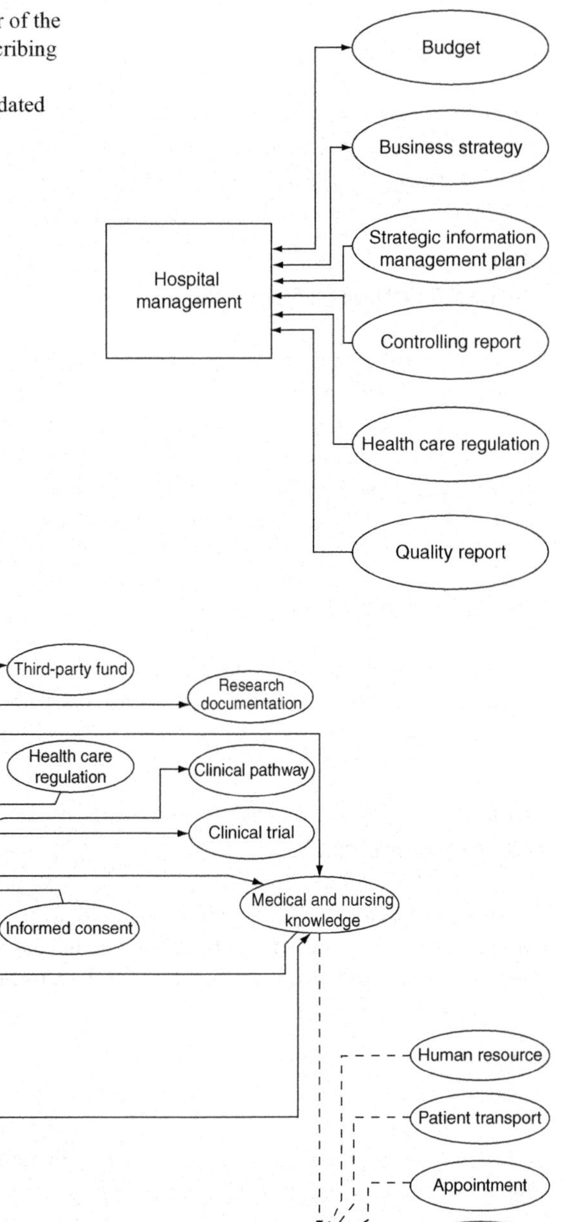

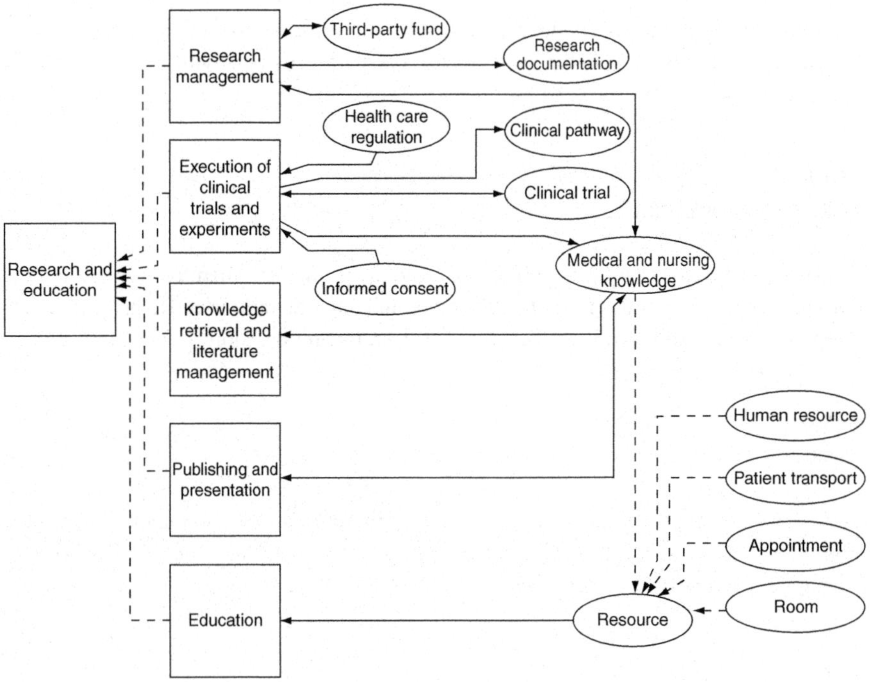

Fig. 6.28 Extract of the domain layer of the 3LGM²-based reference model describing the enterprise function *research and education*, its subfunctions, and interpreted and updated entity types

6.3.5.1 Research Management

Research management is executed in all organizational units of the hospital which decide upon planning, monitoring, and directing research activities. This includes the documentation of research activities as well as the management of third-party funds.

6.3.5.2 Execution of Clinical Trials and Experiments

Experiments and clinical trials are important for the progress in medicine because they update medical and nursing knowledge. Scientific staff must be supported in planning, executing, and analyzing studies and experiments. Planning and execution must conform to legal requirements; for example, patients have to be informed about chances and risks before they can consent to take part in a clinical trial.

6.3.5.3 Knowledge Retrieval and Literature Management

Scientific staff needs access to research-relevant information and general medical knowledge. In addition, doctors and nurses must be provided with specific medical knowledge.

6.3.5.4 Publishing and Presentation

Scientific staff needs to prepare publications and presentations. Therefore, central collections of both the hospital's relevant publications and other literature need to be made available to them and can be arranged according to year, institution, topic, or person.

6.3.5.5 Education

Medical casuistics have to be made available for training and *education* in medical professions. Furthermore, the organization and execution of teaching and exams, for example, by e-learning tools, have to be supported.

6.3.6 Clinical Documentation: A Hospital Function?

It may be surprising that 'documentation' is not listed as a hospital function in the previous sections. In fact, clinical documentation, which comprises medical documentation and nursing documentation, is a time-consuming and often unpopular duty of health professionals in a hospital. Moreover, every hospital function described so far requires a lot of documentation. During *patient admission*, identifying data and general health data about the patient have to be documented, the results of diagnostic procedures have to be written down, discharge summaries have to be documented, and so on. Hence, how does "documentation" fit into our 3LGM²-based view on HIS architectures? As the aforementioned examples show, documentation takes place every time a function is executed, new information is generated, and respective data are stored somehow somewhere.

In Sect. 5.3.2.4 we already described this in a more formal way:

Defining documentation needs at least one function, one entity type, and one application component, which are interrelated as follows: if an entity type E is updated by an enterprise function and this entity type's data are stored in an application component, we call this combination the documentation of entity type E.

Thus, every introduced function which updates an entity type is a documenting function.

6.3.7 Domain Layer: Exercises

6.3.7.1 Differences in Hospital Functions

Look at the hospital functions presented in this section. Now imagine a small hospital (e.g., 350 beds) and a big university medical center (e.g., 1,500 beds). What are the differences between these hospitals with regard to their enterprise functions? Explain your answer.

6.3.7.2 Different Health Care Professional Groups and Hospital Functions

Look at the hospital functions listed in this section. Analyze the relationships between the hospital functions and the different health care professional groups (physicians, nurses, administrative staff, others) working in a hospital. Which hospital functions are performed by which health care professional group?

Create a table with health care professional groups as columns, hospital functions as rows, and the following symbols as content in the boxes:

"++": Enterprise function is primarily performed by this profession.
"+": Enterprise function is also performed by this profession.
"–": Enterprise function is not performed by this profession.
".": Neither "++," "+," nor "–".

6.3.7.3 Support of Hospital Functions

As discussed at the beginning of this section, we have presented the main hospital functions that should be supported by a HIS. Look at a hospital you know and try to find out for each hospital function whether more computer-based or more paper-based information-processing tools are used to support it.

6.3.7.4
The Patient Entity Type

Take a look at the entity type patient interpreted and updated by various enterprise functions. Which enterprise functions update the patient information and which interpret it?

6.3.8
Domain Layer: Summary

The main patient care functions are:

- *patient admission* with *appointment scheduling*, patient *identification and checking for recurrent, administrative admission, medical admission, nursing admission, visitor and information service*;
- *decision making, planning, and organization of patient treatment* with *decision making and patient information*, as well as *medical and nursing care planning*;
- *order entry* with *preparation of an order*, *appointment scheduling*;
- *execution of diagnostic, therapeutic, and nursing procedures*;
- *coding of diagnoses and procedures*;
- *patient discharge and transfer to other institutions* with *administrative discharge and billing, medical discharge and medical report writing, nursing discharge and nursing report writing*.

These patient care functions are typically complemented by enterprise functions such as:

- *supply and disposal management, scheduling and resource allocation, human resources management*;
- *hospital administration with patient administration, archiving of patient information, quality management, cost accounting, controlling, financial accounting, facility management, information management*;
- *hospital management*;
- *research and education*.

These hospital functions describe what a HIS should support. It is not important at this point how they are supported – by non-computer-based or by computer-based information-processing tools.

All hospital functions introduced earlier are summarized on a 3LGM² domain layer in Fig. 6.29.

The hospital functions update and interpret different entity types. The following entity types are related to patient history:

- case, clinical pathway, clinical trial, diagnosis, diagnosis class, discharge summary, external finding, finding, informed consent, medical anamnesis, medical procedure, nursing anamnesis, nursing procedure, order, procedure, patient, patient transport, procedure class, sample, transfer.

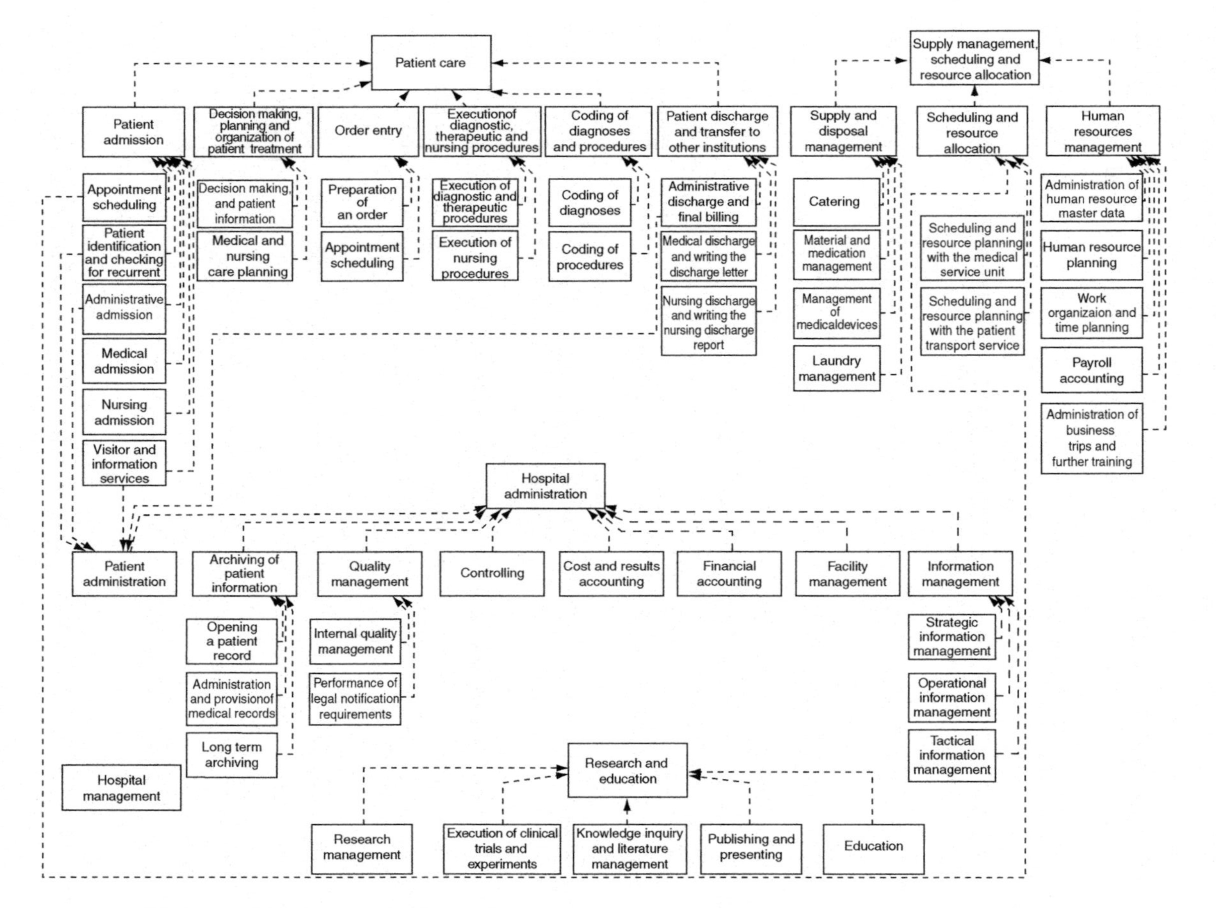

Fig. 6.29 Reference model of the hospital functions on the domain layer

The following entity types represent resources:

- appointment, bed, health care professional, drug, food, human resource, laundry, material, means of transport, medical and nursing knowledge, medical device, room, service.

The following entity types are related to administration:

- patient record archive, classification, classification of diagnoses, classification of procedures, cost unit, bill, budget, information system model, facility and area, notification, service catalog, third-party fund.

The following entity types are important for management:

- business strategy, controlling report, strategic information management plan, health care regulation, KPI, project, quality report.

6.4 Logical Tool Layer: Application Components

After having looked at hospital functions in the previous section we now describe information-processing tools at the logical tool layer of HIS, that is, the application components supporting these functions.

Taking the enterprise functions into account, we will sum up the task of the application components by tables enumerating the supported hospital functions; you may refer to Sect. 6.3 for their detailed descriptions. In addition, for every function we list typical features the application component should offer. A feature is a functionality offered by a software product which directly contributes to the fulfillment of one or more enterprise functions (compare Sect. 5.3.4). We denote features by a short phrase consisting of at least one verb and one noun expressing an ability of the software product, for example, "generate a unique PIN", "provide catalog of diagnoses". Features need not be directly invoked by a person, but can be triggered when using a preceding feature of the software product. The finer the granularity of an enterprise function is formulated, the greater is the probability that the enterprise function semantically corresponds with a feature an application component offers.

Each health institution uses a different set of computer-based and non-computer-based application components (organizational systems) to support its enterprise functions. However, in hospitals typical basic application components supporting specific hospital functions can be identified. In this section, we take a closer look at basic application components used in HIS. In the following section we will then discuss how these basic components can be combined similar to developing a city by stepwise adding new or replacing old buildings.

In spite of the still existing significance of non-computer-based information processing in hospitals we will focus here on computer-based application components. But we will discuss non-computer-based application components as well in Sect. 6.4.16.

Note that we refer to some of the components as "XYZ information system" (e.g., "Laboratory Information System"). Although this sounds contradictory to our definition of the term "information system" we use the terminology in order to integrate popular names.

After reading this section, you should be able to answer the following question:

- What application components are used in hospitals, and what are their characteristics?

6.4.1 Patient Administration System

The <u>*patient administration system*</u> supports the administration of patients and their contacts at the hospital. Especially for *patient admission*, *discharge*, and billing of patients this application component will be used. It must provide correct, complete, and up-to-date administrative patient data for all other application components. In addition, all other application components must be able to transmit relevant administrative patient data (e.g., diagnoses) to the *patient administration system*. Therefore, the *patient administration system* can be regarded as the center of the administrative memory of the HIS.

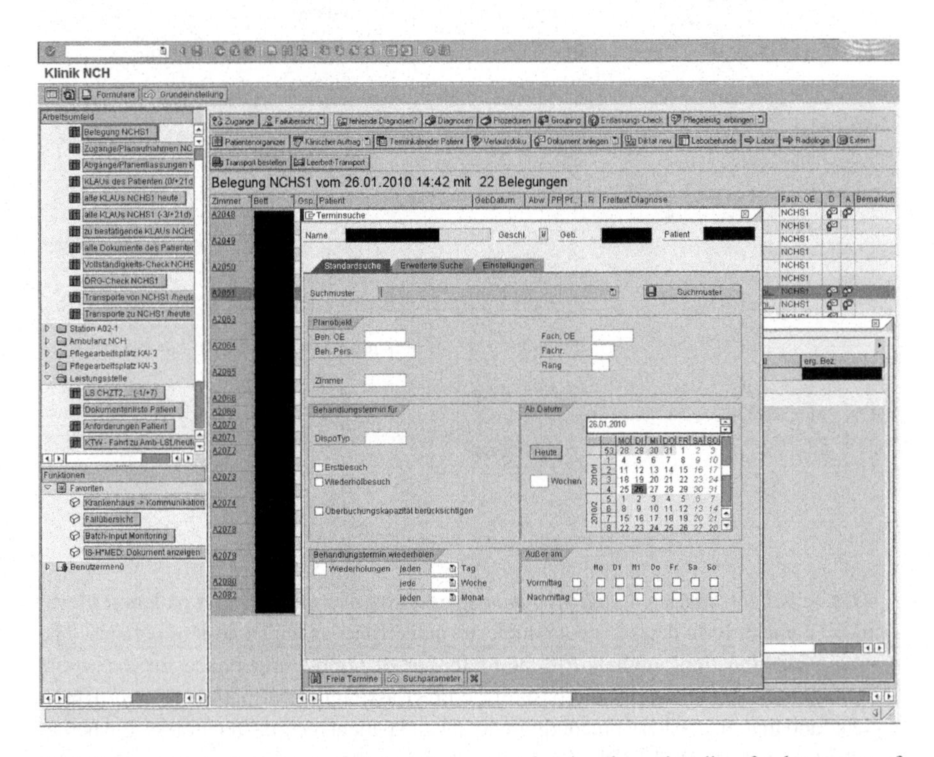

Fig. 6.30 Screenshot of a *patient administration system* showing the patient list of a department of neurosurgery in the background and a window for assigning an appointment to a patient in the front

Table 6.1 Typical supported hospital functions and related features of the *patient administration system*

Hospital function (from Sect. 6.3)	Typical application component features
Scheduling and resource allocation (see Sect. 6.3.2.2)	Provide means for scheduling patients' appointments
	Provide means for ordering transport services
Patient identification and checking for recurrent (see Sect. 6.3.1.1)	Retrieve patient
	Generate a unique patient identification number (PIN) and a case identification number (CIN)
	Administrate the master patient index (MPI)
Administrative admission (see Sect. 6.3.1.1)	Provide forms for entering or updating patient administrative information (name, address, birth date, relatives, admission diagnosis, etc.)
	Merge patient information from two records
	Provide means for ordering patient transfer within the institution
	Admit patients to the ward
	Assign patients to rooms and beds
	Provide means for preparing hospital-wide statistics
Visitor and information service (see Sect. 6.3.1.1)	Provide relatives with information on the location of a patient
Coding of diagnoses and procedures (see Sect. 6.3.1.5)	Provide catalogs and other means for coding patients' diagnoses
	Provide catalogs and other means for coding patient-related procedures
	Provide means for verifying coding done in departments
	Provide forms for preparing a bill for the patient insurance
Administrative discharge and billing (see Sect. 6.3.1.6)	Provide means for initiation of final billing
	Provide reminder for fulfilling of legal reporting requirements

During *patient admission*, *patient administration systems* must support patient retrieval (e.g., by name or birth date) to avoid duplicate and erroneous registration of patients. The resulting identification numbers PIN and CIN are of utmost importance for the whole information system. They are the basis for correct assignment of patient-related data to patients and thus are the very precondition for a valid patient record – regardless of whether it is electronic or not. Without the correct PIN and CIN all the high technology of a modern HIS would be useless.

Application components providing a correct PIN are often called a master patient index (MPI). Hence a *patient administration system* shall contain an MPI. It is essential to have only one MPI in a health information system – regardless of whether it is a HIS or a transinstitutional health information system.

Both PIN and CIN, as well as the related patient information, must be made available to other application components of the hospital. If the patient already has a paper-based patient record, the application component should automatically trigger the transfer of this record from the patient record archive to the unit where the patient has been admitted.

In addition, the *patient administration system* may update patient information in case of changes, or merge patient information from two cases if a new PIN was wrongly assigned to a patient.

The *patient administration system* (Fig. 6.30) is usually not only used by administrative staff but also by nurses and doctors at the ward. In the latter case it also supports daily management activities by health care professionals that occur on a ward. It especially supports the assignment of patients to beds and rooms with the features shown in Table 6.1.

6.4.2 Medical Documentation System

The medical documentation system (see Fig. 6.31) supports specific documentation tasks (e.g., patient history, planning of care, progress notes, report writing). Typically, it contains specialized modules for different medical fields (e.g., ophthalmology, psychiatry,

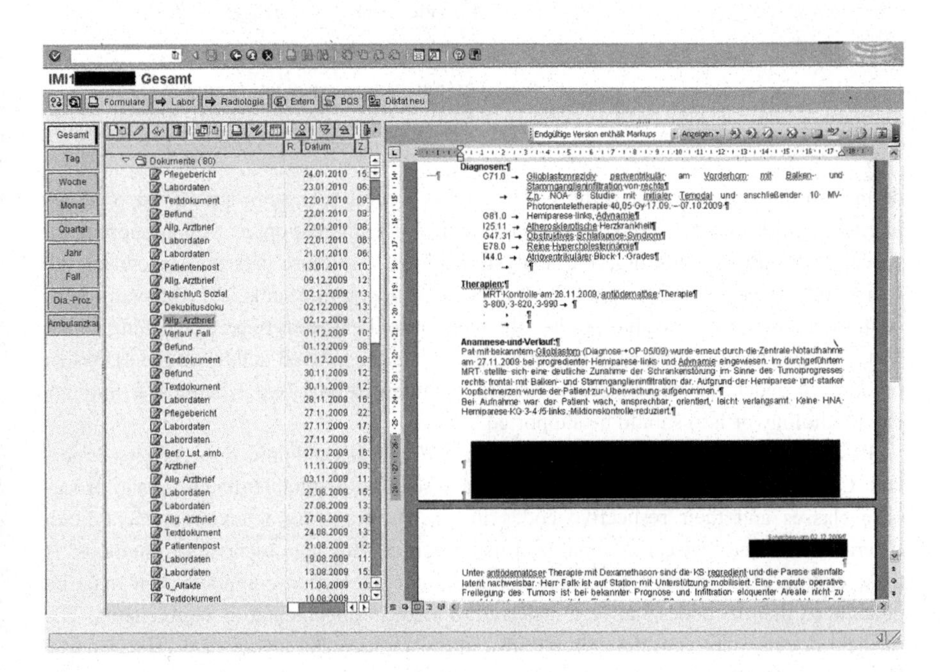

Fig. 6.31 A screenshot of a *medical documentation system* showing a list of patient-related documents on the left and an opened discharge letter on the right

Table 6.2 Typical supported hospital functions and related features of the *medical documentation system*

Hospital function (from Sect. 6.3)	Typical features
Medical admission (Sect. 6.3.1.1)	Provide forms for documenting medical anamnesis
	Provide forms for documenting diagnosis
	Scanning documents from referring physician and other sources
Decision making and planning of patient treatment (Sect. 6.3.1.2)	Provide forms for documenting patient's informed consent
	Provide forms for documenting planned tasks
	Provide guidelines for care planning
	Provide context-related medical knowledge
Execution of diagnostic, therapeutic, and nursing procedures (Sect. 6.3.1.4)	Provide forms for entering clinical data (free-text or structured)
	Provide forms for preparing clinical reports
	Print reports
Patient discharge and transfer to other institutions (Sect. 6.3.1.6)	Provide forms for writing the discharge letter or discharge report
	Provide means for finalizing documentation
Human resources management (Sect. 6.3.2.3)	Provide means for managing ward staff
	Creating a roster
	Assign doctors to patients or rooms

dermatology). They normally offer generic forms for free-text, semi-structured, or structured (e.g., drop-down lists) data entry for medical documentation, as well as support for speech recognition, reporting, and analysis features. The more data are structured, the easier are patient-related computer-based decision support and statistical data analysis. It is important that users are able to adapt the features to their needs (e.g., by defining which items have to be documented, and which constraints the entered data must meet). When reports are generated, the reuse of already-documented data (e.g., diagnoses, findings from radiology or lab) should be supported.

Besides clinical documentation, the *coding of diagnoses* and procedures is very important. Coding components must support the easy search for suitable diagnosis and procedure classes and their respective codes in classifications for a given medical field. Alternatively, free text can be analyzed using natural language recognition methods. If these coding components are separate from the documentation components, it must be guaranteed that the codes can be transferred to medical documentation components. The medical documentation system should also allow an adequate layout of diverse reports. When several persons are involved in the creation of a report (e.g., discharge letters may be dictated by a junior physician, written by a secretary, and approved by a senior physician), the application components should support the management and distribution of different versions of a document having different status (like preliminary or approved).

Medical documentation is the basis for *decision making and planning of patient treatment*. Hence the *medical documentation system* has to support medical staff by providing medical knowledge, which should be preselected using documented data about the patient's conditions; ideally a respective "infobutton"[4] should be implemented.

Table 6.2 sums up the hospital functions being supported and the features usually offered for these functions.

6.4.3 Nursing Management and Documentation System

The *nursing management and documentation system* (see Fig. 6.32) offers similar features as the *medical documentation system*. Nursing is usually oriented toward the so-called nursing process, which mainly comprises nursing patient history, nursing care planning with definition of problems, formulation of nursing aims, and planning of nursing tasks, followed by execution of nursing tasks and evaluation of results. The *nursing management and documentation system* has to support the documentation of all of those steps. To support nursing care planning, the definition and use of predefined nursing care plans (comprising recent problems of the patient, nursing goals, and planned nursing tasks) are helpful.

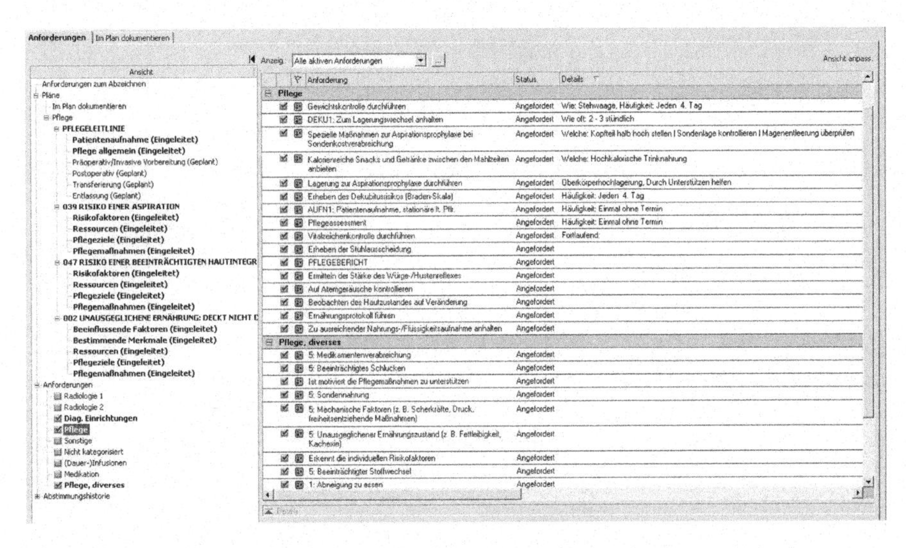

Fig. 6.32 Screenshot of a nursing documentation system. On the left, it shows the selected nursing pathways for the given patient. On the right, it shows the corresponding open tasks that now have to performed

[4]www.dbmi.columbia.edu/cimino/Infobuttons.html

Table 6.3 Typical supported hospital functions and related features of the *nursing management and documentation system*

Hospital function (from Sect. 6.2)	Typical features
Nursing admission (Sect. 6.3.1.1)	Provide forms for documenting the nursing history
Medical and nursing care planning (Sect. 6.3.1.2)	Provide forms for documenting diagnosis and problems
	Provide forms for documenting nursing aims
	Provide forms for documenting nursing tasks
	Support creation of a nursing care plan
Execution of nursing procedures (Sect. 6.3.1.4)	Provide forms for documenting performed tasks
	Provide forms for documenting the outcome of nursing tasks
Coding of diagnoses and procedures (Sect. 6.3.1.5)	Provide catalogs and other means for coding of nursing diagnosis
	Provide catalogs and other means for coding of nursing procedures
Nursing discharge and nursing report writing (Sect. 6.3.1.6)	Provide forms for writing the nursing discharge report
	Provide means for finalizing nursing documentation
	Communicate discharge information
Human resources management (Sect. 6.3.2.3)	Provide means for managing ward staff
	Provide means for creating a roster
	Assign doctors to patients or rooms

The *nursing management and documentation system* offers support for using predefined nursing terminologies and nursing classification such as NANDA, NIC, and NOC.[5]

Table 6.3 sums up the hospital functions being supported and the features usually offered for these functions.

6.4.4 Outpatient Management System

Outpatient care means *patient care* during one or several short visits in outpatient departments (clinics) in a hospital. In most cases, those visits are related to previous or future inpatient stays in the same hospital.

[5]NANDA=North American Nursing Diagnoses Association, the abbreviation is often used synonymously for the international classification of nursing diagnoses; NIC=Nursing Interventions Classification; NOC=Nursing Outcomes Classification

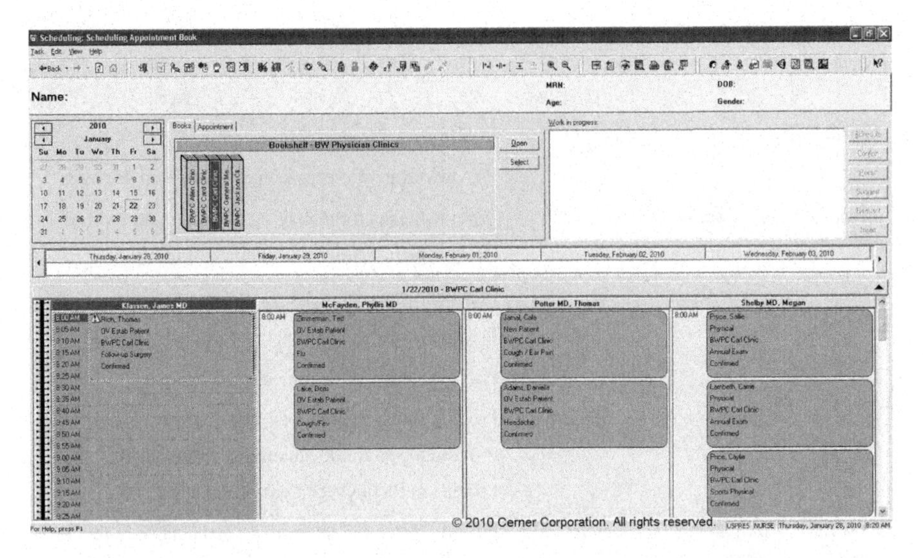

Fig. 6.33 Screenshot of an application component for scheduling in an outpatient unit

The <u>*outpatient management system*</u> is comparable to the *medical documentation system*. Differences exist with regard to a stronger support of *appointment scheduling* (Fig. 6.33) and waiting list management, and stronger work organization support (e.g., task lists, printing of receipts). Additionally many countries have different regulations for in- and outpatient billing. Thus particular features are needed for billing in outpatient departments. These special requirements usually lead to specialized *outpatient management systems* instead of using the *medical documentation system* in outpatient settings.

Upon *patient discharge*, a short report is written and communicated to the institution that continues treating the patient (e.g., the GP or a ward).

Table 6.4 sums up the hospital functions being supported and the features usually offered for these functions.

The functions are similar to functions needed in GPs' offices. Therefore, software products used in GPs' offices are sometimes also implemented in outpatient units in hospitals. These products are attractive, as they offer specific documentation modules for different medical areas (e.g., graphical tools for the documentation of dermatological status for dermatologists). In addition, the software products for billing can also often be transferred easily and cheaply.

However, *outpatient management systems* must be closely connected to other application components used on the ward or in other units in order to support the close cooperation of inpatient and outpatient care. This is often difficult when software products from GPs' offices are used. Therefore, software products from vendors with experience in the area of HIS may be better from an integration point of view. However, in this case, the range of supported functions may not be as broad as if software products from vendors who specialize in the GPs' area are used.

Table 6.4 Typical supported hospital functions and related features of the *outpatient management system*

Hospital function (from Sect. 6.3)	Typical features
Scheduling and resource allocation	Print forms
(Sect. 6.3.2.2)	Provide means for preparing ward-related statistics
Human resources management (Sect. 6.3.2.3)	Provide means for managing outpatient unit's staff
	Assign staff to patients or outpatient units
Medical admission (Sect. 6.3.1.1)	Provide means for check-in of patient
	Provide forms for documenting medical anamnesis
	Provide forms for documenting diagnosis
Decision making and planning of patient treatment (Sect. 6.3.1.2)	Provide forms for patients' informed consent
	Provide forms for documenting planned tasks
	Provide guidelines for treatment planning
Execution of diagnostic, therapeutic and nursing procedures (Sect. 6.3.1.4)	Provide forms for entering clinical data (free-text or structured)
	Provide forms for clinical reports
	Print reports
Patient discharge and transfer to other institutions (Sect. 6.3.1.6)	Provide forms for writing the discharge report
	Provide means for finalizing documentation
Administrative discharge and billing (see Sect. 6.3.1.6)	Provide means for initiating final billing for outpatient treatment
	Provide reminder for fulfilling of legal reporting requirements

6.4.5 Provider or Physician Order Entry System (POE)

A provider or *physician order entry system* (*POE*) (computer-supported POE systems are called *CPOE*) supports *order entry*. This can comprise both *order entry* of diagnostic or therapeutic procedures and ordering of drugs. *POE* systems support formulation of the order, *appointment scheduling*, printing of labels, and the communication of the order to the service unit (Fig. 6.34). In case of ordering drugs, physicians may choose the most appropriate drug or generic drug from drug catalogs. The POE system may then also offer decision-support functionality such as dosage calculation, drug–drug interaction checks, drug allergy checks or drug lab checks to prevent prescription errors. In case of ordering diagnostic or therapeutic procedures, the results (e.g., lab values or an x-ray report) have then to be communicated back to the ordering facility. *POE* systems offer service catalogs that present the available service types of the different service units (e.g., laboratory,

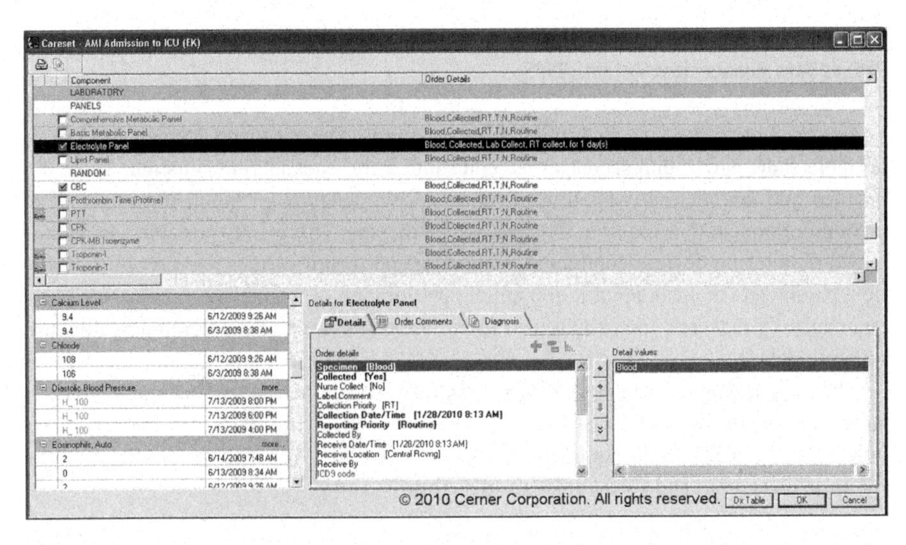

Fig. 6.34 Screenshot of a lab order entry system. An order set of electrolyte has been chosen to see details (lower right). If available, results can already be reviewed (lower left)

Table 6.5 Typical supported hospital functions and related features of the *provider/physician order entry (POE) system*

Hospital function (from Sect. 6.3)	Typical features
Order entry (Sect. 6.3.1.3)	Provide orders for patient-related drugs
	Provide drug catalogs
	Provide means for minimizing adverse drug events
	Calculate dosage of drugs
	Provide orders for patient-related examinations
	Select orders from order sets
	Provide means for scheduling a patient's appointment
	View patient-related appointments

radiology, surgery). Order sets that describe a typical set of combined orders (e.g., a combination of diagnostic procedures that have to be performed in a given situation) can support the ordering process; they are activated and modified by the ordering clinician. Some *POE* systems support receiving and presenting findings. However, this is usually done by other application components like the radiology information system (RIS) or laboratory information system (LIS) .

Table 6.5 sums up the hospital functions being supported and the features usually offered for these functions.

6.4.6 Patient Data Management System (PDMS)

Seriously ill patients are treated in intensive care units. These patients are generally in an unstable state, and within seconds may enter into a life-endangering situation. Thus, the detailed and complete presentation of all vital parameters (e.g., blood pressure, pulse, breathing frequency) is required for a successful therapy. This is only possible when automated monitoring devices continuously measure and record various parameters. In addition, parameters that can point to the initial deterioration of the patient's status should be automatically detected and should lead to an immediate alert of the treating health care professionals.

The *patient data management system (PDMS)* is specialized to automatically monitor, store, and clearly present a vast amount of patient-related clinical data in intensive care units (see Fig. 6.35). It also supports scoring (e.g., TISS,[6] SAPS[7]) and may offer features for decision support and various statistical analyses.

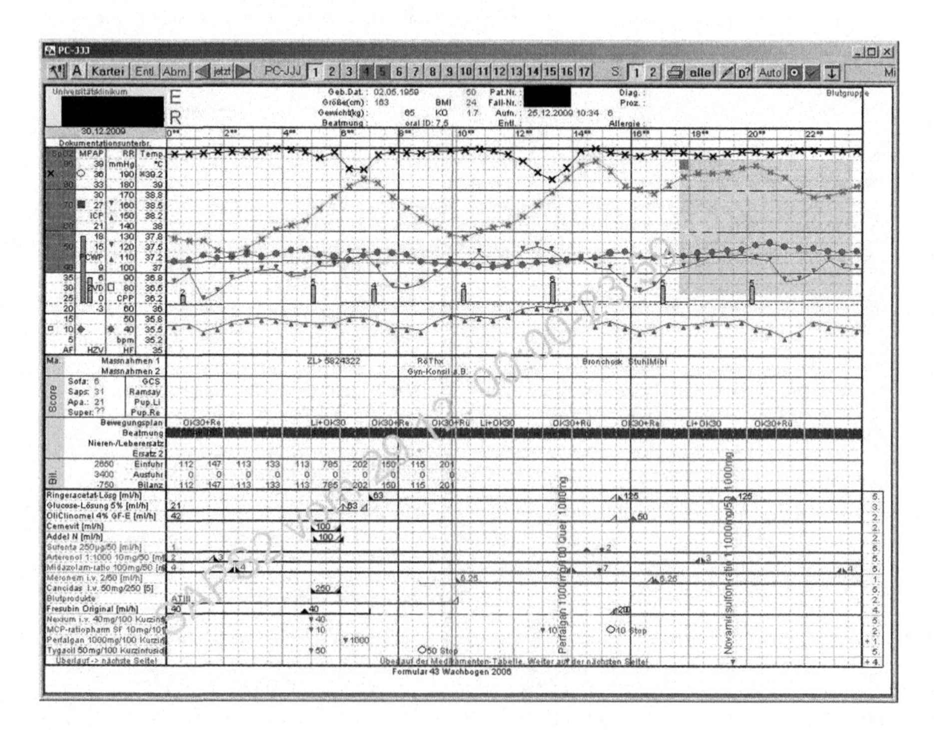

Fig. 6.35 Screenshot of a *patient data management system* showing a patient's vital parameters and given drugs during a day

[6]Therapeutic Intervention Scoring System
[7]Simplified Acute Physiology Score

Table 6.6 Typical supported hospital functions and related features of the *patient data management system*

Hospital function (from Sect. 6.2)	Typical features
Medical admission (Sect. 6.3.1.1)	Provide means for check-in of patient
	Provide forms for documenting medical anamnesis
	Provide forms for documenting diagnosis
Medical and nursing care planning (Sect. 6.3.1.2)	Provide means for preparing a care plan
	Offer decision support for care planning
Execution of diagnostic, therapeutic and nursing procedures (Sect. 6.3.1.4)	Display vital parameters from monitoring devices
	Display warning messages
	Provide forms for documenting clinical procedures
	Provide forms for documenting medications
	Create worklist for a group of patients
	Print forms
	Provide means for creating statistics
Coding of diagnoses and procedures (Sect. 6.3.1.5)	Scoring of the patient (e.g., TISS, SAPSII)
	Provide catalogs and other means for coding of procedures
	Provide catalogs and other means for coding of diagnoses
Patient discharge and transfer to other institutions (Sect. 6.3.1.6)	Provide forms for writing a transfer letter or discharge report
	Provide means for finalizing documentation
	Communicate discharge information
	Provide means for ordering patient transfer to other units
Supply and disposal management	Assign staff to patients or rooms
(Sect. 6.3.2.1), *Scheduling and resource allocation* (Sect. 6.3.2.2)	Provide means for ordering consumables
	Provide means for ordering drugs
	Provide means for ordering laundry
	Provide means for managing medical devices
	Organize patient transport
Human resources management (Sect. 6.3.2.3)	Work scheduling

After transfer to a regular ward, a short summary of the therapy on the intensive care unit should be created and communicated to the application components on the ward. In addition, a connection to the application components for *order entry* and result reporting is necessary. Software for a *PDMS* is sold both by specialized vendors and by vendors that also offer automated monitoring tools.

Table 6.6 sums up the hospital functions being supported and the features usually offered for these functions.

6.4.7 Operation Management System

In ORs, invasive procedures are performed. Usually, patients stay in the OR for only a few hours. During this time, they are prepared for the operation, the operation is performed, and finally, for a period of time after the operation, the patients' state is monitored.

The operation management system supports operation planning and operation documentation as a specialization of *execution of diagnostic and therapeutic procedures*. It allows assigning of operation date and time, and therefore should be available on the wards as well as in the offices and management units of the ORs. Depending on the planned operations, an operation plan can be created for a day or a week (Fig. 6.36). The data necessary for efficient planning are the diagnoses of the patient, the planned operation (medical procedure), the surgeons and other staff (human resources) involved, the planned time

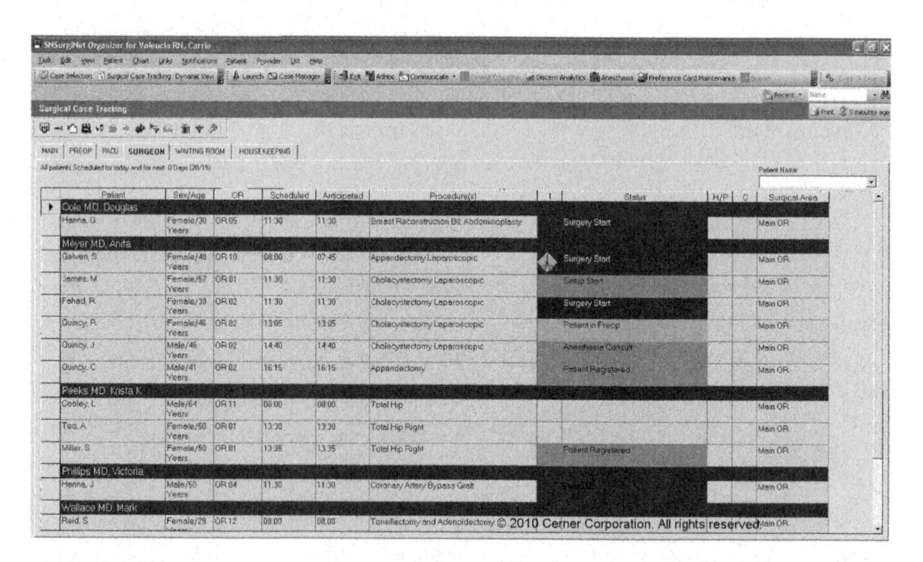

Fig. 6.36 Screenshot of an operation management system, showing the surgeons as well as the patients that are assigned to them. For each patient, the planned procedure and the status of the operation is displayed. The status can also be displayed for each operation room using a time line (not shown)

for operation (appointment), and the available ORs (space). Therefore, the *operation management system* should be closely connected to the *medical documentation system*.

During each operation, a large number of data have to be documented, including the members of the operating team, operative procedure, date and time, duration of the operation, materials (e.g., implants) used, and other necessary data to describe the operation and its results. Surgeons cooperate closely with anesthesiologists during the operation. For their documentation anesthesiologists need a number of data, which have usually to be documented by surgeons and vice versa. To avoid transcriptions, an *operation management system* should therefore also provide supportive features for anesthesiologists in an integrated way.

Table 6.7 Typical supported hospital functions and related features of the *operation management system*

Hospital function (from Sect. 6.2)	Typical features
Medical admission (Sect. 6.3.1.1)	Provide means for check-in of patient
	Provide forms for documenting medical anamnesis
	Provide forms for documenting diagnosis
Decision making and patient information (Sect. 6.3.1.2)	Provide forms for documenting patients' informed consent
Execution of operations (Sect. 6.3.1.4)	Display vital parameters from monitoring devices
	Provide forms for documenting procedures and outcomes
Coding of diagnoses and procedures (Sect. 6.3.1.5)	Provide catalogs and other means for coding diagnoses
	Provide catalogs and other means for coding procedures
	Provide means for creating statistics
Patient discharge and transfer to other institutions (Sect. 6.3.1.6)	Provide forms for preparing operation reports
	Provide means for ordering patient transfer to ward
Supply and disposal management (Sect. 6.3.2.1),	Provide means for managing rooms
Scheduling and resource allocation (Sect. 6.3.2.2)	Provide means for managing appointments
	Provide means for managing medical devices
	Provide means for ordering drugs, materials, and laundry
	Provide means for creating operation plans (daily, weekly)
Work scheduling and time management (Sect. 6.3.2.3)	Provide means for preparing work schedules

Usually, the planning data are taken from the operation planning component to be updated and completed during and after the operation. Based on these data, an operation report can be created, which may be completed with further comments of the surgeons. Therefore, word-processing capability is needed. Operation data needed for billing must be coded and then communicated to the administrative application components. The *operation management system* should also allow extensive data analysis (e.g., operation lists for junior surgeons). It should replace the often-used operation book, where all operations are documented by hand.

Table 6.7 sums up the hospital functions being supported and the features usually offered for these functions.

6.4.8 Radiology Information System

In radiology departments, in- and outpatients are examined. When radiological examinations are needed, the ward or outpatient unit orders them and schedules an appointment. The examination itself may then be done using an analog technology (e.g., x-ray and films) or digital technology (e.g., computed tomography, magnetic resonance imaging, ultrasonography, digital radiography). The tools that generate images are called modalities.

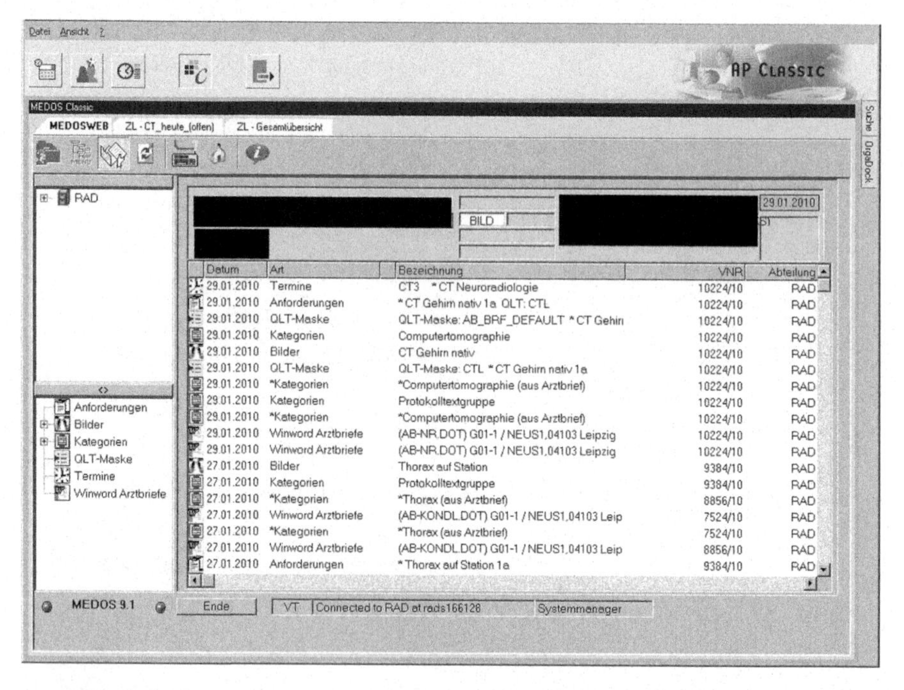

Fig. 6.37 Screenshot of a *radiology information system* (RIS) showing all radiologic documents of one patient

Table 6.8 Typical supported hospital functions and related features of the "radiology information system" (RIS)

Hospital function (from Sect. 6.3)	Typical features
Medical admission (see Sect. 6.3.1.1)	Provide means for check-in of patient
Execution of radiological examinations (see Sect. 6.3.1.4)	Receive orders Assign orders to modalities Provide forms for writing a report
Appointment scheduling (see Sect. 6.3.1.3)	Assign patients to modalities
Coding of diagnoses and procedures (see Sect. 6.3.1.5)	Provide catalogs and other means for coding radiological diagnoses Provide catalogs and other means for coding radiological procedures
Management of medical devices (see Sect. 6.3.2.1)	Manage modalities
Work scheduling and time management (see Sect. 6.3.2.3)	Provide means for preparing work schedules

Based on the generated images, a specialist in radiology creates a report, which is then sent and presented (sometimes together with selected pictures) to the ordering physician. Application components for radiological units therefore comprise features for departmental management, including report writing, image storing, and communication. In this section we will focus on departmental management; Sect. 6.4.9 will deal with image storing and communication.

The radiology information system (RIS) offers features comparable to those of the *outpatient management systems* (see Sect. 6.4.4), that is, features for registering patients, *appointment scheduling*, organization of examinations and staff (workflow management), provision of patient data and examination parameters, creation of radiology reports, documentation and coding of activities, and statistics. A special feature is the close connection to the modalities: The RIS typically provides a working list (i.e., patient name and requested examination) for the modalities, and gets back a confirmation on the completion of a radiologic examination from the modalities. Due to these special features, software for *RIS* typically comes from specialized vendors (Fig. 6.37).

Table 6.8 sums up the hospital functions being supported and the features usually offered for these functions.

6.4.9 Picture Archiving and Communication System (PACS)

In case of analog pictures, so-called *archive management systems* support their archiving (often stored in dedicated picture archives), and their retrieving and lending.

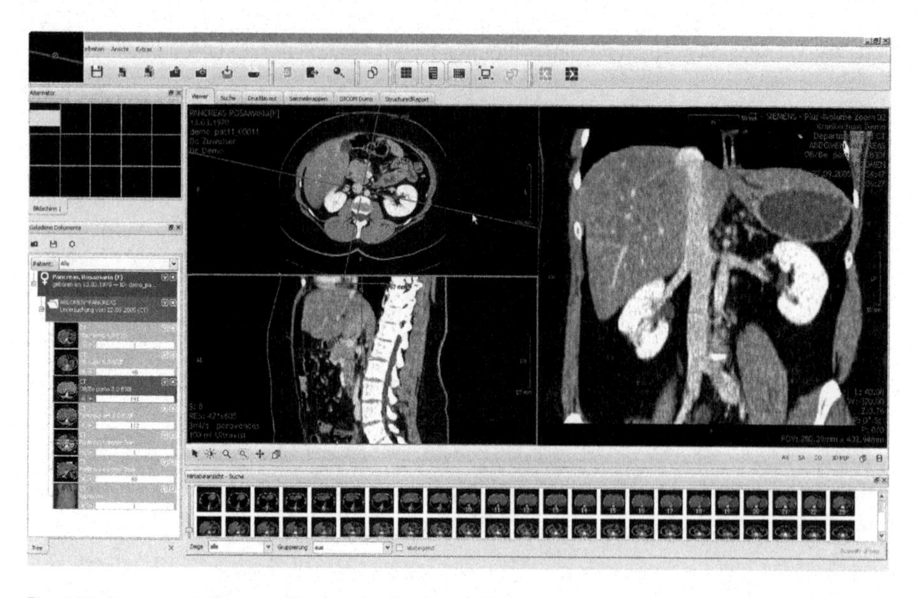

Fig. 6.38 Screenshot from a *Picture Archiving and Communication System (PACS)* application component, presenting different images of a patient

Table 6.9 Typical supported hospital functions and related features of the "radiology information system" (RIS)

Hospital function (from Sect. 6.3)	Typical features
Execution of radiological examinations (see Sect. 6.3.1.4)	Display pictures Modify presentation of pictures Communicate pictures Archive pictures Search for old pictures

By contrast, digital images are stored in the Picture Archiving and Communication System (PACS). This application component allows the storage, management, manipulation, and presentation of large numbers of image data (Fig. 6.38) and their quick communication from the storage media to the attached workstations for the diagnosing specialists or for the ordering departments. Quick communication may require a prefetching strategy to retrieve image data from slower storage devices and to provide it at faster devices well in advance to the situation they will be needed in.

Software products for *PACS* also comprise means for image processing and are often offered by vendors, which also offer physical data processing systems such as storage, networks, and modalities.

Obviously *RIS* and *PACS* should be closely connected. They should also have a close connection to the *patient administration system*, *medical documentation system*, *POE*, and the *PDMS*, in order to allow quick access to reports and imaging pictures from every unit.

Table 6.9 sums up the hospital functions being supported and the features usually offered for these functions.

6.4.10 Laboratory Information System

During execution of lab examinations, specimens of patients (e.g., blood sample, tissue sample) are used. Appointments are therefore not necessary. Depending on the type of laboratory, different examination technologies are used (e.g., chemical analysis of blood samples, microscopical analysis, and tissue samples). Chemical analysis is usually done by automated equipment. Depending on the order, the sample is usually automatically distributed to various analytical devices, which are regularly checked for their precision in order to conform to *quality management* requirements. In addition, the laboratory physician checks all results of a sample for plausibility (so-called validation).

The *laboratory information system* (LIS) supports the management of the whole procedure of analysis: the receipt of the order and the sample, the distribution of the sample and the order to the different analytical devices, the collection of the results, the technical and clinical validation of results, the communication of the findings back to the ordering department, as well as general *quality management* procedures (Fig. 6.39). The validation of laboratory results is more effective when patient-related clinical data (e.g., recent

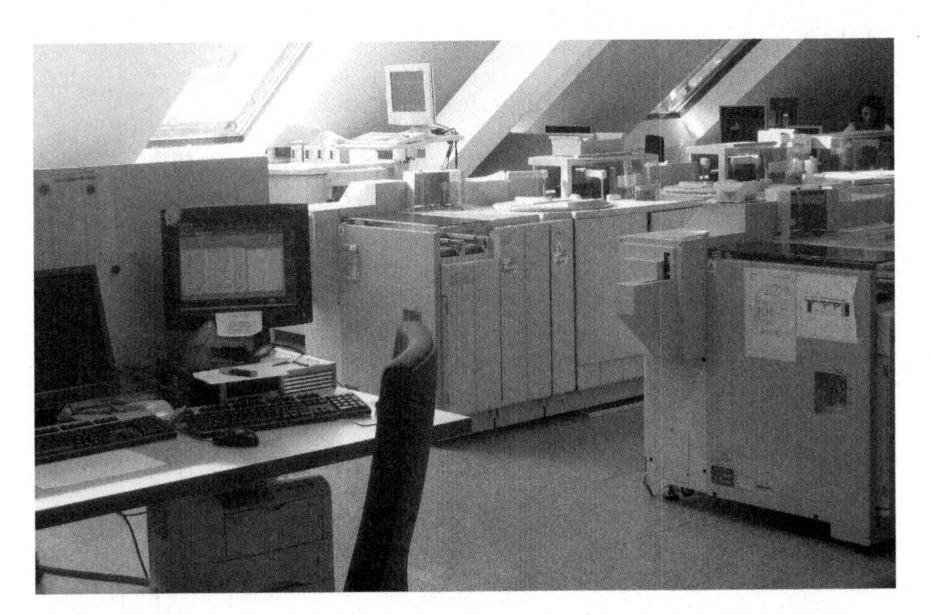

Fig. 6.39 In a laboratory unit. The laboratory information system (LIS; running on the PC in the front) manages the analysis of samples by laboratory devices (in the background)

Table 6.10 Typical supported hospital functions and related features of the *laboratory information system (LIS)*

Hospital function (from Sect. 6.3)	Typical features
Execution of lab examinations	Receive orders
(see Sect. 6.3.1.4)	Receive blood samples
	Assign order and blood samples to devices
	Collect results from devices
	Display earlier lab results of a patient
	Validate results
	Prepare report
	Communicate report to ordering unit
	Provide means for preparing statistics

diagnoses, drug medication) are accessible to the laboratory physician. The *LIS*, therefore, should be closely connected to the *medical documentation system*, *outpatient management system*, *POE*, and *PDMS*. Software for *LIS* is usually also sold by specialized vendors.

Table 6.10 sums up the hospital functions being supported and the features usually offered for these functions.

6.4.11
Enterprise Resource Planning System

The *enterprise resource planning system* (often: *ERP system*) enables a hospital to manage its financial, human, and material resources. It thus supports hospital functions such as *controlling*, *financial accounting*, *facility management*, *human resources management*, *quality management*, and *supply and disposal management*.

A close connection is needed especially to the *patient administration system* but also to the other application components mentioned earlier, in order to obtain, for example, billing data and legally required diagnoses and procedure codes. Most of the software products used for *ERP systems* in hospitals are not specific to hospitals, but are also used in other industries outside health care where similar administrative functions have to be supported.

One major goal of the *ERP system* is the documentation and billing of all accountable services. The types of data needed and the details of billing depend on the country's health care system.

Table 6.11 presents important hospital functions and related tasks with regard to the *ERP system*. The presented table is not exhaustive and just describes a selection of items.

Table 6.11 Typical supported hospital functions and related features of the *enterprise resource planning system*

Hospital function (from Sect. 6.3)	Typical features
Controlling (see Sect. 6.3.3.4)	Provide means for overhead cost management
	Provide means for product costing
	Provide means for cost center accounting
	Provide means for cost element accounting
Financial accounting (see Sect. 6.3.3.6)	Provide means for accounts payable
	Provide means for accounts receivable
	Provide means for general ledger accounting
	Provide means for asset accounting
Facility management (see Sect. 6.3.3.7)	Provide means for preventive maintenance
	Provide means for control of security issues
	Provide means for incident tracking
Human resources management (see Sect. 6.3.2.3)	Provide means for organizing recruitment
	Provide means for organizing training
	Provide means for organizing career development
	Provide means for performance evaluation
Quality management (see Sect. 6.3.3.3)	Provide a collection of internal processes and regulations
	Provide means for editing and graphically illustrating collections of internal processes and regulations
Supply and disposal management	Provide means for managing logistics
(see Sect. 6.3.2.1)	Provide means for stock keeping
	Provide means for order management
	Provide means for managing and monitoring disposal

6.4.12 Data Warehouse System

A *data warehouse system* contains data which have been extracted from other application components. The data have been transferred and aggregated into a suitable format and then actively loaded into the data warehouse (push-principle). A specific request on the data will only access data already loaded into the *data warehouse*.

There are two major fields of application for *data warehouse systems* in hospitals. They can either be used for *hospital management* or for *research*.

For decision-making the management of a hospital needs up-to-date information about the hospital's operating as a whole (Fig. 6.40). The management of a hospital is, for example, interested in answers to questions like these: What are the top ten diagnoses of the patients treated in our hospital? Which department of the hospital causes the highest material costs? In which department do patients stay longest on average?

A *data warehouse system* can help to answer these questions by pooling management-relevant data from other systems such as the *ERP system* and the *CPOE system* and by providing means for analyzing these data by data mining techniques. A *data warehouse system* supporting *hospital management* is often called *business intelligence system*.

In contrast to other enterprises, the *data warehouse systems* in hospitals are not only important for management-related and, thus, primarily cost-related issues, but also for medical issues, especially for clinical trials. If data from the *medical documentation system* have been loaded into a *data warehouse system*, the recruitment of patients for clinical trials as well as the statistical evaluation of patient data can be effectively supported.

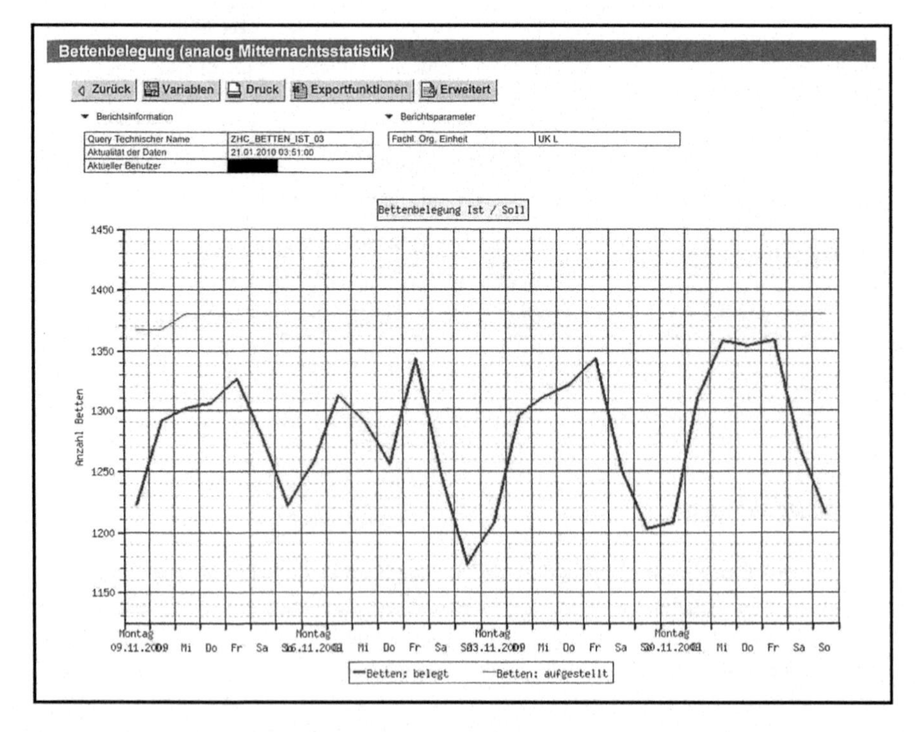

Fig. 6.40 Screenshot of a *data warehouse system*. The diagram shows a target/actual comparison for the bed occupation of a university hospital

Table 6.12 Typical supported hospital functions and related features of the *data warehouse system*

Hospital function (from Sect. 6.3)	Typical features
Hospital management (see Sect. 6.3.4)	Integrate data from different application components
	Structure data
	Analyze data
	Provide means for data mining
Execution of clinical trials and	(see row above)
experiments (see Sect. 6.3.5)	Provide means for recruiting of patients

There is an ISO standard (ISO TR 22221) on "Good principles and practices for a clinical data warehouse (CDW)" which provides implementation guidance for *data warehouses* in a HIS.

Table 6.12 sums up the hospital functions being supported and the features usually offered for these functions.

6.4.13 Document Archiving System

As increasing patient-related data are available in a digital form, the question of long-term archiving has to be solved. Depending upon the type of data and national laws, patient-related data have to be stored up to 30 years. For long-term archiving, confidentiality, availability, and integrity of the data according to the OAIS3[8] (ISO 14721) model must be guaranteed. Availability means that data must be retrievable and readable at any time throughout the archiving period. To ensure integrity, data must be complete and unchanged. In health care, authenticity of the author and the time of the creation of a document are important aspects of integrity. For example, unauthorized alteration of the date of creation results in the loss of integrity of archived data. The conditions of confidentiality, availability, and integrity can hardly be met by individual clinical application components that may not be available in 30 years.

The *document archiving system* offers long-term archiving of patient-related and other data and documents based on sustainable standardized data formats, document formats, and interfaces. The system also provides standardized indexing of document content and regular updates of storage media. Qualified electronic signatures, for example, in compliance with the European guideline 1999/93/EG, can be used to guarantee long-term integrity of stored data in case the *document archiving system* is enabled to renew outdated signatures and hash algorithms. The *document archiving system* is typically closely linked to all application components that generate data and documents which it has to store for a long time. It gets copies of data and documents from those components, indexes them, and

[8]Open Archival Information System 3

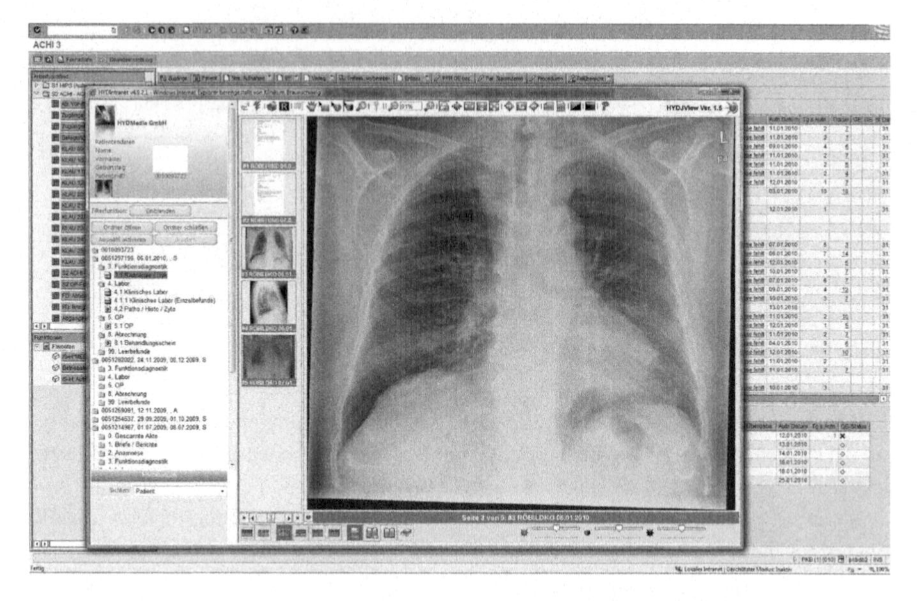

Fig. 6.41 Screenshot of a document archiving system. Besides text documents like findings from the laboratory, operation reports, letters, anamneses, etc., it also contains radiological images

stores them, while enabling fast retrieval. Paper-based documents can be integrated by scanning, which allows for eliminating the physical place needed for paper-based archiving. Typically, *document archiving systems* can archive not only text-related documents, but also images, videos, and other multimedia data (see screenshot in Fig. 6.41). All these documents may be stored using established non-proprietary industry standards such as:

- ASCII (American Standard Code for Information Interchange),
- PDF/A, which is an ISO standard for long-time archiving of documents based on the Portable Document Format (PDF),
- XML (eXtensible Markup Language)
- TIFF (Tagged Image File Format)
- JPEG and MPEG, which are acronyms for the names of the committees who created the standards (Joint Photographic Experts Group and Moving Pictures Expert Group)
- DICOM (see Sect. 6.5.4.3)

In addition, there exists the document format CDA[9], which can be used for structuring clinical documents. Currently, CDA is mainly used for electronic discharge letters and reports. However, it has the potential to become an important standard for document archives because CDA documents include metadata that facilitate the reuse of documents, for example, for decision support systems. Archived XML data (such as CDA) should include the corresponding Document Type Definitions (DTD) in the form of XSD (XML

[9] Clinical Document Architecture, ANSI standard for the structure of clinical documents

Table 6.13 Typical supported hospital functions and related features of the *document archiving system*

Hospital function (from Sect. 6.3)	Typical features
Archiving of patient information (see Sect. 6.3.3.2)	Import documents
	Scan documents
	Index document content
	Manage storage formats
	Manage storage media
	Provide access to archived information
	Attach digital signatures
	Communicate documents to other applications

schema definition), and the layout specification of an XML document in the form of XSL (eXtensible Stylesheet Language) files.

In health care, image data ought to be archived using lossless compression.

Patient-related medical data and documents stored in the *document archiving system* have to be made available to the *medical documentation system* in order to enable their users to directly access information from earlier patient contacts.

Table 6.13 sums up the hospital functions being supported and the features usually offered for these functions.

6.4.14 Other Computer-Based Application Components

In addition to the computer-based application components introduced so far, we can usually find many other, often department-specific application components in a hospital. For example, depending on the size of the hospital, a hospital can have its own pharmacy department, which needs a *pharmacy information system* to supply wards and finally patients with the right drugs in the right dose. Depending on the specializations of a hospital there can be, for example, a *cardiovascular information system* (CVIS) or a *dialysis information system*, which are specialized *medical documentation systems*. Furthermore, there are some application components that are not necessarily department-specific or medicine-related, but support a smooth workflow in different departments of the hospital. An example is a *digital dictation system* which assists doctors in writing discharge letters or reports on diagnostic findings.

Table 6.14 lists some of these specific application components but it is not intended to be exhaustive.

Until now we focused on "classical" application components, that is, software installations in a HIS primarily supporting the hospital functions as listed in Sect. 6.3. But there are increasing installations of software in hospitals which are primarily controlling medical devices. Hence, medical devices can increasingly be considered to be application

Table 6.14 Further specific application components in hospital information systems (HIS)

Application component	Description
Blood bank management system	Supports blood donor services, blood analyses, administration of blood bottles
Cardiovascular information system (CVIS)	Provides many features of a *clinical information system (CIS)* and a *radiology information system (RIS)* while tailoring the special needs of a cardiology department
Decision support system	A knowledge-based system which assists a doctor in finding the right diagnosis or treatment for a specific patient
Dialysis information system	Provides many features of a *CIS* while tailoring the special needs of a dialysis department, has interfaces to hemodialysis machines
Digital dictation system	Offers features for digital voice recording and speech recognition, is often integrated into medical information systems, and supports report, finding, and letter writing
Oncology information system	Provides many features of a *CIS* while tailoring the special needs of an oncology department
Orthopedics information system	Provides many features of a *CIS* while tailoring the special needs of an orthopedics department, can include a computer-aided design (CAD) system for transplant planning
Pathology information system	Has similar features as a laboratory information system (LIS), e.g., receiving orders, writing reports
Pharmacy information system	Supports the workflow in the pharmacy department: receiving drug orders, managing the drug stock, distributing drugs throughout the hospital
Teleradiology system	Enables evaluations of radiological images from (external) radiologists' remote workplaces and may be closely connected to *RIS* and *PACS*

components and in many cases to be specialized *medical documentation systems.* Consequently, they not only provide information (e.g., findings and images) via respective interfaces, but need information from other application components (e.g., patient, case, order) as well. This close interconnection is often referred to by the term "converging technologies" (compare example 9.8.4). Due to the considerable risks for patients' safety reasonable care has to be exercised when integrating these converging technologies into the computer-supported part of a HIS.

6.4.15 Clinical Information System and Electronic Patient Record System as Comprehensive Application Components

Not every HIS contains a *medical documentation system*, an *outpatient management system*, a *nursing management and documentation system*, or a *CPOE* system as separate, identifiable application components. Instead, these components are often closely integrated modules of a so-called clinical information system (CIS). A *CIS* supports the hospital functions as enumerated in Table 6.2 to Table 6.5.

CISs are also often called *electronic patient record systems* (*EPR systems*). As introduced in Sect. 4.4, the electronic patient record (EPR), that is, the *electronic health record* (EHR) in a hospital, is a complete or partial patient record stored on an electronic storage medium. Given this definition, every computer-based application component supporting the *execution of diagnostic and therapeutic procedures* or other subfunctions of *patient care* (e.g., *medical documentation system*, *outpatient management system*, *nursing management and documentation system*, *PDMS*) contains at least a partial EPR. In a *CIS*, these partial EPRs are often integrated and made available to the professionals from all areas of a hospital to provide one harmonized view on the data of a patient. Because of this harmonized view the term *EPR system* as a particular application component has become quite common.

6.4.16 Typical Non-Computer-Based Application Components

Non-computer-based application components contain rules and plans regarding how and in which context what non-computer-based physical tools shall be used in order to support particular enterprise functions.

The coverage of hospital functions by computer-based application components is rising, but most hospitals still have non-computer-based application components and use paper as a physical tool. For example, in a typical medium-sized hospital, parts of clinical documentation while performing hospital functions are still done with paper-based patient records. Thus, despite the growing portion of electronic documents, the "paperless hospital" still seems to be a remote ideal today. There might be a continuing need for some paper-based documents. Typical application components that are still paper-based in a larger percentage of hospitals comprise, for example, the patient chart, the patient record, and clinical textbooks and knowledge sources.

6.4.16.1 The Paper-Based Patient Chart System

The patient chart system supports documentation and presentation of body temperature, blood pressure, pulse, and other vital signs (see Fig. 6.42). It typically also contains physician orders to other health care professionals such as drug orders, orders of examinations, or orders for special dietary. In addition, it may describe executed procedures (e.g., drug is given, examination is ordered) as well as findings (e.g., relevant lab values) and a lot of other clinical information. The patient chart is typically a central interprofessional communication tool that supports quite a lot of enterprise functions and processes that all need to be computer-based before it can be completely replaced. We can denote the application component that builds on the patient chart as *patient chart system*, indicating that it is made up of the patient chart and the organizational rules that define who may use which part of the chart in which situation.

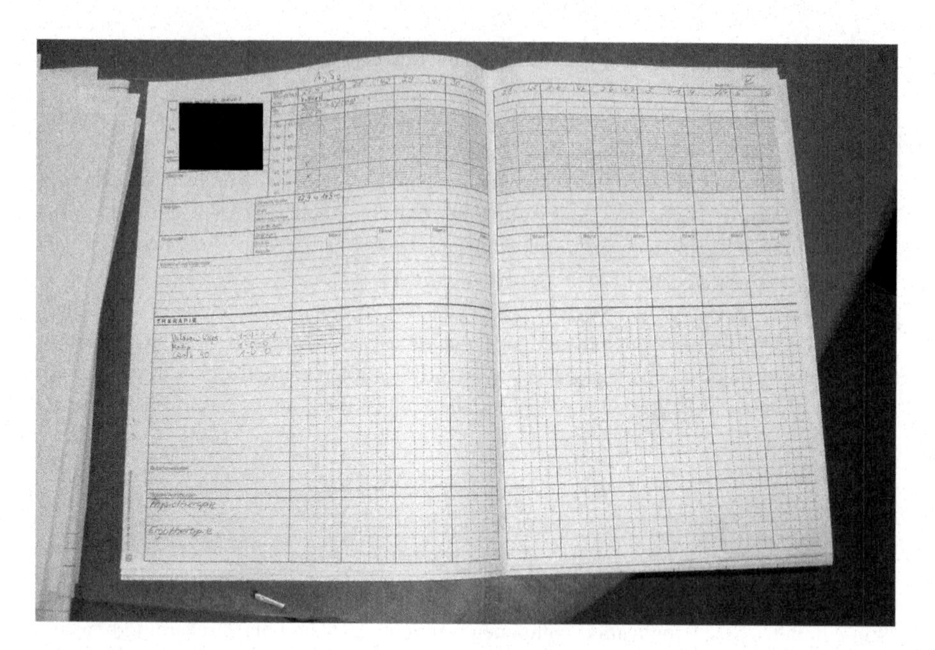

Fig. 6.42 The patient chart

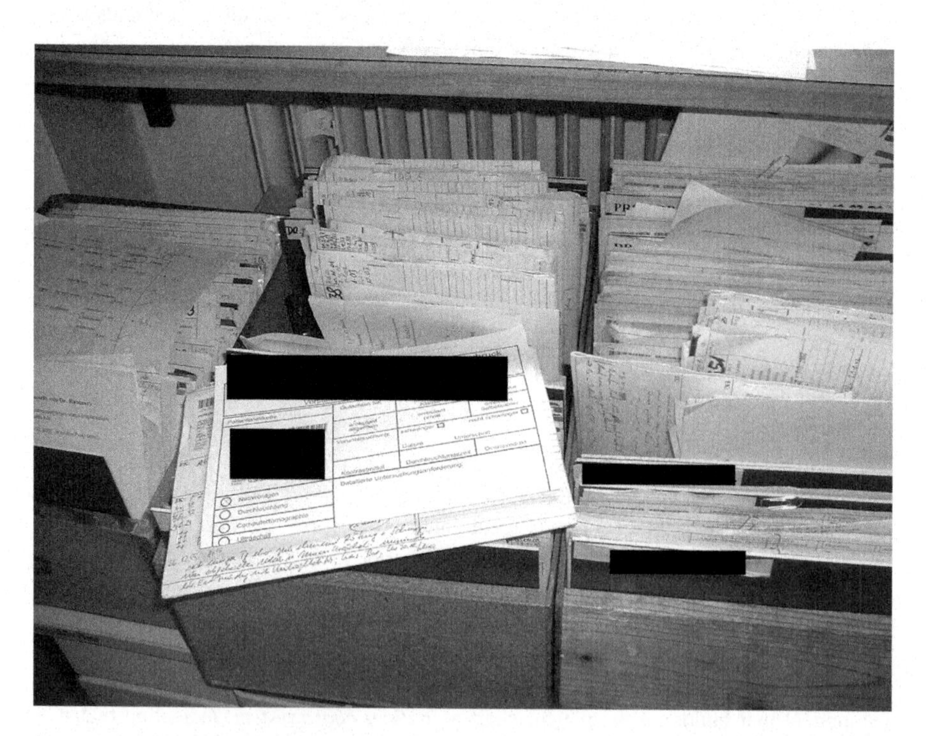

Fig. 6.43 The paper-based patient record

6.4.16.2
The Paper-Based Patient Record System

The paper-based patient record system, comprising a paper file and the organizational rules regarding which papers have to be collected where by whom, serves as a collection of all documents that are either available only in paper-based form (such as the patient chart) or that are printed out by computer-based application components to support easier access to relevant data (such as print-out of new findings) (see Fig. 6.43). As long as not all documents are generated and used only in a computer-based form, the paper-based *patient record system* will remain an important collection for paper-based patient information (by this complementing the EPR, see Sects. 4.4 and 6.4.15).

6.5
Logical Tool Layer: Integration of Application Components

As has been seen, a HIS typically comprises various application components that need to be integrated to achieve high quality of information processing. Integration in general describes a union of parts making a whole, which – as opposed to its parts – displays a new quality. For example, an integrated computer-supported HIS offers better support for enterprise functions and business processes than isolated components, where users, for example, may need to transfer data from one component to another manually.

But besides this meaning as a property of a system, "integration" additionally stands for the actions to be taken in order to achieve this property and thus has a behavioral perspective.

To achieve a high level of integration within a HIS the components need to be able to work together, which means they need to be interoperable. Interoperability in general is the ability of two or more components to exchange information and to use the information that has been exchanged. A component that is called interoperable may, for example, support certain standards for information exchange (compare Sect. 6.5.4) or certain integration technologies (compare Sect. 6.5.5).

In this section, we discuss integration especially with respect to HIS. Please refer to Sect. 7.3.1 for the discussion of integration in transinstitutional health information systems.

HIS at different hospitals usually look different. But there are some criteria helping to categorize the respective architectures. We will first introduce a taxonomy of architectures of HIS, providing criteria at the logical tool layer. In Sect. 6.7.1 we will continue this taxonomy in order to comprise criteria at the physical tool layer as well.

Regardless of what kind of architecture has been chosen for a HIS, integrity, that is, the correctness of data, has to be ensured. We will explain necessary conditions for integrity of data in a HIS, which have to be met in any architecture. Integrated HIS means that all necessary measures have been taken to ensure integrity of data by integration. But it turns out that "integration" is a difficult term with many facets. Therefore we will then discuss types of integration, which shall hold in any architecture. Afterwards we will introduce standards and typical technologies used in HIS to ease integration. But despite there being standards and technologies available to support integration in HIS, a lot of effort is still required. Thus it is not surprising that hospitals tend to have HIS architectures containing very few components. We will discuss related approaches at the end of this section.

After reading this section, you should be able to answer the following questions:

- How can architectures of HIS be categorized?
- What differentiates integrity from integration?
- What are the standards and technologies available to support the integration of HIS?
- How can integration efforts be reduced by decreasing the variety of application components in a HIS?

6.5.1 Taxonomy of Architectures at the Logical Tool Layer

As defined in Sect. 3.3.4, the architecture of an information system describes its fundamental organization, represented by its components, their relationships to each other and to the environment, and the principles guiding its design and evolution. The components of a HIS comprise hospital functions, business processes, and information-processing tools.

With regard to the hospital functions, there is nearly no difference between individual HIS, as the hospitals' goals and thus the hospitals' functions are in general the same. All hospital functions presented in Sect. 6.3 should thus be supported by any HIS. Remember, from our point of view, these hospital functions can be supported by non-computer-based or computer-based information-processing tools.

However, there are significant differences in HIS architectures with respect to the types and relationships of information-processing tools used and the way they are integrated. We will introduce a multidimensional taxonomy, which can be used to characterize different styles of architectures. This taxonomy will help to describe real HIS architectures, to compare them, and to assess them.

We first look at the logical tool layer, and later at HIS architectural styles at the physical tool layer (see Sect. 6.7.1). Doing this, we concentrate on the computer-based part of HIS.

Architectural styles at the logical tool layer of the computer-based part of HIS are characterized by:

- Number of databases being used to store (especially patient-related) data
- Number of application components used to support the hospital functions
- Number of different software products and vendors used to install the application components
- The patterns of communication links between the application components used
- The types of integration which could be achieved

These facets will be introduced as semantic dimensions which can be used to categorize HIS architectures.

6.5.1.1 Number of Databases: Central Versus Distributed

Application components of a HIS may store data about certain entity types persistently (see Sect. 5.3.2.2). Usually a database is used for this. We will use the number of databases storing data in a HIS as the basis to distinguish possible data distribution styles at the logical tool layer of a HIS: the DB^1 and the DB^n style.

DB^1 Style

If a HIS (or its subinformation system) comprises only one database to store all patient-related data, we call this the DB^1 style. This single database is often called the central database.

The precondition for the DB^1 style is that all computer-based application components store their data only in the central database. This is only possible when the database schema of the central database is known, together with the methods that are available to access and store data there. This is usually only the case if the software products of the application components originate from the same vendor, who designed the database, or if they are all self-developed by a health care institution or if they have been developed particularly for this health care institution.

If self-development of software products is considered to be too expensive, commercially available software products may be used, and in most cases they will stem from different vendors. In this case, DB^1 style is only possible if the central database provides not only standardized interfaces but a standardized database schema as well. Even though there are promising developments in the related field of service-oriented architectures (SOAs; see Sect. 6.5.5.3), those standards are hardly implemented yet.

The DB^1 style therefore can be found mostly in HIS or in their subinformation systems where application components are used that are based on homogeneous software products (either self-developed or purchased from the same vendor; see Sect. 6.5.1.3). If application components from different vendors are used, the so-called DB^n style can usually be found.

DB^n Style

In HIS that are based on commercial software components of many different vendors, we can usually find the DB^n style. This means that several application components store data about certain entity types persistently and contain their own databases. Figure 6.44 presents this style.

As a consequence of this style, patient-related data are stored redundantly in different application components. For example, data about the entity types patient and case may be stored in different application components, such as the *patient administration system*, *LIS*, and *RIS*.

Therefore, in this architecture, great emphasis has to be placed on the consistency of redundant data. For example, the architecture must define which system is the responsible source for which data elements. It may be useful to state, for example, that data about patient and case may be created and changed only by the *patient administration system* (however, the other components may locally store and use a copy of these data). We will discuss these topics in more detail in Sect. 6.5.5.2.

In the case where different computer-based application components are not at all connected, and data storage is organized completely independently, there is no way to guarantee integrity and consistency of data. This application of the DB^n style would have negative consequences for data quality. It would lead to redundant data entry and erroneous data. Thus, this HIS style usually indicates that information management has to be improved.

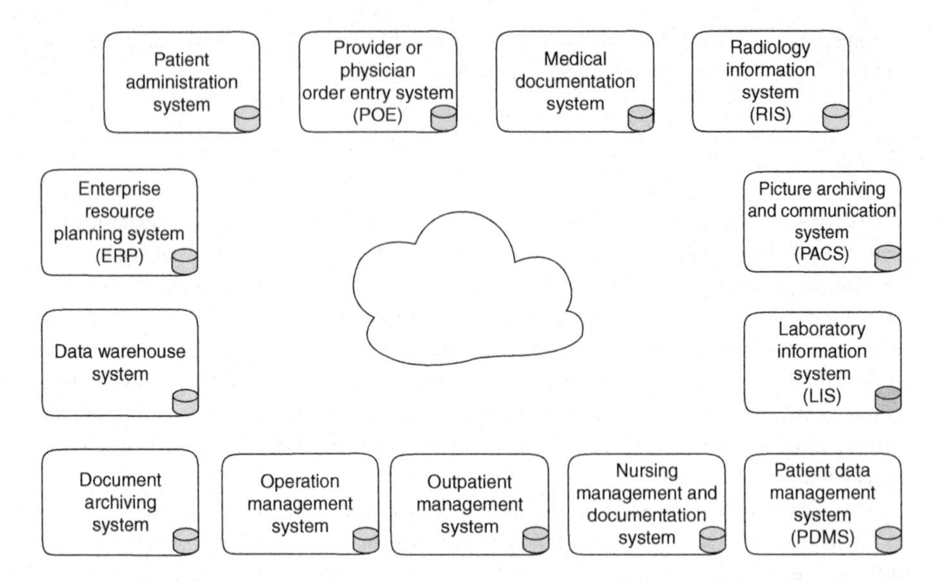

Fig. 6.44 DB^n style with multiple computer-based application components, each with its own database system, using $3LGM_2$ symbols. The cloud in the center indicates that some as yet unknown means is needed to link the components

Mixed DB^1/DB^n Style

In practice you will hardly find HIS with pure DB^1 style. Even if one central application component with the central database has been installed in order to support the hospital functions, it is hardly possible to stop implementation of further application components with integrated databases. Hence, even if a considerable part of these HIS is DB^1-styled, they are in fact DB^n-styled. See Sect. 6.5.6.1 for a typical example.

On the other hand, even DB^n-styled HIS contain subinformation systems which are DB^1-styled. We discuss these architectures in Sect. 6.5.6.1. We will refer to this mixed style by the string "DB^1/DB^n."

6.5.1.2
Number of Application Components: Monolithic Versus Modular

In the simplest case, the overall HIS consists of only one computer-based application component, which supports most of the enterprise functions. This application component looks like the one rock on which the whole hospital rests. Respective HIS are commonly called "monolithic." We will refer to this style by the string "AC^1." Of course this application component contains the central database and AC^1 correlates with DB^1. A graphical representation of such a (DB^1, AC^1) architecture is presented in Fig. 6.45.

However, one application component is usually not sufficient to support the different hospital functions. Since information and communication technology increasingly intrudes in

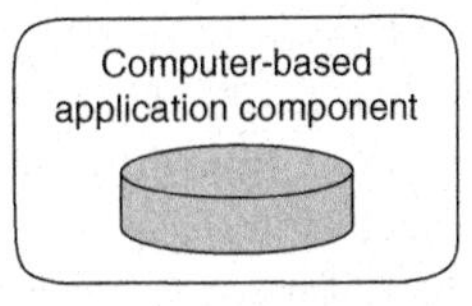

Fig. 6.45 (DB^1, AC^1) architecture using $3LGM^2$ symbols. The gray rectangle denotes the computer-based application component that contains a database system (denoted by the cylinder)

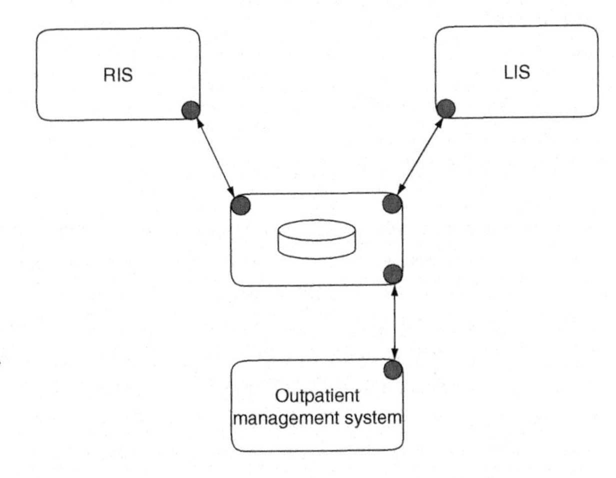

Fig. 6.46 (DB^1, AC^n) architecture with multiple computer-based application components, using $3LGM^2$ symbols. Only one computer-based application component (in the center) contains a database system

health care, an increasing number of specialized computer-based application components as introduced in Sect. 6.4 will be needed. This leads to architectures with a multiplicity of application components, which can be denoted by "AC^n" and are called modular architectures.

However, it can also be a DB^1 architecture: for example, the *RIS*, the *LIS*, and the *outpatient management system* share one single database management system in a certain application component (see Fig. 6.46). This (sub-)information system could be described by (DB^1, AC^n). Anyhow there is a widespread use of a combination of many application components and many databases, that is, of (DB^n, AC^n) architectures.

6.5.1.3 Number of Software Products and Vendors: All-in-One Versus Best-of-Breed

The terms "homogeneity" and "heterogeneity" are commonly used to describe whether a HIS consists of somewhat similar components or very different ones. A practical measure is the number of software products installed or the number of vendors delivering these products to an HIS. We denote a homogenous (sub-)HIS, that is, a (sub-)HIS with software from only one vendor as "V^1." Consequently, independent of the number of application components, V^1-HIS use only software products that all come from the same vendor. On the contrary, heterogeneous HIS comprise software from several vendors; they are denoted as "V^n."

Obviously, (DB^1, V^1) architectures are more common than (DB^1, V^n) architectures.

An (AC^n, V^n) architecture where the different application components are based on software from different vendors is commonly denoted as "best-of-breed," pointing to the fact that the hospital combines the "best" software products from different vendors. This best-of-breed architecture is typically DB^n.

On the contrary, a monolithic (AC^1, V^1) architecture and even an (AC^n, V^1) architecture emphasizes that the hospital selected only one product from only one vendor to support as many hospital functions as necessary. This homogeneous architecture is also called "all-in-one".

6.5.1.4 Communication Pattern: Spaghetti Versus Star

Application components being part of an AC^n architecture have to be connected to achieve integration. One way would be to directly connect those application components that need to exchange certain patient-related data.

For example, if data about the entity types patient and case are needed in the *patient administration system*, in the *RIS*, and in the *LIS*, direct communication interfaces between these components seem to be a possible solution. Hence, a communication interface allowing for the transfer of patient data between the *patient administration system* and the *RIS* may be introduced. Consequently, when connecting several application components, this will lead to an increasing number of bidirectional communication interfaces. This architecture is called "spaghetti" style. All these different interfaces must be supported and managed. As the number of application components rises, the number of interfaces grows nearly exponentially. The maximum number of communication interfaces between n application components ($n \geq 2$) is $\sum_{x=1}^{n-1} x$.

We denote architectures with this "spaghetti-styled" communication pattern as "CP^n". Figure 6.47 presents a (DB^n, AC^n, V^n, CP^n) architecture.

To reduce the large number of interfaces, one can use smarter methods and tools to organize and realize the interoperability of application components – that is, middleware approaches (see Sect. 6.5.5.3).

For example, most HIS following the DB^n style use a communication server. By using a communication server, no direct interfaces between application components are needed. Interfaces are needed only between the application components and the communication server. The number of interfaces that must be managed can consequently be low – ideally, only n interfaces exist for n application components.

We call this style "star architecture" and denote it as "CP^1." Figure 6.48 presents a (DB^n, AC^n, V^n, CP^1) architecture. Note that star architectures do not necessarily contain communication servers, as the center of the star may also be a database. Consequently (DB^1, AC^n) architectures will also be CP^1 architectures. Furthermore, we may call a SOA with one application component serving as a broker or as a service bus a CP^1 architecture as well. But for AC^1 this concept obviously does not make sense and neither CP^1 nor CP^n should be applied.

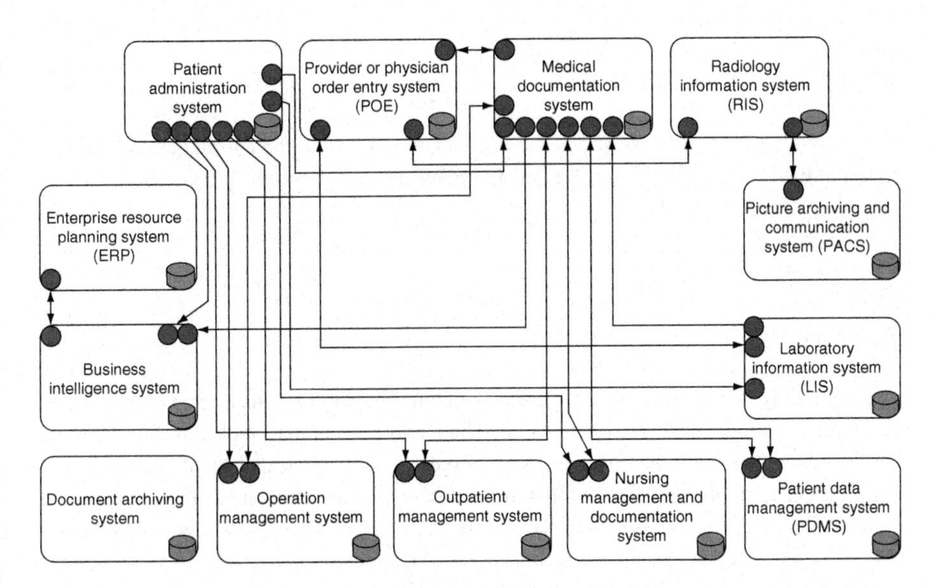

Fig. 6.47 (DB^n, AC^n, V^n, CP^n) architecture with multiple computer-based application components, using $3LGM^2$ symbols, with several bidirectional communication interfaces. This representation is also called a "spaghetti" architectural style

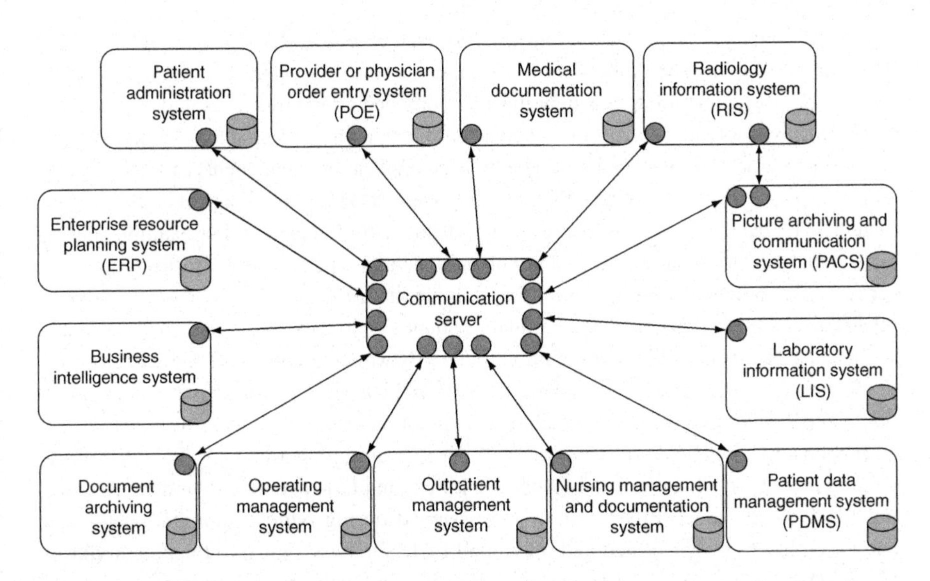

Fig. 6.48 (DB^n, AC^n, V^n, CP^1) architecture with multiple computer-based application components connected by a specific application component, using $3LGM^2$ symbols. This representation is also called a "star" architectural style

6.5.2 Integrity

In a HIS, integrity in the broadest sense is understood to mean the correctness of the data stored in the HIS. Object identity, referential integrity, and consistency are important conditions for integrity in HIS.

6.5.2.1 Object Identity

Object identity comes from object-oriented programming and means that an object has an existence that is independent of its value. Thus, two objects may look the same, that is, have the same value, but be different. Applying this to the representation of entity types in a database leads to the requirement that the representation of every entity must be uniquely identifiable. In a HIS, this is especially important for entity types like patient and case but also for finding, order, and all other entity types. This identity is needed, since all medical data need to be assigned to a particular patient and his or her cases.

Experience has shown that object identity of the entity type patient can be guaranteed only when every patient receives a unique number, the PIN. The PIN should have no internal meaning. That is, it is created continuously and is usually numerical. Past attempts to generate a PIN from data collected from the patient, for example, from the date of birth and the name, have led to considerable problems that absolutely need to be avoided. Problems that arise include, for example, if a date of birth is corrected, the PIN must also be changed. In this case, object identity could be compromised.

Similar actions should be taken for the entity type case. A CIN, which should also have no apparent meaning, should be assigned for every case. A CIN cannot change, as opposed to the PIN, whose relation to a patient must be corrected after a misidentification has taken place. However, after the correction of a misidentification of a patient, it may be necessary to assign a particular CIN to a different patient. If all application components of the HIS guarantee that a case identified with a CIN is always assigned to the correct patient in its database, then the CIN can be used as a distinguishing identifier for the patient. For example, during *order entry* the case identifier is used to uniquely identify a patient on the forms requesting, for example, laboratory testing. Then, for example, the *LIS* can use its database system to relate the CIN to the PIN, and thereby find the patient's data. It must be assumed, though, that the actual assignment of the case identifier to the PIN was communicated to the LIS.

Assigning a PIN and a CIN to a patient is part of the hospital function *patient identification and checking for recurrent*, which is a subfunction of *patient admission*.

In a hospital, a patient will receive his or her PIN during the first visit. This PIN has to be used in all parts of the hospital for the identification of the patient and will be used during future visits. Since PIN and CIN are assigned during *patient admission*, only one admission has to be performed and only one PIN has to be assigned to the patient during his or her visit. This works well if there is exactly one dedicated application component supporting patient *admission*, namely the *patient administration system*. The *patient administration system* must have direct access to a database that holds data allowing the

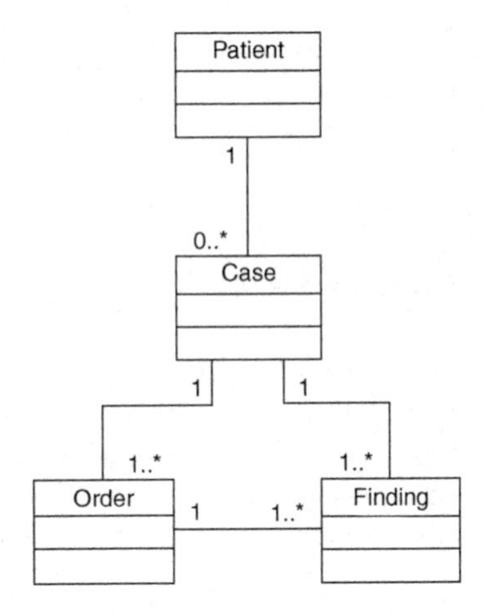

Fig. 6.49 Assignment of findings to orders and to cases, and of those cases to a particular patient, in a UML-based data model

reidentification of all past patients and cases in the hospital. To have this MPI as part of the *patient administration system* is an obvious choice.

6.5.2.2 Referential Integrity

Referential integrity means the correct assignment of entities, for example of cases to a certain patient, or results to the cases, (see the UML diagram in Fig. 6.49). Object identity is needed for referential integrity. Thus findings and orders need strict appliance of unique identifiers as well as patient and case.

Ensuring object identity for patients and cases is the basic duty of a HIS, regardless of whether it is computer-supported or not. Without object identity there is no referential integrity, and without referential integrity it cannot be ensured that results can be related back to the correct patient. Without the correct distribution of the PIN and CIN, the installation of communication networks and computer systems is practically useless.

6.5.2.3 Consistency

In DB^n-styled information systems patient data and data of other objects are often stored redundantly, that is, there are copies of data representing the same information about one particular object. Obviously these copies are supposed to be identical at all sites where they are stored. In other words, even redundant data must not be contradictory. We denote this type of integrity consistency. However, if the data are not identical and thus representing contradictory information, we call these data inconsistent. These potentially inconsistent copies of the same data are called duplicates. Transaction management (see

Sect. 6.5.5.2) tries to make sure that data are consistent – we then talk of replicates, meaning that copies of data are automatically held consistent. In DB^1 architectures, no redundant data exist as all data are unicates.

6.5.3 Types of Integration

Even if the application components at the logical tool layer are linked (or networked) together through interfaces in order to cooperate, there may be different types of integration. In the following paragraphs, we will introduce seven types of integration, namely data integration, semantic integration, access integration, presentation integration, contextual integration, functional integration, and process integration.

6.5.3.1 Data Integration

Data integration is obtained in a HIS when data that have been recorded are available wherever they are needed, without having to be reentered. Thus, each data item needs to be recorded, changed, deleted, or otherwise edited just once – even if it is used in several application components. Data integration reduces efforts to collect data, it helps to increase the quality and consistency of data, and it helps to reduce unnecessary double examinations. In DB^n architectures, communication interfaces in the computer-supported part of HIS are required, and ways to print out data (e.g., labels, order entry forms) or scan data in order to provide communication between the computer-based and the non-computer-based parts of HIS.

Assume your child was treated in the pediatrics department and a detailed patient history was collected and saved. Now, the child has to go for a hearing examination at the ear, nose, and throat department of the same hospital. If the patient history needs to be collected again because the document from the pediatrics department cannot be accessed, there is no data integration. Data integration is possible even when data items are stored redundantly.

6.5.3.2 Semantic Integration

Like data integration, semantic integration is concerned with data. Semantic integration is guaranteed if different application components use the same system of concepts, that is, they interpret data the same way. For example, when the sending application component uses the abbreviation "GOT" for a lab parameter, but the receiving application does not know this code but uses "ASAT" instead for the same concept, then semantic integration is violated.

Semantic integration between different application components using different systems of concepts can be achieved by implementing a mapping for the mutual translation of the concepts between the different application components, or by using the same system of concepts. An example for a system of concepts in medicine is the ICD (currently most prevalent in version 10). If the same ICD10[10] catalog is available in both the *patient administration system* and the *RIS*, then they interpret diagnoses in the same way and semantic integration with respect to diagnoses is guaranteed. Other examples of systems of concepts are SNOMED[11] for medical terms, ATC[12] for medications, NANDA[13] for nursing diagnosis, LOINC[14] for encoding laboratory procedures, lab results, and diagnostic procedures, and the UMLS metathesaurus[15] which links different systems to each other.

Semantic integration can be supported by medical data dictionaries (MDDs) elegantly and thoroughly. MDDs are central catalogs of medical concepts and terms that offer the possibility of representing the semantic relationships among all data stored in a HIS, and of linking that local vocabulary to internationally standardized nomenclatures and knowledge sources. MDDs can be independent application components or part of existing application components.

6.5.3.3 Access Integration

Access integration is guaranteed when the application components needed for the completion of a certain task can be used where they are needed. If, for example, the *patient administration system* is needed for *patient admission*, then the *patient administration system* should be accessible at all workstations where *patient admission* has to take place: central admission areas, wards, outpatient units, the radiological outpatient unit, emergency department, etc.

6.5.3.4 Presentation integration

Presentation integration is guaranteed when different application components represent data as well as user interfaces in a unified way. So, for example, different application components at a workstation should display the name of the patient who is currently being processed at nearly the same place on the interface, and icons for patients should code gender with the same colors.

[10]http://www.who.int/topics/classification/en/

[11]Systemized Nomenclature of Medicine (SNOMED). College of American Pathologists. http://www.ihtsdo.org/snomed-ct/

[12]Anatomical Therapeutic Chemical (ATC). WHO Collaborating Centre for Drug Statistics Methodology. http://www.whocc.no/atcddd/

[13]North American Nursing Diagnoses Association (NANDA). http://www.nanda.org/

[14]Logical Observation Identifier Names and Codes (LOINC). http://loinc.org/

[15]Unified Medical Language System (UMLS). National Library of Medicine (NLM). http://www.nlm.nih.gov/research/umls

6.5.3.5
Contextual Integration

High quality of the HIS is achieved when data, semantic, access, and presentation integration are realized. However, at the workstation of a staff member the user and patient context may get lost through the change from one application component to another. Contextual integration means that the context is preserved when the application component is changed. Or, more generally, the aim is that a task that has already been executed once for a certain purpose, such as login to a component, or selecting a patient, does not need to be repeated again in the information system, in order to achieve the same purpose.

Assume that a nurse first wants to order a lab examination for the patient Peter Maier using the *POE* application component, before documenting certain nursing procedures in her *nursing management and documentation system*. She would first login to the *POE*, search the patient Peter Maier, and then order the requested examination. Then, without context integration, she would have to start the *nursing management and documentation system*, login again, and select again the patient before being able to document the nursing procedures. Context integration would be achieved when both login (then also called "single-sign-on") and patient selection do not have to be repeated again, even when changing the application component. A standard that supports context integration is Clinical Context Object Workgroup (CCOW) (see Sect. 6.5.4.5 for details). In literature, this type of integration is also referred to as visual integration, where, however, emphasis is put on the fact that the integration of application components within a graphical user interface is dealt with.

6.5.3.6
Functional integration

Functional integration means that features needed in several application components are implemented only once and can be invoked by other application components. In a hospital, *coding of diagnoses and procedures*, for example, is an enterprise function which should be supported by the *patient administration system*, the *operation management system*, the *RIS*, the *LIS*, etc. The HIS would be functionally integrated with respect to *coding of diagnoses and procedures* if only one application component (e.g., the *patient administration system*) provides the features needed for coding diagnoses and procedures and all other application components can invoke and use them. A current approach allowing for functionally integrated information systems are SOAs (see Sect. 6.5.5.3).

6.5.3.7
Process Integration

Process integration is guaranteed when business processes are effectively supported by a set of interacting application components. Typically, as we have seen, hospital functions are supported by many different, yet interrelated application components. A user thus has to use different application components for one task. For example, during radiological report writing, the radiologist may need access to patient data in the *CIS*, the *RIS*, and the *PACS*. These components should interact as transparently and smoothly as possible. This means that all integration qualities introduced so far contribute to different extents to process integration. For example, data integration avoids the need for the user to reenter available data; access integration makes sure that he has the needed tools available for his tasks; and context integration reduces the need for double login and patient selection in different application components. Additionally good process integration prevents users from transcriptions and media cracks (see Sect. 4.5). Altogether, process integration describes a situation where different components cooperate in an optimal way, so that business processes are best supported.

6.5.4 Standards

Regardless of the technology for integration used application components have to communicate if they shall be integrated. A consensus must exist about the syntax and semantics of the data and messages that are to be exchanged. Costs of the implementation and running of communication links can be significantly reduced when standards are put in place.

For health information systems there are communication standards, documents, and health record standards available. The most important standards for communication inside HIS are HL7, DICOM, and CCOW. While HL7 and DICOM mainly support data integration, CCOW is a means for enabling contextual integration. For the exchange of bio-signals and vital parameters between point-of-care devices the ISO/IEEE[16] family of standards is available. These standards also support data integration. IHE provides guidelines for applying HL7 and DICOM properly but does not consider itself to be a separate standard. Like the other communication standards EDIFACT supports data integration but is focusing on message exchange between health care institutions. CDA is a standard for structuring medical documents and contributes to data integration, but in combination with the systems of concepts mentioned in Sect. 6.5.3.2 it contributes to semantic integration as well.

6.5.4.1 Health Level 7 (HL7) Version 2

Health Level Seven (HL7)[17] Version 2 is the most implemented communication standard in HIS for the transfer of messages with data about the entity types patient and case and the other entity types of Sect. 6.2, but excluding image data. It has been developed by the HL7 organization. HL7 describes events and dedicated message types that are exchanged between application components.

HL7 assumes that a message is sent from application component A to another application component B through the occurrence of an event (see Fig. 6.50). The message type

[16] http://www.iso.org/iso/catalogue_detail.htm?csnumber=36347

[17] Health Level Seven. HL 7. http://www.hl7.org

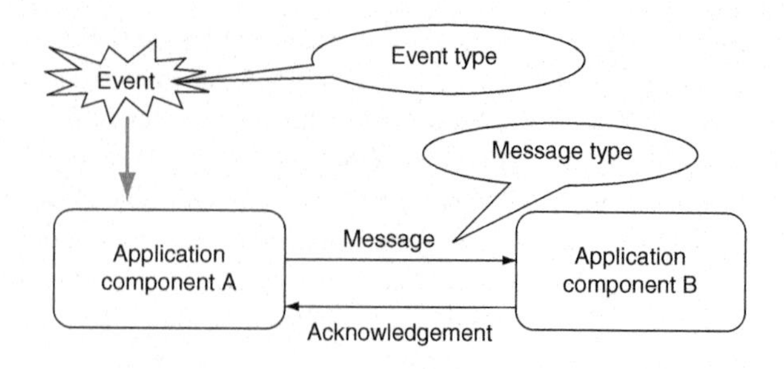

Fig. 6.50 Event-driven communication with HL7

that is used for the message depends on the occurring type of event. It describes the structure of the sent message and determines the meaning of the individual parts of the message (see Sect. 5.3.3).

Following the arrival of the message, application component B confirms the receipt of the message through a receipt message (ACK) that is sent back to application component A. If a communication server such as the one described in Sect. 6.5.5.3 is used to send a message from the *patient administration system* to the *LIS*, then the communication server first takes over the role of the receiving application component B. As a second step, the communication server as the sending application component A sends the message to *LIS*, which takes over the role of B.

HL7 possesses an extensive catalog of event types. For example, A01 describes the event "admission of a patient," A02 "transfer to another organizational unit," A03 "discharge of a patient," and R01 "completion of an examination result."

In addition, HL7 provides a list of standardized message types, such as ADT for messages related to *admission*, *discharge*, and transfer of a patient. Other message types are ORM for a general order message (e.g., ordering a radiological examination), ORU for an unsolicited observational result (e.g., a radiology report), and BAR for a patient accounting message.

Message types are assigned to event types. For example, if the *LIS* in the laboratory of a hospital registers the occurrence of an event of type R01, then it can send a message of message type ORU.

All HL7 V2 messages are structured into segments, with each segment containing fields. For example, the ADT message contains at least the following segments: Message Header (MSH); Event Description (EVN); Patient Identification (PID); Patient Visit Information (PVI). With each segment, the relevant information is provided in different fields, each of them separated by "|". The following example shows a very simplified pattern of an ADT message where a patient is admitted to a specified ward:

MSH|SENDING COMPONENT|RECEIVING COMPONENT|DATE OF MESSAGE|

PVN|A01|DATE OF EVENT|

PID|PATIENT IDENTIFIER|NAME^FIRST NAME|BIRTH OF DATE|SEX|

PVI|PATIENT CLASS|WARD ID|DATE OF ADMISSION|

Despite this standardization, the use of "plug and play" equipment is often not possible due to various reasons. On the one hand, HL7 leaves users with freedom with regard to the definition of terms, that is, the concepts, to be conveyed. In this case, consensus must exist between the communicating application components, whether, for example, the choices "male," "female," "other," and "unknown" for gender can be documented as "m," "f," "o," and "u," with "0," "1," "2," and "3," or in some other fashion. On the other hand, manufacturers of software products sometimes offer HL7 interfaces to their products that cannot send or receive all required event types and/or all necessary message types. In this case, a thorough analysis is necessary before deciding on a purchase. For existing implementations, there furthermore exists the problem of the comparison of catalogs. For example, if a *CIS* wants to order a radiological examination, it must have an up-to-date copy of the service catalog of the radiological unit. Finally, there exist different subversions of HL7 V2 (2.1, 2.2, 2.3, 2.4, 2.5) which partly differ in their definition of message content.

When a message was constructed in accordance with the previous explanations, it is up to the particular implementation as to how communication between the physical data-processing systems will occur. A message can then, for example, be written in a text file or can be transported by a disk or through an FTP file transfer. The exchange format and protocol on the physical tool layer is to be decided on in every single data transmission connection.

6.5.4.2
Health Level 7 (HL7) Version 3

Health Level 7 Version 3[18] is the newest version of HL7. Unlike version 2, which was developed in a rather pragmatic way, messages in version 3 are derived from a well-defined information model, the so-called HL7 Reference Information Model (RIM),[19] leading to much more precisely defined message semantics and a finer-grained message structure (i.e., less optional fields in each message definition). The message encoding is based on XML. The following example[20] shows a very simplified extract of an HL7 V3 message, representing a lab result message. The elements specify the type of observation (glucose), the ID, the time of the observation, and the status (the observation is completed). The value for the actual result is shown in the value element, and the data type is PQ = physical quantity.

```
<observationEvent>
    <id root="2.16.840.1.113883.19.1122.4">
    <code code="1554-5" codeSystemName="LN"
        codeSystem="2.16.840.1.113883.6.1"
        displayName="GLUCOSE^POST 12H"/>
    <effectiveTime value="200202150730"/>
    <statusCode code="completed"/>
    <value xsi:type="PQ" value="182" unit="mg/dL"/>
</observationEvent>
```

[18]http://www.hl7.org/implement/standards/v3messages.cfm
[19]http://www.hl7.org/Library/data-model/RIM/modelpage_mem.htm
[20]Adapted from http://www.ringholm.de/docs/04300_en.htm

Since HL7 version 3 is not compatible with version 2, and a "translation" between both formats is not trivial, version 3 has seen only limited uptake in those fields where version 2 is already successfully established. HL7 Version 3 is primarily used for transinstitutional message exchange for which version 2 is not well suited. Both HL7 versions can be expected to coexist for a long time.

6.5.4.3 Digital Imaging and Communications in Medicine (DICOM)

Digital Imaging and Communications in Medicine (DICOM)[21] is a standard maintained by the International DICOM Committee that addresses the integration requirements of the medical imaging sector. The standard comprises file and message formats for all types of medical imaging modalities (e.g., computed tomography, digital x-ray, magnetic resonance imaging, ultrasound, nuclear medicine imaging, etc.), a network protocol (see Sect. 6.7.2), and a set of well-defined services. These services permit, for example, an imaging modality to retrieve a "worklist" describing the patients to be examined from the *RIS*, to transmit the images and x-ray dose information created during an examination to the *PACS*, to confirm that the images have been archived successfully (and can thus be deleted locally), and to notify the *RIS* that the imaging procedure has been completed. Other services permit an application component supporting image-based diagnostics at a respective workstation to retrieve current and prior imaging studies, to print a hardcopy on a medical printer, or to store a report and results of measurements performed on the images. Unlike HL7, the DICOM standard defines a complete network protocol stack (based on TCP/IP, see Sect. 6.7.2) using efficient binary encoding and optionally image compression techniques. The capabilities of two systems (such as the services and encodings supported by both sides) are dynamically negotiated whenever a new network connection is initiated, which permits a tight integration because systems can to some degree adapt to the capabilities of their communication peers. DICOM has gained widespread acceptance in the medical imaging sector and all medical disciplines heavily relying on digital images (in particular radiology and cardiology).

It should be noted that the *RIS* application component (see Sect. 6.4.8) is also dependent on messages from the *patient administration system* and must also send, for example, billing data there. As discussed above, this communication should be carried out on the basis of HL7. Orders from wards and outpatient units will also most likely reach radiology as HL7 messages, whereas the results and images will come back as DICOM messages. The common initiative Integrating the Healthcare Enterprise (IHE)[22] (see below) has taken on the task of settling this complex interplay.

[21] http://medical.nema.org/

[22] IHE. Integrating the Healthcare Enterprise. http://www.rsna.org/IHE/index.shtml

6.5.4.4
ISO/IEEE 11073

The ISO/IEEE[23] family of standards defines a communication protocol for the exchange of bio-signals and vital parameters between various point-of-care devices. Furthermore, the standard enables a dynamic exchange and reconfiguration of devices and remote control, for example, of infusion pumps. The protocol can be used to display data from infusion pumps, respirators, ECG, etc. on patient monitors in the intensive care unit, but also for personal health applications. ISO/IEEE 11073 defines a complete communication protocol stack, with various cabled or wireless options on the lower layer, and a binary encoding optimized for near real-time transmission and small embedded devices on the upper layers, thus enabling a true "plug and play" operation.

6.5.4.5
Standard for Contextual Integration

Contextual integration requires the synchronization of application components at the workstation. The "Clinical Context Object Workgroup" (CCOW)[24] has developed standards for the synchronization of application components of different vendors on one client computer. In one of the first versions of the standard, a process, referred to as "Patient Link", is described for the synchronization of application components with regard to a chosen or identified patient. When the user of an application component changes the chosen patient at the client, all other application components on this client follow this change. This is amended through a process that passes the data about the patient to the other application components.

A similar method is used to eliminate annoying multiple user logins for different application components by passing data about user authorization to the other application components when the user has logged in at an involved application component ("single sign-on").

It can be expected that CCOW will see increasing acceptance, especially in (AC^n, V^n) architectures.

6.5.4.6
Integrating the Healthcare Enterprise (IHE)

Integrating the Healthcare Enterprise (IHE)[25] is an organization founded by medical professional societies together with the health care IT industry with the aim of improving the interoperability of application components in health care (in particular within the hospital). The approach taken by IHE is to analyze typical work processes occurring in health care, and to identify the application components involved in these processes as well as the

[23] http://www.iso.org/iso/catalogue_detail.htm?csnumber=36347

[24] Clinical Context Object Workgroup (CCOW), http://www.hl7.org/special/Committees/ccow_sigvi.htm

[25] http://www.ihe.net/

information that should be exchanged between these application components to support the diagnostic and therapeutic processes as well as possible. IHE then selects existing standards, that is, especially HL7 and DICOM, for each "transaction" (information exchange between application components) and restricts the options offered by these standards for each transaction such that plug-and-play interoperability becomes possible. IHE furthermore offers comprehensive test software enabling vendors to test their products' interfaces for IHE compliance and organizes large cross vendor testing events called "IHE connect-a-thon" (from "connection" and "marathon"). IHE is not a standards body as such, but fills a very important gap by selecting the most appropriate set of standards for a typical clinical workflow. It reduces the indeterminacy of the way of interaction, for example, between HL7 and DICOM, by proposing clear rules for their joint use. The resulting technical specifications are published annually as the "IHE Technical Framework."

6.5.4.7 Electronic Data Interchange for Administration, Commerce, and Transport (EDIFACT)

EDIFACT[26] is a message format developed and maintained by the United Nations Centre for Trade Facilitation and Electronic Business (CEFACT) as a standard format for electronic data interchange in electronic commerce (e.g., purchase orders, dispatch/delivery information, and inventory reports). EDIFACT somewhat resembles HL7 version 2: it specifies a message format, not a complete protocol stack (see Sect. 6.7.2), and the message format is text-based, using segments containing a list of elements each, separated by separator characters defined at the top of the message. The European Committee for Standardization (CEN) has developed a number of standards for message interchange based on the EDIFACT syntax, including messages for the exchange of laboratory information (EN 1613), patient transfer and discharge (EN 12538), and request and report messages for diagnostic service departments (EN 12539).

In health care, EDIFACT is mostly used for communication between health care institutions in transinstitutional HIS or between health care institutions and business partners. Within institutions other communication standards such as HL7 version 2 are used instead.

6.5.4.8 Clinical Document Architecture (CDA)

Also derived from the HL7 RIM (see Sect. 6.5.4.2) is an HL7 document format called the Clinical Document Architecture (CDA). Unlike HL7 messages, CDA documents are persistent records of medical information (such as diagnostic reports, discharge summaries, or lab reports), also based on an XML encoding. CDA supports free text as well as fully

[26]http://www.unece.org/trade/untdid/welcome.htm

structured, machine-processable information. Document templates (so-called implementation guidelines) define CDA-based document structures for specific use cases such as a discharge summary or a radiology report (see also Sect. 6.4.13).

6.5.5 Integration Technologies

To achieve integration within DB^n architectures, several integration technologies are used within a HIS. For closer coupling of application components, we will first introduce federated database systems. For looser coupling, we will look at the possibilities of transaction management in DB^n architectures and then introduce middleware approaches such as asynchronous communication by communication servers, synchronous communication by remote function calls/remote procedure calls, and SOAs and portals.

6.5.5.1 Federated Database System

A federated database system is an integrated system of autonomous (component) database systems which are part of respective application components. The point of integration is to logically bring the database schemata of the component database systems to a single database schema, the federated database schema, in order to attain data integration even when there are redundant data in HIS with a DB^n architecture. This virtual federated database schema should be able to be accessed by application components as though it were a real database schema.

When a federated database system has been implemented for a given set of application components, software can be developed that can have read access and, if applicable, write access on the corresponding data described by the federated database schema. This has a major consequence.

This method allows for developing new application components "on top" of existing ones. The existing ones are sometimes called "legacy systems." If the aim is to continuously use the legacy systems by their users as before, this is not an appropriate means for realizing data integration between these legacy systems. This holds because the integrational effect is only achieved at the new application component "on top" of the existing legacy ones. Hence the use of the method of federated database systems should be restricted to situations, when new application components, which shall reuse data out of legacy systems, are implemented.

6.5.5.2 Transaction Management: 2-phase commit protocol and master application components

Transaction management in databases but also in sets of distributed databases ensures that every update of data, which are consistent, will lead to another state in which data are consistent again. This turns out to be not trivial especially for complex update operations, so-called transactions. It is even more complicated in settings of more than one database than in DB^n architectures. Transaction management guarantees consistency of data (see Sect. 6.5.2.3) by **a**tomicity, **i**solation, and **d**urability of any transaction (ACID conditions). Atomicity guarantees that either all of the tasks of a transaction are performed or none of them are; isolation makes intermediary updates of data inside the transaction invisible and durability stands for persistence of the transaction's results.

The "2-phase commit protocol" was developed for transaction management in DB^n architectures. In the initial phase, this protocol checks if the transaction can be carried out by all affected database systems. Only if the changes are possible everywhere, they are actually carried out in a second phase in all database systems. For carrying out the protocol, the database systems must be tightly coupled by synchronous communication, and the database schemata of all involved database systems must be known. For an application component in a HIS this means that an interface must be provided where changes as well as the cancellation of these changes are possible. This is not the case for commercial application components available today. Generally, the individual database schemata of each component are also not known.

Due to these reasons, the 2-phase commit protocol to ensure consistency has usually not been implemented within a HIS yet. Nevertheless, to guarantee consistency the following more asynchronous approach is typically chosen within a HIS.

For every redundantly stored entity type, an application component is determined as the master application component for this entity type. Thus, data about entities of this type can only be inserted, deleted, or changed in this master application component. For example, typically the *patient administration system* is master for the entity types patient and case. Consequently data about patients and cases can be created, deleted, or changed only in the *patient administration system*. Therefore this application component is sometimes called the "leading system".

Transactions in a database of the master application component are carried out without regard to whether the corresponding operations can also be (immediately) carried out in the databases of the other affected application components. *Patient admission* is thereby carried out through the *patient administration system* independent of, for example, what is going on in the *RIS*. It may happen that the *RIS* is not capable of inserting corresponding data about the patient or case which have been sent by the *patient administration system* into its database at the same point in time. The *RIS* is then obliged to catch up on database operations at a later point in time.

6.5.5.3 Middleware

The very basis for integration is proper communication between application components. In this section we will explain the most important methods and tools used for communication and thereby achieving integration of HIS with a DB^n architecture.

Generally the term middleware describes the software components of a computer-based information system that serve for the communication between application components.

Middleware can be considered as the “glue” in between application components, that is, in the “middle” of a set of components.

Message Exchange by Communication Servers

A quite simple way of communication between application components is the asynchronous exchange of messages. Asynchronous communication means that the application component sending a message will continue its tasks without interruption even when awaiting a response message from the communication partner. Message exchange generates queues of messages that have to be managed. Besides direct, point-to-point communication between two application components, middleware tools for managing message queuing can be used. These so-called queue managers support the sending of messages from the sender to the receiver and the distribution of a single message to numerous receivers (multicasting).

In HIS, queue managers are typically referred to as communication servers. A communication server is an application component standing at the center of the logical tool layer of a HIS (see Fig. 6.44 in Sect. 6.5.1.1). Corresponding software products are offered by different manufacturers. This architectural principle can be found in most HIS with the DB^n architecture.

Generally speaking, a communication server is used for the asynchronous sending, receiving, and buffering of messages. It can also be used to monitor the traffic between application components. An application component can relay or send a message to the communication server over its communication interface. The communication server will then relay the message to the one address or many addresses (multicasting) when these application components are ready to receive. In the meantime, the communication server buffers the sent messages in a queue (message queuing).

In the case that the receiving application component is awaiting messages in a different format than the sending application component sends, the communication server can translate the sent message.

The communication server is in this way a tool with which asynchronous communication can efficiently be supported in order to provide data integration in a HIS of (DB^n, AC^n) architecture. It supports a rather loose coupling between autonomous application components. Specific application components can be more easily exchanged, thus supporting the expandability of the HIS architecture. Furthermore, communication servers prevent (DB^n, AC^n) styled HIS from spaghetti architectures and support CP^1 architectures.

With the communication server software available today, message sending can also be done as synchronous communication (see next section). For this, the communication server is configured so that the sending application component is blocked from the time that it sends a message to the time that it receives a response message. This way, communication servers can be used to provide functional integration as well.

Applying a communication server in order to integrate application components as in Sect. 6.4 (see Fig. 6.51) is popular in many hospitals worldwide.

The application components have to provide communication interfaces for sending and/or receiving messages to/from the communication server. As can be seen in Fig. 6.51

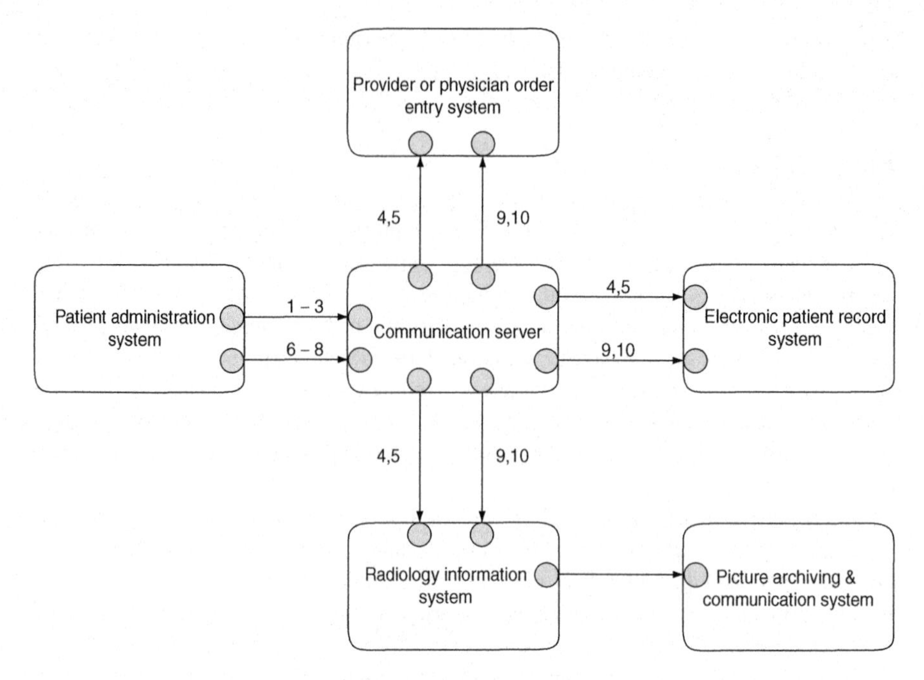

Fig. 6.51 DB^n architectural style with multiple computer-based application components, each with its own database system, using 3LGM symbols. A communication server links the components

the *PACS* is typically connected to the *RIS* directly, that is, without using the communication server. While communication to/from the communication server is usually based on HL7 or proprietary formats being able to translate to HL7, the communication between *RIS* and *PACS* is based on DICOM.

In HIS with DB^n architecture and redundant data storage the application components store all the data needed for supporting their enterprise functions by themselves. This holds especially for data about the entity types patient and case. Consequently the communication server is used to ensure that every application component will find these data in its database system whenever the data will be used without needing to request for these data in some central database system. Therefore the following communication processes are of utmost importance:

After *patient admission*:

1. If the enterprise function *patient admission* has been performed at a certain time for a certain patient, this results in an event called "A01" by HL7. Since the *patient administration system* is a master application component for the entity types patient and case, *patient admission* is exclusively supported by the *patient administration system* (see Sect. 6.5.5.2).
2. In case of "A01" the *patient administration system* arranges data about the entity types patient and case in a message, for example, according to the rules of HL7.
3. The *patient administration system* sends the message to the *communication server*.

4. The *communication server* multicasts this message to all application components, which may need data about the entity types patient and case during the stay of the admitted patient. Usually this holds for nearly all application components of the HIS.
5. All application components receiving the message will store the data about the entity types patient and case in their database system in order to have them ready in case they are needed.

After update of data during performing any other enterprise function:

6. Since the *patient administration system* is a master component of patient and case, all updates of related data have to be done using the *patient administration system*. Updating data about patient and case results in an event called "A08" by HL7.
7. In case of "A08" the *patient administration system* arranges the updated data in a message, for example, according to the rules of HL7.
8. The *patient administration system* sends the message to the communication server.
9. The communication server multicasts this message to all application components, which already received data about the entity types patient and case. Usually this holds for nearly all application components of the HIS.
10. All application components receiving the message will update the data about the entity types patient and case in their database system according to the received message. Afterwards data integrity is provided and application components will have actual data ready in case they are needed.

Remote Function Calls

Middleware components for remote procedure calls (RPCs) or remote function calls (RFC) enable the execution of a procedure that can run on a remote computer through a process that is running on a local computer. Synchronous communication is thereby carried out, meaning that the process in the initiating application component, following the initialization of communication with another application component, is interrupted as long as response data from the partner are not obtained. Using this method, a user of one application component can use a procedure provided by another component. For example, a user of the *outpatient management system* can use a procedure supporting *patient admission* provided by the *patient administration system*. In this example, the *outpatient management system* may call the function *patient admission* of the *patient administration system*. As long as *patient admission* is not finalized, the *outpatient management system* has to wait. After termination of *patient admission*, the patient and case identifier may be communicated back to the *outpatient management system*, and it can continue with the procedures (e.g., supporting patient scheduling).

RPC and RFC are classical means for providing functional integration. They provide a secure and technically well-supported way of synchronous communication between closely coupled application components. However, the calling application component is dependent on the successful response of the called component, and the exchange of an application component is typically more difficult than using asynchronous message exchange.

Service-Oriented Architectures (SOAs) and Portals

In the history of system integration there have been several paradigms to describe how application components exchange data and interoperate. As already discussed, earlier approaches based on the idea to exchange messages and to invoke features of a remote application component by remote function or procedure calls. In parallel to the paradigm of object orientation in software engineering, system integrators as well considered application components to be objects. Based on that understanding, application components would provide so-called methods, which can be used in order to manipulate (data of) certain objects.

The most recent paradigm is that of service orientation. It emerged in parallel to the introduction of web services, which can be combined or orchestrated in order to create new applications. In so-called service-oriented architectures (SOA) an application component is considered to provide and/or to invoke services (compare Sect. 5.3.4).

Some software products to support combination and orchestration of services are commercially available. They are usually called integration platforms. Similar to communication servers, they are used both at construction time to construct integrated application components and at run time to manage and control communication and interoperation between connected application components.

Using integration platforms, portals can be constructed that not only allow access to certain features, that is, services of the hospital's application components, but can also retrieve data, compute it, and use the results as input for the invocation of another service of another application component. Thus, especially functional, presentation, and contextual integration can be achieved.

The more standardized the services and the more providing and invoking interfaces are, the easier is the realization of the different integration qualities (Sect. 6.5.4) in a HIS. In 2005 the Healthcare Services Specification Project (HSSP) was initiated as a joint initiative between the Health Level 7 (HL7) organization and the Object Management Group (OMG). Up to now the project defined functional specifications through HL7 for four services: the decision support service; the entity identification service; the clinical research filtered query service; and the retrieve, locate, and update service. Technical specifications and commercial implementations have been developed as well within OMG.

SOA is a promising approach for providing not only data integration and functional integration but presentation integration and access integration as well.

Whether or not these standardized services and interfaces will be widely used in HIS in future will depend on the marketplace. The question is, whether vendors are interested in selling rather small application components providing standardized services instead of "integrated information systems" as described in Sect. 6.4.15.

6.5.6 Logical Tool Layer: Example

6.5.6.1 Typical Realizations: Centralized, Monolithic and All-in-One HIS

The most effective (but not necessarily most efficient) strategy of reducing integration efforts in a hospital is to strive for a HIS with one database, one application component, and software from one vendor, that is, a (DB^1, AC^1, V^1) or centralized, monolithic, and all-in-one architecture. This strategy would enable to transfer the efforts for ensuring the necessary types of integration (see Sect. 6.5.3) from the hospital to the software vendor or developer. Experiences show that the centralized database, that is, the DB^1 architecture, is the most important factor for reduced integration efforts.

DB^1 architectures have been the basis for the realization of the computer-supported parts of some very successful HIS in the 1970s and 1980s (e.g., DIOGENE of the University Medical Center of Geneva, Switzerland). Those HIS first started with mostly self-developed computer-based application components that facilitated easily connecting them in a DB^1 architecture (DB^1, V^1). Nowadays you can hardly find "pure" DB^1-styled information systems.

Moreover, hospitals typically buy software products for their application components, and they buy it from different vendors. Nevertheless, there are two typical situations where software for particular components comes from the same vendor. In either case, the application components will usually share the same database system. And thus the group of the respective application components can be regarded as a subinformation system having (DB^1, V^1) architecture. We will have a look at two typical situations of this in the next paragraphs. Since (DB^1, V^1) architectures reduce integration efforts in the hospital significantly, vendors often emphasize the lower integration efforts. They talk of an "integrated information system," meaning that their software already has tightly integrated modules supporting several enterprise functions in more than one area and for more than one professional group.

One situation of a (DB^1, V^1) architecture of a subinformation system is when the *medical documentation system*, the *nursing management and documentation system*, the *outpatient management system*, and the *POE* are based on one software product from one vendor. These four application components can be considered to be modules of a super component, which is then often called (integrated) *CIS* (Fig. 6.52). In this case, the major medical professional groups on all wards and outpatient units work with the same component that presents the specific features for the different areas. This integration has the advantage that major parts of the clinical data are available in one application component; this eases the development of an EPR. An example is the *CIS* of Chiba University Hospital, Japan. In Chiba, a MUMPS[27] database system has been used for a long time and even today a couple of different application components access that database system. See Fig. 6.53 for Chiba University Hospital's DB^1-styled subinformation system. Besides the central component,

---

[27] Massachusetts General Hospital Utility Multi-Programming System, a database management system developed in the 1960s for hospital data management

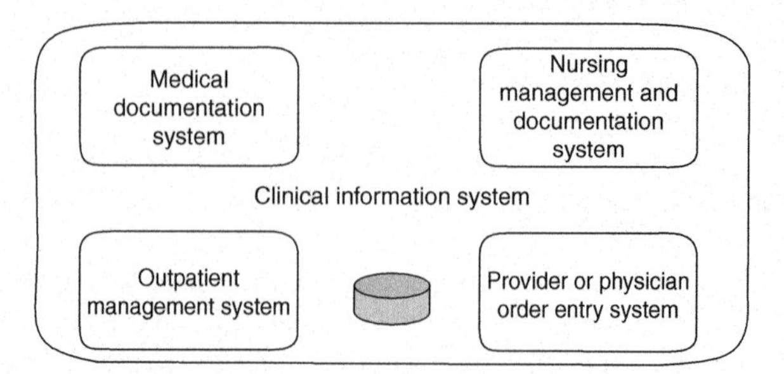

Fig. 6.52 An integrated *clinical information system (CIS)* as an example for a (DB^1, V^1) architecture. The CIS often contains the *medical documentation system*, the *nursing management and documentation system*, the *outpatient management system*, and the *physician or provider order entry system (POE)* as modules

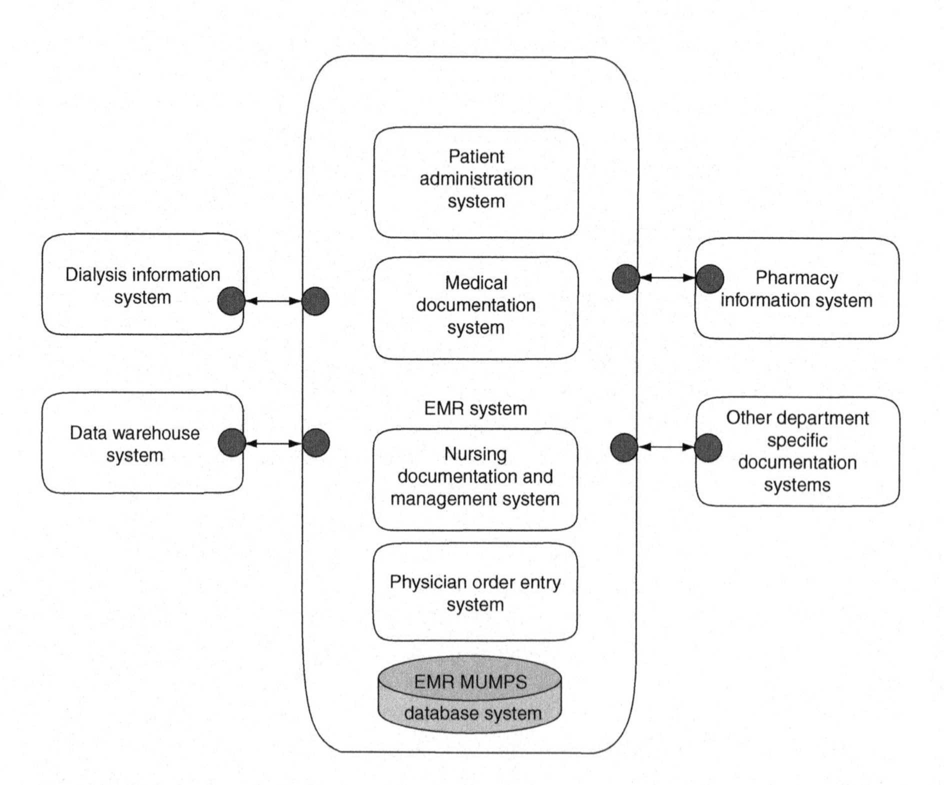

Fig. 6.53 A (DB^1, V^1)-styled subinformation system at Chiba University Hospital, Japan. The central electronic medical record (EMR) system has a database which can also be accessed by other application components

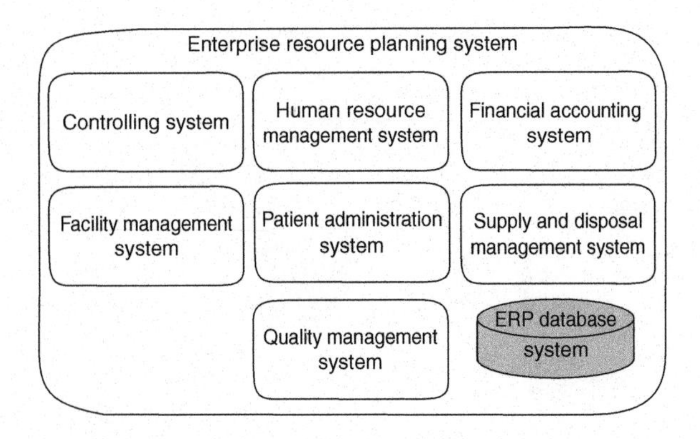

Fig. 6.54 A typical situation in German University Hospitals: the enterprise resource planning (ERP) system includes a component for *patient administration*

called "EMR system" (electronic medical record system), it includes a *patient administration system*, a *medical documentation system*, a *nursing documentation and management system*, and a *POE*, and is used both in inpatient and outpatient units of the hospital. The application software for these components has been developed by one vendor especially for Chiba University Hospital.

Another situation of a (DB^1, V^1) architecture of a subinformation system is when the *patient administration system* and the *enterprise resource planning system* come from the same vendor. This is a typical situation, as *patient administration* can then closely be linked to *financial accounting* and *controlling*. See Fig. 6.54, which demonstrates that situation which is quite typical for German university hospitals.

These central, all-in-one (sub-)information systems help to reduce the effort for integration, but as drawback, hospitals tend to be more dependent on one or two major vendors.

6.5.7 Logical Tool Layer: Exercises

6.5.7.1 Data Distribution Style at the Logical Tool Layer

Look at Fig. 6.48. It shows a specific representation of a (DB^n, AC^n, V^n, CP^1) architecture. Describe this architectural style. How is it distinguished from (DB^1, AC^n, V^n, CP^1) architecture? What are its advantages and disadvantages?

6.5.7.2 HIS Infrastructures

Look at Figs. 6.55–6.58 taken at an ophthalmology unit of the Plötzberg Medical Center and Medical School (PMC). Describe the individual information processing tools on it. Then summarize the typical HIS infrastructure for a ward in this hospital.

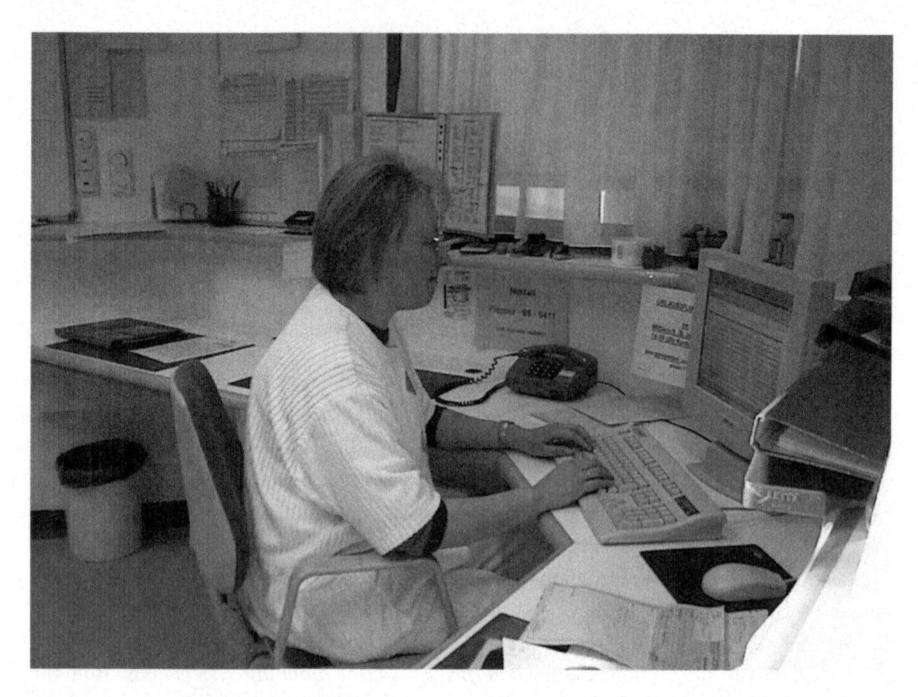

Fig. 6.55 At an ophthalmology unit (1)

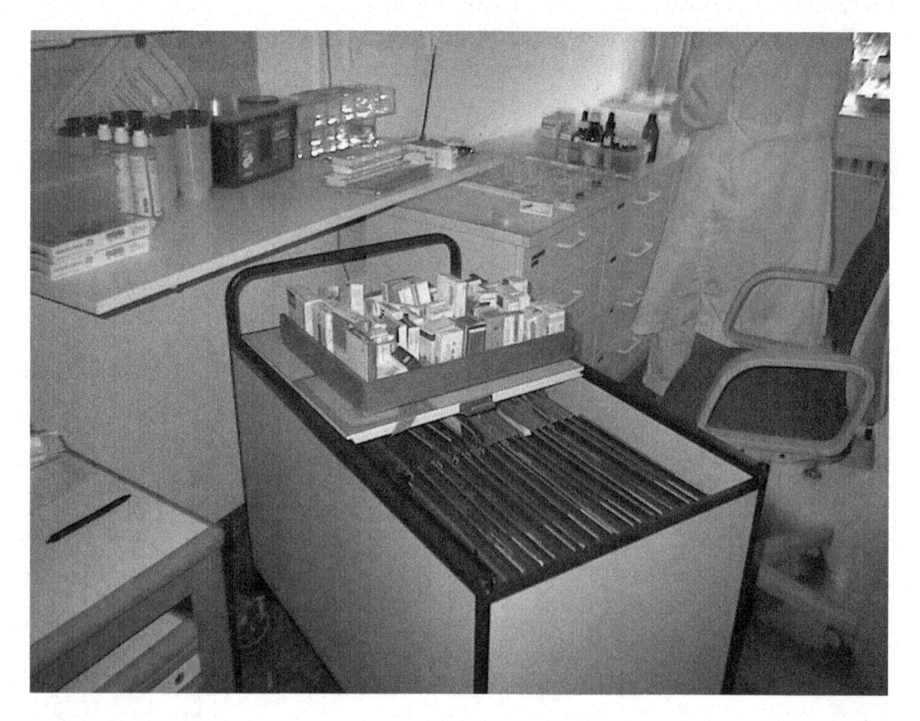

Fig. 6.56 At an ophthalmology unit (2)

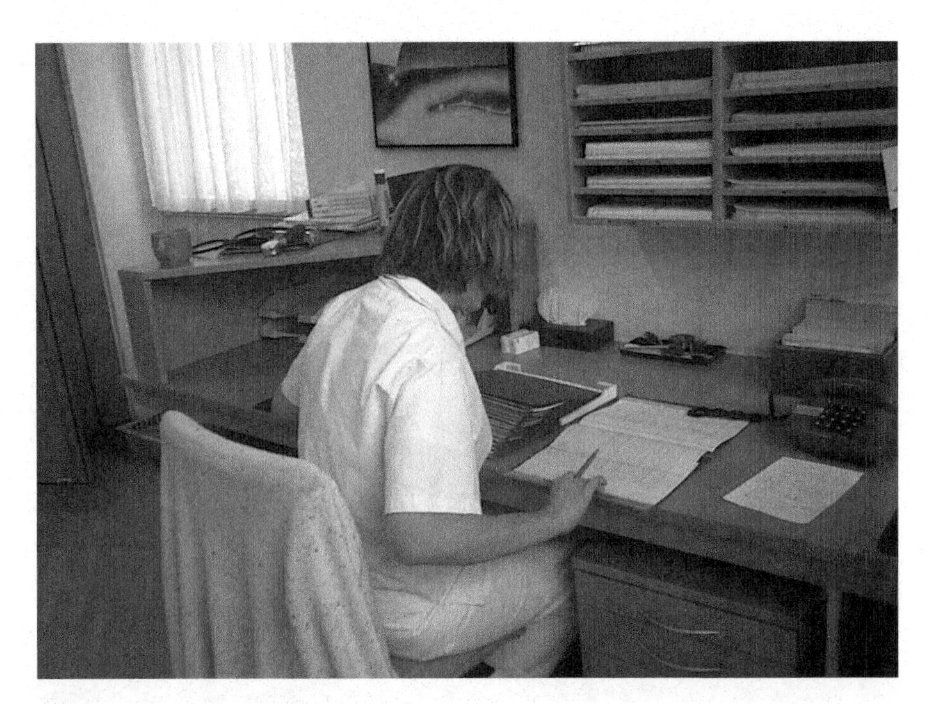

Fig. 6.57 At an ophthalmology unit (3)

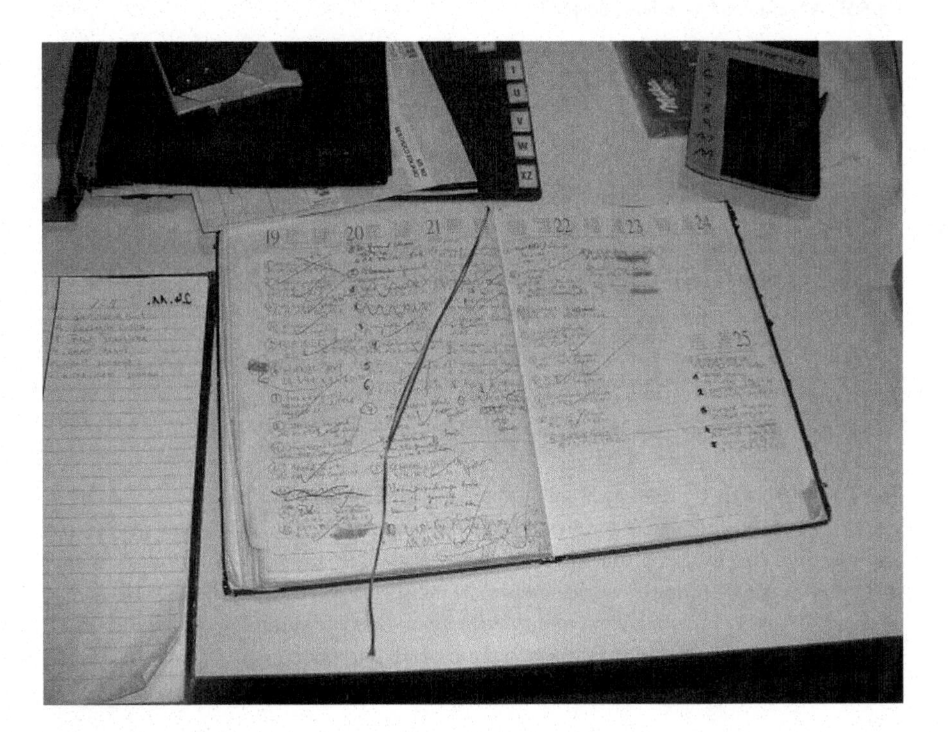

Fig. 6.58 At an ophthalmology unit (4)

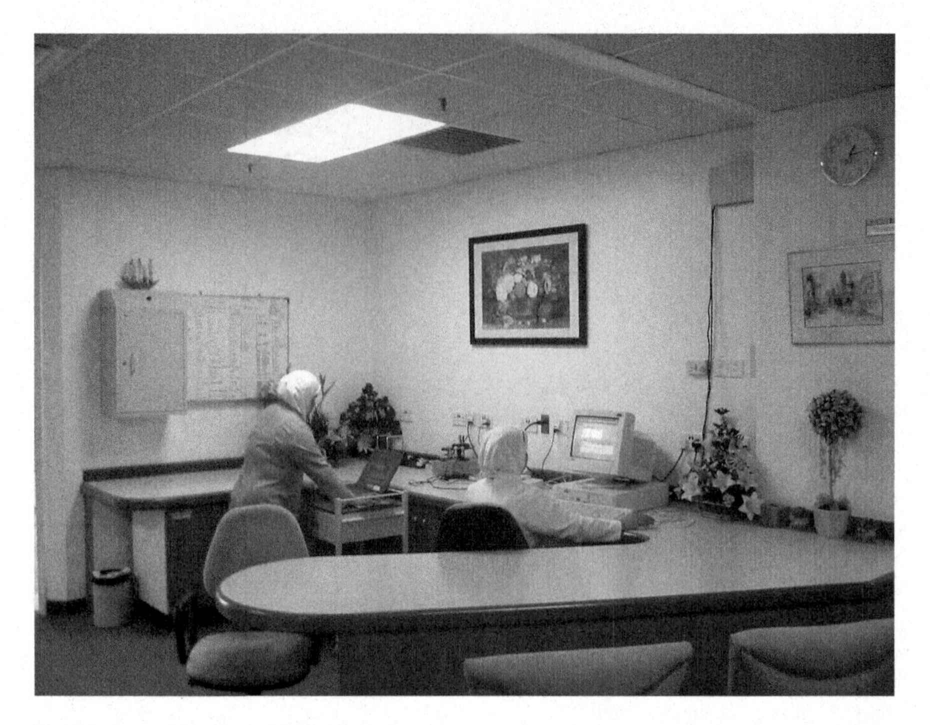

Fig. 6.59 A ward in a "paperless" hospital

6.5.7.3
A Paperless Hospital

Look at Fig. 6.59 and compare the HIS infrastructure with that from the ophthalmology unit in exercise 6.5.7.2. What is the main difference? Do you think a completely paperless hospital is really an aim that can be and should be achieved?

6.5.7.4
Introducing a Departmental Computer-Based Application Component

The Department of Cardiology wants to buy and introduce a new cardiologic computer-based application component for their wards and outpatient units. The hospital already has an integrated *CIS* in use in other departments, but the Department of Cardiology argues that this *CIS* is not sufficiently oriented toward the special needs of cardiology. If you had to decide: Would you allow them to introduce a new specific cardiologic computer-based application component, or would you recommend introducing the hospital-wide *CIS* instead? Please justify your choice.

6.5.7.5
Loose and Close Coupling

Message sending is typically referred to as "loose" coupling, while remote function calls are referred to as "close" coupling. Which type of coupling do you find more helpful when you want to have an architecture where components can be easily exchanged? And which type of coupling do you prefer when you want to have the *RIS* being able to support *patient admission* as well, although the *patient administration system* already provides a related feature and you want to avoid functional redundancy?

6.5.7.6
Integrating Nursing Documentation

Imagine you want to transfer administrative patient data from the *patient administration system* to a *nursing management and documentation system* where they are needed to identify patients. How would you realize this? Which standards for integration would you chose? Explain your solution.

6.5.8
Logical Tool Layer: Summary

At the logical tool layer, a HIS comprises dedicated application components to support hospital functions in different units of a hospital. Typically there are the following application components:

- *patient administration system;*
- *medical documentation system;*
- *nursing management and documentation system;*
- *outpatient management system;*
- *provider/physician order entry system;*
- *patient data management system;*
- *operation management system;*
- *radiology information system;*
- *picture archiving and communication system;*
- *laboratory information system;*
- *enterprise resource planning system;*
- *data warehouse system;*
- *document archiving system.*

An integrated *clinical information system (CIS)* combines several application components such as a *medical documentation system*, an *outpatient management system*, a *nursing management and documentation system* and a *CPOE* system in one component. *CIS* are also often called *electronic patient record (EPR) systems*.

Information managers have to keep in mind that besides computer-based application components, even today there are a lot of important non-computer-based application components such as the paper-based patient chart system and the paper-based patient record system.

A major challenge for information management is to integrate these application components in order to achieve and maintain integrity. In a HIS, object identity, referential integrity, and consistency are important aspects of integrity. Since there are different ways of integration and different constraints in different hospitals, different architectures of HIS may result. A taxonomy taking the number of databases, number of application components, number of software products, and communication patterns into account is helpful for describing architectures.

Integration of application components encompasses different aspects such as data, semantic, access, presentation, contextual, functional, and process integration. A well-integrated HIS should implement all of them.

Using standards can reduce integration efforts and result in better reliability. In HIS, communication standards like HL7, DICOM, ISO/IEEE 111073, and EDIFACT are of outstanding importance for data integration. IHE defines how HL7 and DICOM can be used in combination. CCOW supports contextual integration and CDA provides a standard for structuring medical documents.

Several integration technologies are used within a HIS. The concept of federated database systems can be used as a basis for the development of a new application component in a HIS. This can be complemented by a 2-phase commit transaction management. Since this is often not possible, master application components have to be defined in many cases. According to the requirements, different middleware concepts are applicable to implement interfaces and communication. Communication servers are most popular but often complemented by remote function calls. SOAs may emerge to replace these technologies.

6.6 Physical Tool Layer: Physical Data-Processing Systems

Application components are logical tools and they cannot exist without physical tools as a basis. In an information system we can describe this basis by the physical data processing systems at the physical tool layer. As said earlier physical data processing systems can be human actors, non-computer-based physical tools, or computer systems. We will now have a closer look at typical computer-based physical data processing systems in a hospital.

After reading this section, you should be able to answer the following questions:

- What computer-based and non-computer-based physical data processing systems can be found in hospitals?
- What is meant by the term “infrastructure”?

6.6.1
Servers and communication networks

Servers are used to provide sophisticated features to clients (see Sect. 6.6.2). Servers can run databases (database server), they can run the back-end part of application software (application server), or support printing (printer server). Terminal servers run the front-end part of application software, which traditionally has been implemented on and run by clients. If terminal servers are used, mere terminals (see Sect. 6.6.2) for displaying output and receiving input are sufficient. Further server types are name servers (for DNS name management), DHCP servers (for dynamic IP assignment), mail servers (for e-mail services) and web servers (for Web site management).

There is a strong trend to virtualize servers. One "real" server, that is, a physical server, can simulate lots of so-called virtual servers. Every virtual server runs a particular instance of an operating system and can be used to implement application software. Thus, these virtual servers behave nearly identically to physical servers. This approach makes computing power in a computing center much more flexible and scalable. It fosters the use of large multipurpose central computers instead of smaller departmental and dedicated servers in the past (see also Sect. 6.7.1).

Virtual servers also result from coupling physical servers in order to maximize availability by redundancy. Those coupled servers are called a server cluster. It makes sense to localize the members of the cluster at different sites of the computing center (see Sect. 6.7.3).

Servers are part of, and connected by, larger intra- and interhospital communication networks. Communication networks can be implemented by optical fibers, copper cables, and wireless LAN technologies. Different communication protocols such as Ethernet or token-ring can be used.

6.6.2
Clients

Clients comprise all data processing tools that are immediately available to the various user groups within a hospital, for example:

- a stationary personal computer located at a defined place in a unit (e.g., the personal computer in the ward office);
- a mobile computer such as a laptop or tablet-pc used for mobile information access (e.g., a tablet-pc used by health care professionals on a ward) (see Fig. 6.60);
- mobile devices such as a personal digital assistant (PDA) or a mobile phone to support mobile personal organization and information access;
- a terminal (also called thin client) which has only functionalities for displaying and for data entry, but has no storing capability;
- a beamer used for projecting radiological images onto a wall in order to support a conference of physicians discussing a difficult case jointly (see Fig. 2.1).

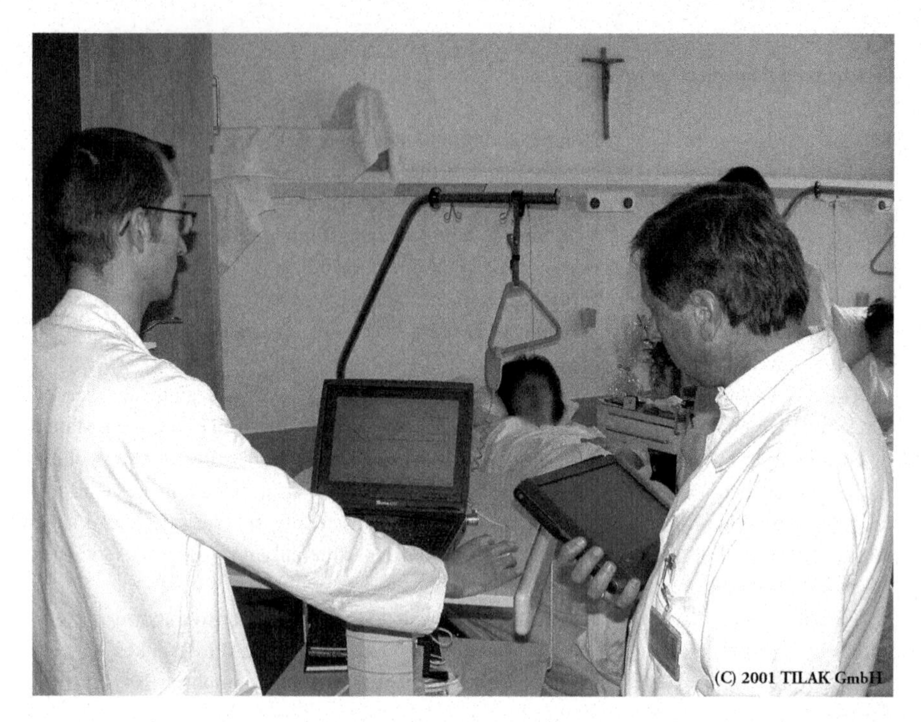

Fig. 6.60 A health care professional accessing patient information

6.6.3 Storage

Not only huge amounts of data but also very important data, which may be crucial for patients' health and life, have to be stored in HIS (compare example 6.7.4.1). This needs storage devices of high capacity and high reliability. Storage media used range from magnetic disks for random access to magnetic tapes and optical media for backup and archiving.

Nowadays storage devices regardless of the media used are not specifically attached to, and exclusively used by, certain servers. Moreover so-called storage area networks (SANs) provide storage services of different kinds to all servers integrated in this network. This technology allows for scaling up and down quite easily the storage capacities depending on actual storage needs. Additionally, SANs support to maximize availability by redundancy. It makes sense to localize the members of the SAN at different sites of the computing center (see Sect. 6.7.3).

6.6.4 Typical Non-computer-Based Physical Data-Processing Systems

Computer-based data processing systems such as servers and clients as described above are often in the center of interest for information management. However, in typical institu-

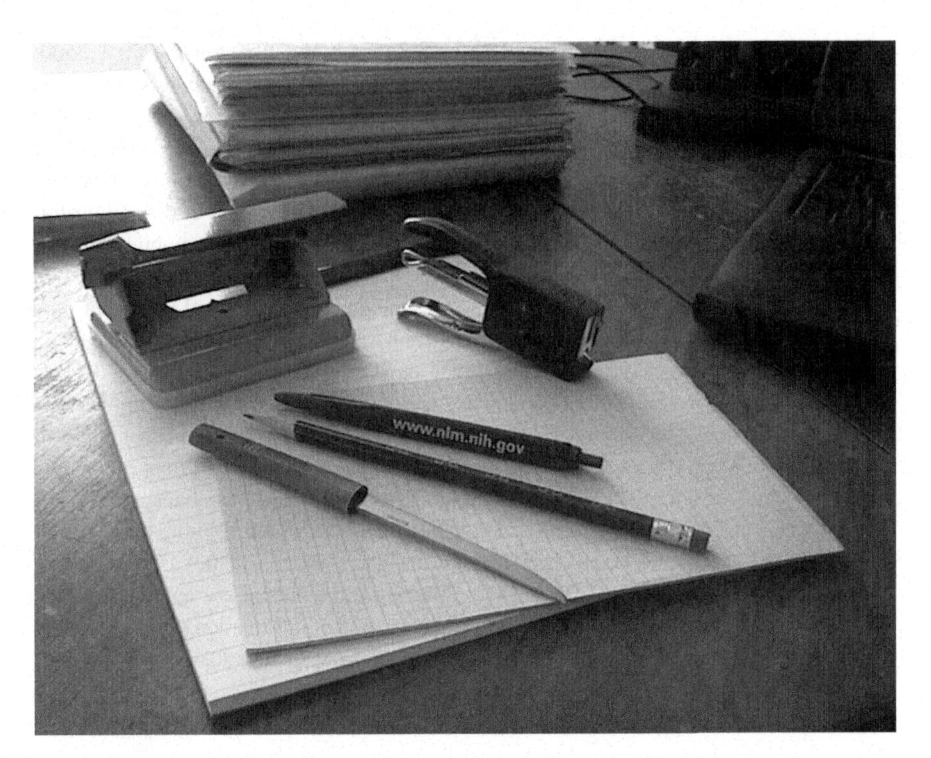

Fig. 6.61 Typical paper-based physical data processing systems

tions, a large number of non-computer-based physical data processing systems are also in use. A clinical user may, for example, use pencil and paper, telephones, mobile phones, pagers, typewriters, fax machines, and even fork lift and cars (e.g., for transportation of patient records) as typical non-computer-based components (Fig. 6.61). Besides, paper-based folders may be in use as basis for the paper-based patient record and the paper-based patient chart (see Sect. 6.4.16 for details). It is important to take those non-computer-based systems into account when building and managing a health information system – only coordination of all tools will appropriately support the clinical and administrative business processes.

6.6.5 Infrastructure

The set of all physical data processing systems in a health care institution is called the infrastructure of its HIS. This infrastructure can be described by the overall number of physical data processing systems, by the average number of physical data processing systems per unit (e.g., two personal computers and one laptop per ward), or per staff member.

The infrastructure of a given HIS can comprise primarily paper-based physical data processing systems, primarily computer-based physical data processing systems, or a mixture of both. Typically, you will find such a mixture in hospitals.

For example, a typical scenario could be the following: The infrastructure for a 1,500-bed university hospital may comprise about 4,000 clients (personal computers) and 3,000 telephones. At least two to four personal computers and two laptops are usually installed for use in each ward and outpatient unit (in intensive care units, there is one computer for each patient's room). Every physician may have access to a personal computer. One personal computer may also be available in each OR and for each member of the administrative staff. At least two telephones may be available in each unit, and a mobile phone or pager for approximately half of the staff members (mainly physicians).

Despite the fact that "Green IT" seems to be a commercial buzzword in current fairs and far from the interest of academic medical informatics, it has a considerable impact on medicine and health care. Taking the above-mentioned infrastructure into account, it needs not only resources for administration, maintenance, and reinvestment, but also tremendous energy. For the above-mentioned 4,000 clients we can assume a power consumption of approximately 300 W for each PC. This results in a total consumption of approximately 1.2 MW (Mega Watt) for the PCs. For two redundant computing centers housing the servers an additional 0.5 MW have to be added. Altogether, this would be more than enough power to heat 170 detached houses even in coldest winter times. It is quite easy to calculate the considerable amount of annual costs resulting from the related energy consumption. These numbers emphasize the need for close collaboration of information system planning and *facility management* in technical departments in order to find solutions for energy recycling, for example, to support hot water supply.

6.7 Physical Tool Layer: Integration of Physical Data-Processing Systems

If application components, which exchange data and interact with each other, are installed on different physical data processing systems at the physical tool layer, these physical data processing systems have to communicate as well, that is, integration is needed. Similar to the logical tool layer, we categorize architectures and discuss integration at the physical tool layer.

After reading this section, you should be able to answer the following questions:

- How can physical data processing systems be grouped and arranged in order to support application components in an optimal way? What architectures can result?
- What is meant by physical integration?
- How do modern computing centers look?

6.7.1 Taxonomy of Architectures at the Physical Tool Layer

There are no remarkable differences between the physical tool layer of a hospital and the physical tool layer of any industrial enterprise. At both settings we can find clients, that is, personal computers and terminals, servers, storing media, and communication networks. And in both settings there are different ways of sharing tasks between clients (terminals, PCs) and servers or mainframes. We continue our taxonomy of architectures taking this aspect into account.

6.7.1.1
Distribution of Computing Power: Mainframes vs. Client-Server

From their beginnings in the middle of the twentieth century, computer-based HIS were based on centralized mainframes in a computing center. In a mainframe architecture, all computer-based application components are installed on one or multiple mainframe system(s) to which various terminals are attached. The terminals cannot execute applications or store data, that is, they only serve for data input and output. Until the late 1980s mainframe architectures had been predominantly in hospitals. We will refer to these 1-tier architectures with one centralized physical data processing system as "T^1."

Note that the architecture of the physical tool layer can be chosen independently of the architecture of the logical tool layer. Thus, you can find for example (AC^1, T^1) architectures as well as (AC^n, T^1) architectures.

Since the 1990s mainframes have been considered as legacy systems, that is, they are out of date. However, the concept of terminals as so-called thin clients has continued into the era of client-server architectures.

In decentrally styled or so-called distributed physical tool layers, sets of clients and sets of servers can share their tasks in different ways. This became possible with the coming up of PCs, which could take over a part of program execution, which allowed for graphical user interfaces (GUI), for example.

In a 2-tier architecture, there is a server that serves both as application and database server. The program execution can partly or completely be given to the client PCs. We will refer to these architectures as "T^2."

In a 3-tier architecture, there is a separate application server and a separate database server. The database server is responsible for storing the data, and on the application server the application components are installed and executed. This requires communication between the three components during runtime. We will refer to these architectures as "T^3."

During the 1990s, the low costs of hardware have led to an increased use of client-server architectures in hospitals, with various clients and servers distributed over different units. However, these T^2 and T^3 architectures have engendered high costs for maintenance and support of the servers and of the clients, and have made data security and server availability difficult to guarantee. To solve this problem, the different servers have been recentralized in one computing center, hoping to reduce costs for server maintenance. A collection of servers at one site also allows for the improvement of data security and availability (e.g., by clustering servers). In addition, hard disks and CD/DVD drives are often removed from the personal computers as clients, in order to reduce costs for maintenance and support of clients. Moreover, during the last years the number of PCs in client-server architectures has decreased in favor of thin clients. Similar to the terminals of the mainframe era, thin clients are only used for data input and output, but they have enough processing power for running a GUI. In addition to a database server and an application server, a terminal server is necessary (see Sect. 6.6.1). But if we again take the above-mentioned strong trend towards virtualization into account, the differentiation into different servers and server types becomes increasingly irrelevant. Moreover, the park of servers and the storage area network in a computing center can be considered to be only one big server. And hence we are back where we started decades ago: at T^1 architectures.

6.7.2 Physical Integration

The types of integration introduced in Sect. 6.5.3 relate to the logical tool layer and, more precisely, to sets of computer-based application components. Let us supplement this catalog of integration types by physical integration.

Physical integration is guaranteed if there exists the physical communication network for any kind of data exchange. In other words, physical integration between different physical data processing systems is a prerequisite for data integration between application components.

Physical integration needs not necessarily be achieved by connecting different physical data processing systems such as servers by a communication network (see Sect. 6.6.1). It can also be achieved by installing two different application components on the same physical data processing system.

If different physical data processing systems have to be connected by a communication network, the network topology has to be considered. In general, we can distinguish logical and physical network topologies. Please note that both topologies correspond to the physical tool layer in the 3LGM metamodel.
There are six basic physical topologies:

- Bus: Every physical data processing system is directly connected to the shared transmission medium called bus. There are no other active devices between the devices and bus.
- Ring: Every physical data processing system has exactly two neighbors for communication purposes. Finally the physical data processing systems are interconnected to form a ring. Data are passed from one system to the other in the same direction (either "clockwise" or "counterclockwise") as long as they reach their destination.
- Linear: Two physical data processing systems are interconnected in order to form a line. Data are passed from one physical data processing system to the other as long as they reach their destination.
- Star: All physical data processing systems are connected via a two-point connection to a central system which handles data transmission.
- Tree: Practically speaking, the tree topology hierarchically connects two or more star topology networks by connecting the central physical data processing systems.
- Mesh (partially connected or fully connected): Each physical data processing system is connected with one or more devices; if each device is connected with all other devices on the network the mesh is said to be fully connected.

By contrast, the logical topology is the way in which physical connections (topology) are used or signals transmitted. The logical and the physical topology can be chosen independently from each other. For example, Ethernet can physically be implemented on a physical Bus or Star topology but logically Ethernet is clearly a Bus topology. The same is true for Token Ring which is logically a Ring but may physically be organized as a Star using so-called Multi Station Access Units. Note as well that all these combinations of topologies at the physical tool layer can be combined with every communication pattern at the logical tool layer as described in Sect. 6.5.1.4.

In order to best describe standards for data exchange on a network and their different functions it is useful to consider the ISO/OSI reference model. This reference model provides a framework for describing communication between computers at seven levels. Standards for the respective communication protocols such as TCP/IP are available for each level. With respect to $3LGM^2$ these seven levels interconnect the physical with the logical tool layer of a HIS. Level 7 may be considered as the logical tool layer which corresponds to the name of the communication standard HL7 (see Sect. 6.5.4.1). A set of protocols for each of the seven levels is called a protocol stack.

6.7.3 Computing Centers

Regardless of whether you choose a T^1, a T^2, or a T^3 architecture, the servers must fulfill special requirements related to availability, stability, performance, maintainability, and redundancy. When T^2 and T^3 architectures came up, servers in hospitals were often installed near the departments where the application components running on these servers had to be used. This was due to the lack of high-performance communication networks and relatively low prices of these servers. The last years showed clearly that these solutions are not economically sound. Hence there is a strong trend back towards centralized computing centers. But note that this centralization goes well with any of the T^1, T^2, or T^3 architectures.

The reliability of the computing center with all its equipment and physical data processing systems is the very basis for the reliability of the HIS as a whole. Although system stability of application components deals with the quality of the software used, system stability has to be enhanced by redundancy. However, redundancy is not needed at the logical tool layer but at the physical tool layer.

Hence, computing centers are required providing at least two redundant sites, with mirrored servers and storage devices at each site, stable energy supply, high-capacity air-conditioning, server rooms that are burglar-proof and disaster-proof, and effective means for fire protection. Even if an information management department cares for an effective backup, the continuous operation of the computing center by appropriate redundancy is of utmost importance. It may need 3–4 weeks to restore image data from a *PACS* if the respective storage device has crashed and no mirrored, redundant device had been provided.

People working here need software tools for supervising proper operation of servers, communication network components, PCs and terminals, and the application components running above these physical tools. See Fig. 6.62 for a computing center's server room.

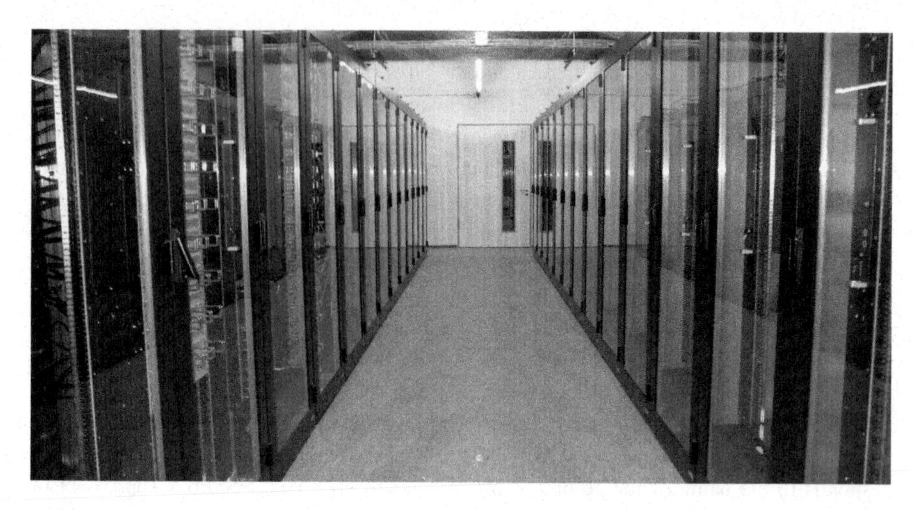

Fig. 6.62 A modern server room in a computing center of a university hospital

6.7.4 Physical Tool Layer: Example

6.7.4.1 The Amount of Data to Be Processed at a Hospital's Computing Center

The amount of digital data a hospital has to manage depends, for example, on the hospital's size, the medical services offered, and the existing IT infrastructure. Let us consider a particular university hospital with approximately 1,200 beds, which provides maximum medical care and is also responsible for *research and education*.

The server infrastructure is operated at two different sites, that is, there is a redundant computing center. Besides physical redundancy, virtualization is an important concept of the server hardware at the university hospital. Currently, 40 terabytes of the storage area network (SAN) are needed for the server infrastructure. Services for the *CIS* and the *ERP system*, exchange services, non-DICOM images and a variety of other application components are implemented or stored on these servers. Backup is done with a deduplication appliance using 20 terabytes at each site and a compression rate of 6:1.

For imaging during radiologic diagnostics, three image servers, each having 4 terabytes of fast cache, are available. Tape libraries with a current volume of 100 terabytes are used for long-term archiving of radiologic images. The estimated medium-term capacity amounts to 230 terabytes.

The overall data volume is expected to grow by 10–15 terabytes a year. It is hard to estimate this number more precisely because the modalities and, thus, the images generated get more sophisticated. Additionally, each single user's demand for storage space grows rapidly.

6.7.5 Physical Tool Layer: Exercises

6.7.5.1 HIS Infrastructure

Look at a hospital you know. Answer the following questions concerning HIS infrastructure:

- What kind of non-computer-based and computer-based data processing systems are used in the hospital?
- How many personal computers are used?
- What kind of communication network is installed? What logical and physical topologies are used?
- How many sites does the computing center have? Do they have more than one computing center?
- How are findings transported from laboratory to the ward physically?

6.7.6 Physical Tool Layer: Summary

At the physical tool layer, a HIS comprises data processing systems which are quite similar to those of information systems of enterprises in other industries. Consequently, similar servers, clients, and communication networks connecting them can be found. But especially in health care institutions non-computer-based data processing systems such as pencil, telephone, and paper-based patient charts are still of considerable importance. And presumably they will be. The set of all data processing systems in a health care institution is called its information system's infrastructure.

Similar to the components of the logical tool layer the physical data processing systems of the physical tool layer have to be integrated. And again there are different ways and styles to do this. The taxonomy of architectures as introduced for the logical tool layer therefore has been expanded to cover 1-, 2-, or 3-tier physical architectures as well. Physical integration roughly means that data can be exchanged between physical data processing systems.

A well-organized computing center consisting of two redundant sites is the very prerequisite to ensure availability, stability, and performance for the computer-supported part of a HIS.

6.8 Summarizing Example

6.8.1 Health Information Systems Supporting Clinical Business Processes

In this example, typical activities and processes during a patient's stay in the Plötzberg Medical Center (PMC) and Medical School (PMC) are described by means of a fictional example. It is demonstrated how clinical business processes can be supported by advanced HIS. This example presents a more dynamic view of the process starting at a physician's general practice and ending with *discharge* from PMC.

Patient Treatment at a Physician's General Practice

Dr. Healthy, a physician in general practice, diagnoses the patient Tom Bender, 62 years old, with a transient ischemic attack and suspected stenosis of the internal carotid artery, based on the reported symptom of an amaurosis fugax – a transient blindness – on the left side. He would like to hospitalize Mr. Bender for further examination and treatment.

While Mr. Bender is in the doctor's consulting room, Dr. Healthy calls the nearest hospital, the PMC, for the purpose of an *admission*. The physician carrying out the *admission* at PMC consults a clinical guideline that shows that about 7 days of treatment will have to be planned. He can see that a bed is vacant and proposes an immediate hospitalization. Dr. Healthy agrees. The physician performing *admission* documents Mr. Bender's name, date of birth, and the diagnosis for hospitalization. Dr. Healthy gets an automatic confirmation of this appointment which he prints out, along with further information on the PMC, for this patient.

Dr. Healthy selects recent clinical documents of his patient (e.g., a recent ECG and a list of recently prescribed drugs) and marks them as "available" for the hospital physician. As soon as Mr. Bender is at the PMC, the hospital physicians can access this information in their *CIS*.

Administrative Admission

Mr. Bender arrives at the PMC and the employee in the patient administration department sees that a reservation has been made and she admits Mr. Bender to the neurology department as a new patient. Mr. Bender gets a wristband carrying a bar-code that can be used to uniquely identify Mr. Bender. After completion of the *administrative admission*, Mr. Bender is taken to his ward.

Arrival at ward

On the ward, Mr. Bender is welcomed by the nurse, Mrs. Weber. He tells her that he would like to have a single room. Mrs. Weber can see from the ward monitor that a single room is available, and brings him to his bed. The patient terminal at his bedside allows Mr. Bender to access selected parts of his medical record. He can, for example, review the ordered medications and his latest lab values. He can also access general medical information for patients that have been checked for quality and clarity.

Nursing Admission

Mrs. Weber carries out the *nursing admission*. After talking to Mr. Bender, she defines the relevant nursing diagnosis and then reviews the automatically proposed nursing care standards that match the situation of Mr. Bender. She selects two standards and adapts them to the situation of Mr. Bender. She also notes that Mr. Bender has false teeth and limitations in movement.

Medical Admission

Dr. White, the attending neurologist, screens the available electronic information from Dr. Healthy, the GP, and from other physicians who have treated the patient before. The most important data from the medical history and the essentials on the previous treatment of hypertension are automatically copied to the EPR. Dr. White reviews this information and then conducts a physical examination of Mr. Bender. The findings that he dictates during this examination are automatically transcribed and entered in the patient record.

Medical Care Planning and Order Entry

Dr. White then selects the clinical guideline "suspected stenosis" and, based on the diagnoses of the patient, automatically gets a proposal for a treatment plan for the next days. Based on this treatment plan, Dr. White confirms the proposed administration of heparin from the standard spectrum of therapies that, in conjunction with the regular checking of coagulation factors, shall be carried out. He also orders medications to treat the hypertension of the patient. Each of his medication orders is automatically checked for errors such as overdosing, drug allergy or drug–drug interaction that may harm the patient. In case of errors, the physician gets an alert message and a proposal for an alternative medication.

In addition, Dr. White confirms and finalizes proposed orders for a color duplex sonographic examination for the assessment of the stenosis, a cranial computed tomography for exclusion of infarction, and a blood test to analyze blood lipid concentration and coagulation factors.

During the ward round, Dr. White uses a tablet computer to instruct that, as a nursing procedure, regular blood pressure measurements have to be taken, based on the information he has on hand regarding the patient's hypertension. He also orders a low-salt and diabetic diet for Mr. Bender.

The nurse, Mrs. Weber, documents Mr. Bender's meal request. The selection that is available for him is restricted as a result of the diet that has been ordered, and the choice of food is automatically adapted to the requirements of diabetes and hypertension.

Execution of Diagnostic, Therapeutic, and Nursing Procedures

In the morning, Mrs. Weber prepares Mr. Bender's medication based on the medication orders documented by the physician. She uses a drug-dispensing machine that automatically prepares the drugs for Mr. Bender. To assure that the drugs are given to the correct patient, she scans the barcodes of the drugs as well as the wristband of Mr. Bender before giving him his medication.

Mrs. Weber reviews the series of further measures that have been ordered by the physician for her patient. She activates a reminding function to make sure that she does not forget any of the regular blood pressure measurements that have been ordered.

The nurse prepares the catheter and the syringe for heparinization. Dr. White inserts the catheter to which he connects the automatic syringe containing the prescribed dose.

During the period for which the checking of coagulation factors has been ordered, a request for a blood test is automatically prepared every day and put into the worklist of the responsible nurse, Mrs. Weber. She then takes the blood sample, adds a patient label that she automatically gets printed, and then sends the blood sample to the laboratory.

Mrs. Weber also orders color duplex sonographic and CCT examinations as requested by the physician. On this occasion, she uses the automatic scheduling function to set up a date for each examination. Those dates are automatically documented in the patient record, sent to the transportation unit to organize the transport of the patient, and also made available to the patient for information. In addition, Mrs. Weber can easily review the status of each order (ordered, scheduled, in progress, report being written, finalized).

Review of Findings

As soon as the results of the orders (lab report, CT report, CT images) are available, an automatic note is put in the patient record to inform the treating physician. Findings not yet reviewed are highlighted. The laboratory results can be displayed in various ways, for example, by displaying the time line of selected lab parameters. Pathologic values are highlighted. The CT report and the CT images, as well as results of earlier examinations, can be displayed side by side. As far as the CT result is concerned, Dr. White can view a reference x-ray image selected by the radiologist.

Decision Making

After having reviewed all findings, Dr. White decides that the stenosis should be removed by vascular surgery. For support in his decision-making process, he can electronically consult recommendations provided based on the clinical data of the patient and most recent evidence-based clinical guidelines.

Stress and excitement about the forthcoming procedure leads to an increase in Mr. Bender's blood pressure, a circumstance realized by Dr. White during his ward round from the profile of blood pressure values automatically shown on his mobile tool. He therefore orders an increase in the dose of the antihypertensive drug. This change in medication is recorded and will be taken into account during the next dispensing of medicine.

Organization and Scheduling of Patient Treatment

For scheduling of the surgical procedure, Dr. White contacts the Department for Vascular Surgery of the PMC and discusses Mr. Bender's case with the surgeon, Dr. Sunny, on the basis of all information contained in the EPR. They both agree on a date for the procedure. Dr. Sunny uses the resource management functions to make the reservations for a bed and OR. Dr. White orders, as an administrative measure, the transfer of Mr. Bender on the agreed date.

Transfer to Another Department

On the date of transfer, Dr. White again reviews both Mr. Bender's therapy and the state of health. He can easily limit the presentation to those values most relevant for this case, which are coagulation factors, blood pressure, and diabetes control.

During his ward rounds, Dr. White confirms the transfer scheduled for that day. Thereafter, all the services provided to the patient are ceased and documented for billing purposes. A transfer service is requested for taking him to the department performing further treatment.

The nurse automatically generates a final nursing report, based on the documented data, which she completes and signs, using her health care professional card for authentication.

The final nursing report, the epicrisis (on the treatment given by then), and other essential documents are automatically made available to the Department for Vascular Surgery.

Discharge from Hospital and Aftercare

As the procedure engendered no complications, Mr. Bender remains in the surgical department for a few more days of observation. The physician in the neurology department is automatically informed about the outcome of the operation and the progress of recovery.

Mr. Bender is discharged from the PMC a short time later. Before leaving the hospital, Mr. Bender calls on the neurology department where the dates for postoperative care are set up. A (standard) plan for aftercare is proposed to Dr. White which he, together with Mr. Bender, adapts to the patient's requirements and desires. To counteract further progression of the atherosclerosis which caused the arterial stenosis, Mr. Bender enters a rehabilitation exercise training program funded by his insurance company. He is also equipped with a small wearable sensor device that monitors his daily physical activity level and provides individualized feedback and training recommendations.

After completing the measures requested for Mr. Bender and documentation of the results, Dr. White dictates a discharge report that is automatically transcribed. He completes the document and electronically signs it. The report is then transmitted to his senior physician for approval. The final discharge report is automatically transmitted to Dr. Healthy, the referring physician.

All of the information required for billing is automatically extracted from the documented patient data. An invoice of the services supplied is automatically sent to the insurance company.

After completion of the case, the EPR is archived in electronic form. Should Mr. Bender be readmitted to the PMC for treatment at a future time, this archived information is immediately available.

6.9 Summarizing Exercises

6.9.1 Hospital Functions and Processes

Look at the process presented in example 6.8.1. Match the different steps of the patient's stay at PMC with the hospital functions presented in Sect. 6.3.

6.9.2 Application Components and Hospital Functions

Look at the process presented in example 6.8.1. What application components of Sect. 6.4 do you suggest to support the functions you found in exercise 6.9.1?

6.9.3 Multiprofessional Treatment Teams

Look at the process presented in example 6.8.1. Describe the different health care professionals who are involved in *patient care*. What are their roles in the multiprofessional treatment team? Which health care professional groups are also important for *patient care* but not explicitly mentioned in the process description?

6.9.4 Information Needs of Different Health Care Professionals

Look at the process presented in example 6.8.1. What are the most important information needs of the different health care professionals involved? Use the entity types as introduced in Sect. 6.2 to describe the needs.

6.9.5 HIS Architectures

Look at the different architectures on the logical and physical tool layers described in Sects. 6.5.1 and 6.7.1. Which architectures at the logical tool layer are typically matched to which architectures at the physical tool layer? Discuss your findings.

6.9.6 Communication Server

Imagine that you want to model the information system's architecture of a given hospital. You expect that there may be a communication server that organizes the communication between most of the computer-based application components.

- How can you find out whether there is a communication server in the given HIS? Is a site visit on various wards useful to find a communication server?
- Where will you model the communication server in your HIS model: at the domain layer, at the logical tool layer, or at the physical tool layer? Explain your answer.
- What can happen when you overlook a communication server? How will your model change? Which (wrong) communication pattern would you model?

6.9.7 Anatomy and Physiology of Information Processing

If the architecture of a HIS can be compared to the anatomy of information processing, what could the physiology of information processing be? It may help to look up the terms in an encyclopedia.

6.10 Summary

The architecture of a HIS can be described using three interconnected layers.

At the domain layer we describe the information to be processed in a hospital as entity types. There are entity types related to *patient care*, administration and management, and resources. These entity types are interpreted and updated by hospital functions. Since the HIS comprises all areas of a hospital, these functions do not deal only with *patient care* but also with *supply and disposal management*, *hospital administration*, *hospital management*, and *research and education*.

The logical tool layer presents the application components used to support the functions and to store the data of the entity types. Typically there are a lot of different computer-based application components in a hospital such as a *patient administration system*, a *RIS*, and a *LIS*. Sometimes some of them are integrated to a so-called *CIS*. All these application components form the basis of an EPR. But it shall not be forgotten that there are still non-computer-based application components in hospitals.

A major challenge for information management is to integrate the different application components. Here, integrity as well as different types of integration needs to be achieved. Different standards such as HL7 or DICOM as well as integration technologies such as middleware can reduce integration efforts. The architectures of a HIS can be described based on the number of databases, the number of application components, the number of software products, and the used communication patterns.

The physical data processing systems needed to install the application components on are described at the physical tool layer. It turns out that this layer is not very specific for hospitals, since servers, personal computers, and networks are also used in other industries. But again non-computer-based systems have to be taken into account at this layer. Availability, stability, and performance of the overall computer-based part of the information system significantly depend on a well-organized computing center.

7 Specific Aspects for Architectures of Transinstitutional Health Information Systems

7.1 Introduction

Although this book focuses on hospital information systems, it is important to understand that institutional information systems, in general, and hospital information systems, in particular, are parts of larger, cross-linked systems.

Given the demographic change in most countries we can assume that in future the number of chronically ill patients will increase. The medical treatment of chronic diseases typically involves many different actors over a long period of time, including hospitals, medical practitioners, specialists of different medical fields, nurses of home care services and even relatives. Since relevant information should be available whenever and wherever it is needed, we need to understand and design transinstitutional information systems (see Sect. 4.3) that efficiently support transinstitutional care processes, that is, continuity of care.

Hospitals are the most complex institutions in health care and the architectures presented for their information systems are valid also for transinstitutional health information systems. However, with the extension of our perspective beyond one institution, the complexity raises and the challenges for health information systems (see Sect. 4.5) are even intensified.

In this chapter, we first discuss the influences of these challenges to the three layers of transinstitutional health information systems. Since electronic health records (EHRs) are the major concern of these systems, we will then introduce different strategies on how to organize responsibility for these records in this highly distributed environment.

After reading this chapter, you should be able to answer the following questions:

- How do architectures of transinstitutional health information systems differ from those of hospital information systems?
- What additional challenges do we have to cope with?
- Which strategies are appropriate for maintaining electronic health records in a transinstitutional health information system?

A. Winter et al., *Health Information Systems*,
DOI: 10.1007/978-1-84996-441-8_7,

7.2 Domain Layer

Since a transinstitutional health information system can be considered as the entirety of all institutional information systems of a health care network (see Sect. 4.3), it has to support all the enterprise functions to be performed in the member institutions. If hospitals are part of this health care network, at least the hospital functions introduced in Sect. 6.3 have to be supported and data about the entity types in Sect. 6.2 have to be stored, communicated, and processed.

But in the context of transinstitutional collaboration of health care providers, further specific aspects have to be considered. Additional enterprise functions and entity types have to be taken into account, if health insurances and governmental authorities are members of a transinstitutional health information system.

7.2.1 Specific Aspects for Hospital Functions

7.2.1.1 Patient Admission

As mentioned in Sect. 6.3.1.1 *patient admission*, among others, aims at correctly identifying each patient, and assigning a unique patient and case identifier (Fig. 7.1).

Considering a single health care institution, for example, a hospital, a *patient* will receive his or her PIN during the first visit to the hospital. This PIN has to be used in all parts of the hospital for the identification of the patient. Since PIN and CIN (case identification number) are assigned during *patient admission*, only one *admission* has to be performed and only one PIN has to be assigned to the patient during his or her visit. This works well, if there is exactly one dedicated application component supporting *patient admission*, namely, the hospital's *patient administration system* with its master patient index (MPI).

In transinstitutional health information systems the situation turns out to be more complicated. Object identity (see Sect. 6.5.2.1) can be guaranteed only if a patient will receive his or her PIN during the first visit to one of the health care network's institutions. Again this PIN has to be used in all parts of the health care network for the identification of the patient and will be used during future visits regardless of the visited institution. This could simply be realized by using exactly one dedicated *patient administration system* throughout the network. In many countries however, nationwide PINs have been or will be introduced shortly. Usually, smart cards are used to bear these PINs. The PINs can be used during *patient admission* instead of self-generated PINs and every institution can use its own *patient administration system* for *patient admission*, if preferred. If both solutions are not available, one master patient index for this transinstitutional health information system should be used; see Sect. 7.3.1 for more details

Regardless the technology used, data recorded at *patient admission* and especially PIN and CIN have to be made available to all enterprise functions needing them throughout the transinstitutional health information system.

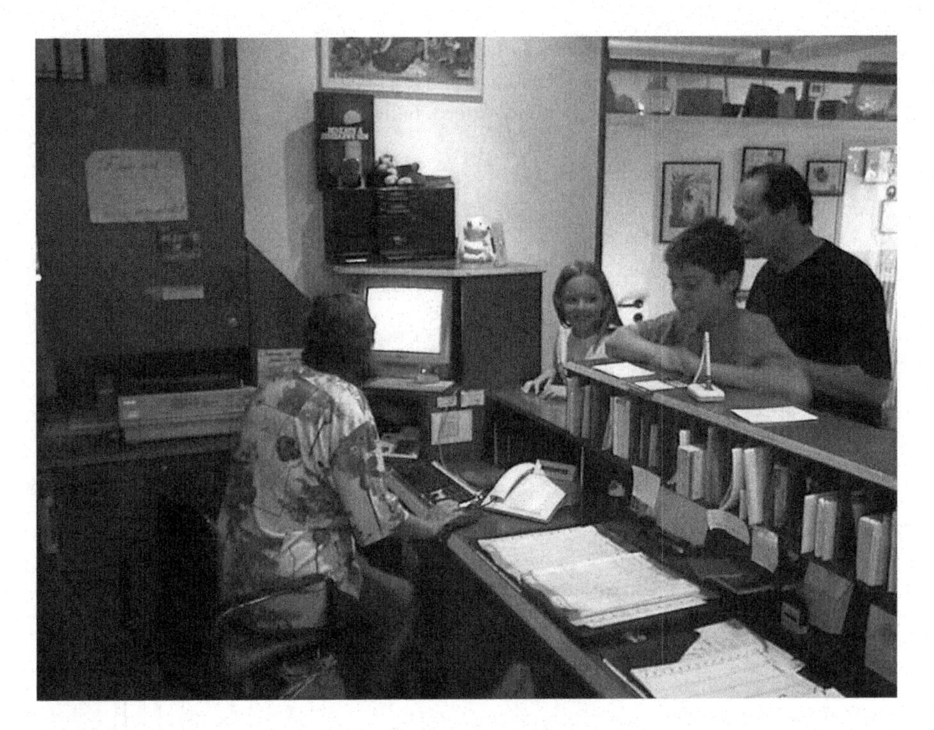

Fig. 7.1 *Patient admission* in the office of a general practitioner

7.2.1.2
Decision Making, Planning, and Organization of Patient Treatment

Realizing that a hospital is part of a health care network provides new opportunities for better and more efficient *decision making, planning and organization of patient treatment*, and thus new chances for continuous and better care.

Quality of decisions on diagnoses and appropriate therapies can be improved by incorporating experts in other organizations into the decision process. Teleconsultations using means for video conferencing and exchange of patient's documents are more and more used. Transfer of rights to access to the patient's record in parallel to the patient's path from one care provider to the next and of course their ability to access the records are prerequisites for this kind of joined decision making.

7.2.1.3
Execution of Diagnostic and Therapeutic Procedures

In health care networks, not only can expertise in decision making be shared, but resources for diagnostic and therapeutic procedures are also shareable.

For example, a radiology expert in one hospital may supervise modalities at other hospitals as well and be in charge of radiological diagnostics. She or he may do this by using teleradiology equipment for digital transmission of image, finding, and worklist data.

A pathologist in one hospital may examine tissue in other hospitals using telemicroscopy technology. A small rural hospital may transport patients to the operation room of a second hospital for some specialized surgical procedures but will care for recovery and rehabilitation afterward.

7.2.2 Additional Enterprise Functions

As mentioned before, not only hospitals and other health care providers may be part of a health care network and thus incorporated within one transinstitutional health information system. Additional institutions may be health insurances and governmental authorities for example. Besides their general administration functions, they have to perform specific enterprise functions.

A health insurance company, for example, has to develop insurance plans, to advise its clients, to receive and pay bills from hospitals and practitioners. More specifically they have to take responsibility for disease management. That is to support their clients – the patients – in finding a path, which is best suited for her or his special health care needs. Performing functions like this, the insurance company needs a lot of data from attached hospitals. This holds not only for entity types related to administration and management, but also for those related to *patient care* (see Sect. 6.2). Additionally, these hospitals need respective data from the insurance companies.

Governmental authorities, for example, have to care for the health care system as a whole. Hence they take responsibility for the availability of health care providers of different kind at any place in a region. They need data about incidence and prevalence of diseases in order to plan for care resources meeting the needs of the people. In case of disasters they have to coordinate help for the people involved. Furthermore they observe epidemiologic development of diseases in order to detect or better to prevent epidemics and pandemics. Diagnoses are therefore needed from any health care provider across all relevant health care networks.

7.3 Logical Tool Layer

The logical tool layer of a transinstitutional health information system consists of the application components of all involved institutional information systems.

7.3.1 Integration of Application Components

The challenge of data redundancy is reinforced in a network of institutions. In different institutional types, such as rehabilitation centers, ambulatory care providers or private practices, different "best-of-breed" solutions have been used in the past and lots of vendors can be found in the markets. Hence, all transinstitutional HIS do have (DB^n, AC^n, V^n) architectures.

Standards for integration, such as HL7, DICOM, and EDIFACT (see Sect. 6.5.4), become even more important against this background. Integration needs communication links between the respective application components. Of course the standards introduced in Sect. 6.5.4 and the integration technologies of Sect. 6.5.5 can be applied for transinstitutional HIS as well.

Especially important in this context is the IHE Technical Framework (see Sect. 6.5.4.6). The IHE Cross-Enterprise Document Sharing (XDS) Integration Profile focuses on providing standard-based specifications for transinstitutional sharing of medical documents. The content of the documents is not limited to textual information but also comprises images and coded clinical information. In IHE XDS, a document repository is responsible for storing the documents in a secure, reliable and consistent way and responds to retrieval requests that can be submitted by any connected institution. In the document registry, information about these documents is stored so that they can be found and selected irrespective of the repositories where they are physically stored. The idea of the IHE Patient Demographics Query (PDG) Integration Profile is to implement a central patient information server that is queried by other application components and retrieves the patient's demographic and visit information. The query can be based on the partial or complete patient name, a patient ID, date of birth, age range, or bed ID.

In many areas standardization initiatives are either at the beginning or heavily influenced by local governance. Hence, standards are not always scalable to an international scale. Additionally, the following two problems are reinforced in transinstitutional information systems:

- Encryption: Those messages transferred during communication in the context of notifications, teleconsultations, or teleconferences, and for the global use of patient records, have to be protected from unauthorized third party access. Encryption procedures based on public key infrastructures exist for these cases. They are sufficiently secure and can be obtained as commercial encryption software. A problem in this case, however, is the correct identification of the respective communication partner. A remedy in this case could be electronic identification. In health care, the so-called health care professional card (HPC) is currently being tried out, which uniquely identifies a specific health care professional. In Germany, a so-called Telematic Infrastructure is currently under construction, which combines such HPC with smart cards for patients, called electronic health cards. Both elements shall enable secure data interchange in health care.
- Patient identification: We have already determined that patient-based communication within a hospital is only possible when a patient is identified uniquely by his or her PIN. The proper assignment of a PIN to patients within a transinstitutional health information system is only possible if there is only one application component used for *admission* in the health care network or if all application components that are used for *admission* have access to one central master patient index (MPI). In case of MPI, manually or semiautomatically found relationships of PINs from different institutions are saved in one network MPI and are made available to all member institutions. IHE PDG may be used to query the MPI.

- This difficult process of patient identification is a huge barrier for the establishment of a regional or even national patient health record. As an interim solution for notifications, teleconsultations, and teleconferences, patient identification can also be achieved through the personal agreement of the involved parties.

In transinstitutional information systems, communication links between application components in different organizations are means for providing access to distributed patient data. Beside this, communication also enables the direct usage of a hospital's application component at a remote site. The use of portals, as discussed in Sect. 6.5.5.3, enables a physician at his own practice to easily and cost-effectively read and update medical data in an electronic patient record of a hospital. For example, this record may include the images that are managed in the hospital's radiology department. But note that this (simple) way of access integration will expect doctors to use different portals for every hospital they are in contact with. This might reduce acceptance in a network of positively collaborating institutions.

Since institutions used to work as a "closed world" from *patient admission* to *discharge and transfer* (see Sect. 6.3.1) many functions are carried out redundantly in transinstitutional health information systems leading to functional redundancy (see Sects. 5.3.2.4, 8.5.4, 8.7.4). Well-organized patient identification and encrypted communication may open potential for sharing application components and to give up components turning out to be redundant in the context of the transinstitutional health information system. Two hospitals in a network may, for example, share one *patient administration system* or *RIS* or *PACS* instead of operating one at each site.

Unfortunately, computer-based application components supporting transinstitutional data exchange are still exceptional. This poor transinstitutional integration results in the challenge of transcription because the documents have to be printed out, sent by mail, and retyped or scanned.

Electronic documents must contain structured information in order to be processed automatically. Often, the semantics differ between institutions which results in the challenge of terminology and thus leading to the need for semantic integration. This challenge is picked up by the openEHR initiative[1]. OpenEHR defines onotologies and provides open source software tools for maintaining and managing patient-centric electronic health records (compare Sect. 7.3.2.2). It contains clinical models of content and processes, which are known as archetypes.

7.3.2 Strategies for Electronic Health Record Systems

Besides the intensified integrational challenges transinstitutional information systems have to cope with specific problems regarding the ownership and organization of the electronic health record (EHR). As discussed above transinstitutional health information systems are characterized by (DB^n, AC^n, V^n) architectures and thus are very heterogeneous and highly

[1]http://www.openehr.org

redundant. One important question is how an EHR can be organized in a way that the complete set of relevant patient data is available whenever and wherever it is needed. To achieve this goal the responsibility for completeness and availability could be assigned to one actor in the health care system. In the following section, different strategies[2] of transinstitutional health information systems are discussed that are distinguished by the responsible role. Note, that the introduced strategies may appear combined in reality.

7.3.2.1 The Provider-Centric Strategy

In the provider-centric strategy the medical records are kept by the institution that created them and are made available to other organizations on request. This model supports a process-oriented health care approach, which is central to such organizational types as managed care, integrated delivery systems, and disease management programs. However, this model has also some disadvantages. First, the information about a patient remains dispersed between different institutions. The EHR can only be assembled virtually and is likely to be incomplete, for example, if one institution that holds information about a patient is not available. Second, the participating institutions have to agree on semantic standards in order to achieve semantic integration (see Sect. 6.5.3.2). Since semantics is often heavily influenced by historically grown and institution-specific documentation processes, transinstitutional alignment of semantics causes huge efforts. Third, the provider-centric strategy does not neutralize the challenge of competition between the institutions on the one hand and the need to cooperate in order to establish a complete EHR on the other hand (see Sect. 10).

7.3.2.2 The Patient-Centric Strategy

A second strategy that is implemented today is the patient-centric strategy. In this strategy, the patient is perceived as the primary owner of his data. A patient can set up a record on an internet portal or on other appropriate media. The record is filled by the patient and practitioners or other physicians may support him or her. The patient decides which information should be included and which persons can access the record. This type of patient-owned electronic record is also called Personal Health Record (PHR). The disadvantages of this model are the supposed incompleteness of the record, the perception of the record by health workers as "unprofessional," as well as the unsolved problem of accessing data in emergency situations. In order to compensate for these disadvantages, the patient-centric strategy is often combined with the provider-centric strategy, that is, a health care provider manages the PHR on behalf of the patient.

---

[2]The presented strategies of EHRs are based on: Shabo A. A Global Socio-economic-medico-legal Model for the Sustainability of Longitudinal Electronic Health Records. Part1: Methods of Information in Medicine 45(3):240–245. Part 2: Methods of Information in Medicine 2006;45(5): 498–505.

7.3.2.3 The Regional- or National-Centric Strategy

In the so-called regional- or national-centric strategy, the EHR is maintained centrally by a public institution. This can be on a regional or nationwide level. Although this strategy has some advantages that are based on the legal authority of public services, the centralized operation might lead to inefficiency. Second, many ethical questions regarding the problem of "Orwellization" remain unsolved.

7.3.2.4 The Strategy of Independent Health Banks

Finally, the non-centric strategy of "independent health banks" can be identified, although this model has not been implemented yet. This strategy stands out, because it is not centered on the mentioned stakeholders in health care. Comparable to normal banks, there are lots of independent health banks being responsible for managing lifetime EHRs without having any control over other parties. Since these banks are not part of the health care system, they remain neutral. In health care institutions, there would be no need to maintain archives of medical records. This is similar to taking money to the most trusted bank instead of keeping it in one's own safe. This bank will also take care, that only authorized parties will get (part of) the money.

7.4 Physical Tool Layer

At the physical tool layer a transinstitutional health information system depends on a trustworthy and secure communication network. Installing and operating dedicated hardware and, especially, exclusively used wires, cables, or radio-relay links to connect institutions of a health care network could provide excellent potential for high performance and protection from illegal intrusion. But since these are quite expensive solutions, usually the public infrastructure of the Internet is used.

Providing trustworthiness and security while using Internet-based communication networks demands particular endeavors. An exclusively used communication network can be simulated by virtual private networks (VPN), which are based on encryption technologies. But in most cases communication is needed not only to partners being connected by the VPN but also to others. Therefore, institutions have to install so-called firewall hardware to monitor and check data exchange between inside and outside the institution's information system. Thus an internal intranet is built, which is clearly separated from the Internet. Servers hosting data, which shall be easily accessed by other institutions and do not represent sensitive information, can be placed outside the intranet; thus they form a so-called demilitarized zone. Obviously installation and operation of such technologies require considerable technical know-how. In case of small institutions, for example, medical practices, particular support is needed. If in doubt it may be necessary to disconnect computers connected to the Internet physically from those storing sensitive data.

7.5 Examples

7.5.1 "Gesundheitsnetz Tirol (GNT)": The Tyrolean Health Care Network

7.5.1.1 Background and Overall Functionality

The state of Tyrol is located in the western part of Austria, with an alpine topography. Twelve hospitals all over the state including the University Hospital of Innsbruck and about 1,500 general practitioners or outpatient units provide medical care for about 700,000 citizens. In 2008, the "Gesundheitsnetz Tirol (GNT)" (Tyrolean Health Care Network) project – was started, driven by the eHealth Action Plan of the European Union[3] and the Austrian e-Health Initiative.[4]

Basically, the GNT network allows health care institutions (and later also patients) to share documents (such as discharge summaries, nursing summaries, laboratory findings, radiologic findings) as well as radiological images. The document formats conform to the CDA Level 1 standard (XML with structured header information and with an embedded PDF/A document). Participating organizations and professionals can make documents available within the GNT. Other organizations and professionals can search for documents or images and retrieve them. All available documents and images are indexed in a dedicated application component, called registry which is using standardized metadata (e.g., metadata describing author and type of document).

7.5.1.2 System Architecture and Workflows

The GNT network is basically an IHE XDS Affinity Domain,[5] meaning that each hospital keeps its own document or image repository (provider-centric strategy). The distributed, local application components are linked together by the following set of central application components, allowing the localization and the access of the distributed data:

- The master patient index (conform to the IHE PDQ integration profiles)
- The XDS document registry (conform to the IHE XDS integration profile)

[3]http://www.good-ehealth.org/about/ehealth_action_plan.php
[4]http://ehi.adv.at
[5]http://www.ihe.net/IT_infra/committees/index.cfm

- An audit record repository (for logging every transaction in this network)
- A gateway for communication with other IHE XDS Affinity Domains in Austria

The software products are designed as modular components using web service technology. The product family is called "sense® – smart eHealth solutions."[6] Figure 7.2 shows an illustration of the architecture.

To make a document or image (e.g., based on DICOM) available within the GNT, the document is automatically submitted from the *clinical information system* of a participating organization (called "document source") to the Source Adaptor which triggers the following IHE Transactions (see Fig. 7.2, dark-gray numbers):

1. Adding patient identification to the master patient index (PIX/PDQ) (using several identification characteristics and sophisticated matching algorithms)
2. Submitting the document to the own institutional application component, where the document will be stored (XDS document repository)
3. Submitting metadata to the XDS document registry (to allow later search and retrieval of the document)

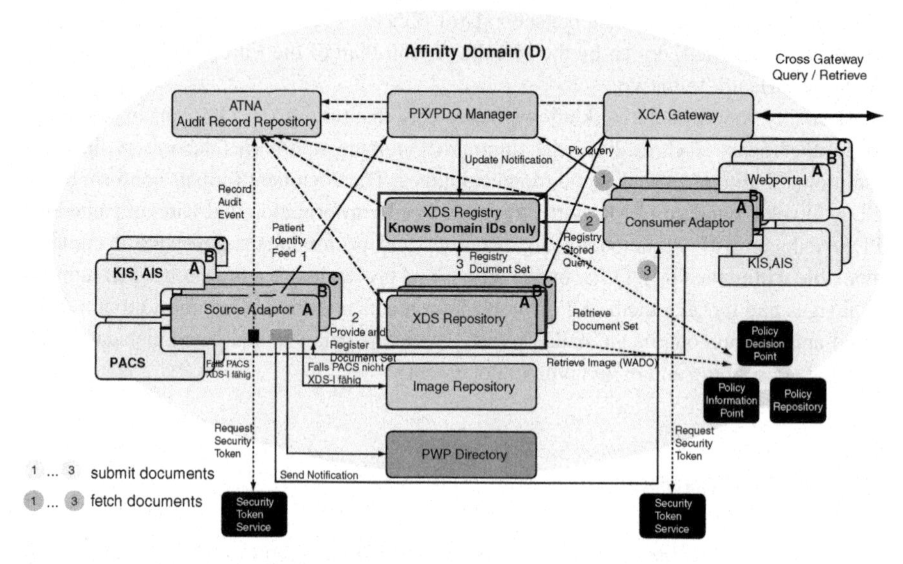

Fig. 7.2 Overview of sense Architecture based on several IHE Integration Profiles. Actors are depicted as boxes and transactions as lines

After this, the submitted document is available within the GNT for other organizations. To retrieve a document, a *clinical information system* uses the Consumer Adaptor which triggers the following IHE Transactions (cf. Fig. 7.2, light-gray numbers):

[6]http://www.ith-icoserve.com/

1. Obtaining patient identification from the master patient index
2. Querying the XDS document registry (using metadata to identify relevant documents)
3. Retrieving the document from one of the local XDS document repositories

Sharing of patient data requires a sophisticated security concept reaching from authenticated and encrypted data exchange to an advanced authorization framework, which – in future – should empower the patient to decide who may access his/her health information.

7.5.1.3 Important Lessons Learned

Prior and during the implementation, a couple of important lessons have been learned, which are of interest to other similar projects:

- The financing and initiation of projects related to eHealth is one of the most difficult tasks. The benefits are mostly realized for public economics, but less for business economics. Consequently, health care institutions are often not willing to invest in such solutions. In addition, health care professionals do not care primarily for overall savings, but try to identify benefits for their personal work. However, these personal benefits of eHealth infrastructures or applications for the individual professional are difficult to be verified. Therefore it is difficult to create acceptance amongst health professionals.
- At the beginning, several independent Tyrolean health care organizations jointly requested a standardized eHealth infrastructure to improve their cooperation. This was the start of the Tyrolean eHealth initiatives. A Tyrolean working group ("ARGE GNT") for common coordination, consisting of all participating health care institutions (CEOs/CIOs of hospitals), was established in 2008, and has successfully served as moderator and initiator of eHealth projects since then.
- The introduction of standards for medical document formats and for metadata was one of the most labor intensive steps. With currently available technology such as the Clinical Document Architecture (CDA), a very fine-grained structure can be applied to clinical data. Structuring of clinical data influences the workflow of data capturing. This is an organizational rather than a technical challenge, as health professionals must be motivated to switch from flexible free text to a rigid framework for data capturing.
- Austrian data protection regulations require a 2-level access control mechanism. The first level requires that a current treatment relationship exists between physician and patient. This is verified by the so-called e-card (the Austrian health insurance card) that is needed to access data in the GNT. The second level requires that the patient gives his/her explicit consent to document retrieval from the GNT. In the consent document, the patient can restrict access for institutions, departments, document type, and time range (e.g., just allowing the health care professional to search for laboratory findings). At the moment, level 2 restrictions are not supported technically, instead physicians querying for documents have to follow the patient's restrictions when setting search criteria in the GNT

user interface. In order to assure that these restrictions are actually applied, all queries are logged, and health care professionals have to agree to periodic inspections of consent documents to prove that their GNT queries match the written consent of the patient.
- Early usability evaluation revealed that a seamless integration of the GNT application in the clinical information system or the GP system is vital for end-user acceptance. A web portal solution is only the second-best choice due to limited data integration and to transcription.
- Operating the GNT in a dedicated physical network, strictly separated from the Internet, improves security, and, therewith, also end-user acceptance.

7.5.2 Veterans Health Information Systems and Technology Architecture (VISTA)[7]

The VISTA system from the Department of Veterans Affairs, USA (VA) is likely one of the largest transinstitutional health information systems in the world. Its advantage has been nicely demonstrated a few years ago when New Orleans experienced the Kathrina disaster and many people got displaced. The VA system was the only that was able to care for their patients and had all information available at other places.[8]

Since 1999, the VA's 155 hospitals, 881 clinics, 135 nursing homes, and 45 rehabilitation centers in the USA have been linked by a so-called universal medical records network. It allows any authorized person to look at 5.3 million patients' records – everything from a nurse's note written during a hospital stay, to the result of a blood test drawn at a clinic visit, to the moving-picture film of a coronary angiogram done in a cardiology lab.

VISTA is built on a client-server architecture, which ties together workstations and personal computers with graphical user interfaces at Veterans Health Administration (VHA) facilities, as well as software developed by local medical facility staff. VISTA also includes the links that allow commercial off-the-shelf software and products to be used with existing and future technologies. VISTA uses standard coding for much of its data, including ICD-9 and LOINC, and other universal and standards-based coding methodologies.

7.5.3 The Hypergenes Biomedical Information Infrastructure[9, 10]

Health information systems as discussed so far are primarily supporting patient care. But the care related data they store are also needed for clinical research. Related research projects such as clinical trials are often organized multicentric, that is, taking patient data out of many health care institutions into account. Hence, we again come to transinstitutional information systems.

For research purposes the semantic meaning of gathered data has to be known exactly. But, unfortunately, institutional HIS typically contain data and knowledge related to a

[7] http://www4.va.gov/VISTA_MONOGRAPH/
[8] By courtesy of Dominik Aronsky.
[9] http://www.hypergenes.eu/
[10] By courtesy of Amnon Shabo.

specific health domain with idiosyncratic semantics. As such they constitute silos of information and data as well as semantic integration are hard to achieve. *Data warehouses* (see Sect. 6.4.12) are established in an attempt to accomplish such integration and support patient-centric care as well as secondary use of the data such as analysis of aggregated data in the context of clinical research, quality assurance, operational systems optimization, patient safety, and public health. In health care, the emerging concept of personalized care involves taking into account the clinical, environmental, and genetic makeup of the individual. To that end, a *data warehouse* may serve as a main information source for putting together data of patient electronic health records (EHR) in a health care network where consistent and explicit semantics is crucial for machines to reason about the records.

The IBM Haifa Research Lab (HRL) developed a Biomedical Information Infrastructure (BII) as a transinstitutional HIS aiming at the integration of data from the various data sets owned by the partners of the Hypergenes network. The main goal of the Hypergenes project is to integrate the clinical, environmental, and genomics data in order to develop a comprehensive disease model for the essential hypertension chronic disease.

One of the main challenges of data warehousing within biomedical information systems is to achieve semantic integration between its various stakeholders as well as other interested parties. Promoting the adoption of worldwide accepted information standards along with common terminologies is the right path to achieve that. To that end, the HL7 Reference Information Model (RIM) has been used as the underlying model for semantic warehousing aimed at establishing integrity and consistency across a vast and growing number of health domains such as laboratory, clinical health record data, problem- and goal-oriented care, public health, and clinical research. The RIM-based data warehouse provides (1) the means for integration of data and knowledge gathered from disparate and diverse data sources, (2) a mixture of XML and relational schemas, and (3) a uniform abstract access and query capability serving both health care and clinical research users.

Through the use of templates, which are sets of constraints on RIM-based standards, semantic integration was facilitated which would be harder to achieve if only generic standards in use cases with unique requirements would have been used. The semantic data warehousing facilitates the continuum of knowledge, information, and data to enable an infrastructure for analysis tools, decision support application components, clinical data exchange, and clinical application components.

7.5.4 The National Health Information System in Korea[11, 12]

The Korean Ministry of Health and Welfare (MOHW) has been implementing the National health information system (NHIS) as a computer-supported transinstitutional HIS with focus on public health centers since 1995. Unlike other Asian and European countries, public health sector is much weaker than the private health sector. Only 11% of health institutions belong to the public sector. MOHW has introduced NHIS in 1995 based on the

[11] Young Moon Chae, Hae Ja Lee, Kyung Won Cho, Joo Hee Park. Systems analysis and design in Health care, Sumoonsa Publishing Co. Korea, 2010.
[12] By courtesy of Young Moon Chae.

client-server architecture. As a result, all public health institutions (250 health centers, 1,200 health subcenters, and 2,000 health posts) have been implementing institutional computer-based HIS since then.

While the computer-based HIS have helped to reduce workloads of health workers by reducing paper works and improved accuracy and timeliness of health statistics at health centers, there were problems with maintenance of hardware and software for the health centers located in the remote areas and with information sharing among health centers and MOHW. Accordingly, MOHW has decided to convert the client-server based systems in 2005 to the web-based ASP (Application Service Provider) system which means that one central server covers the entire health institutions by its services (compare Sect. 6.5.5.3). In addition, MOHW developed the National Standards for health information and Electronic Health Record (EHR) for community residents.

Hospitals use NHIS to send EHR extracts to health centers for a follow-up care of the discharged patients. And health centers and hospitals also use NHIS to refer their patients to other hospitals. Such information sharing helps reducing duplicate tests and improves continuous care for patients.

When community residents register their information to EHR at a hospital or health center, hospital or health center staffs use it to refer him or her to other health institutions, to provide public health services (e.g., tuberculosis program, health screen, etc.), and to process insurance claims. NHIS is also used by the National Health Insurance Corporation for insurance claim review and by other health institutes for producing various health statistics on cancer, tuberculosis, infectious diseases, etc. Once health center staff has completed the monthly reports on activities, they are sent to MOHW via NHIS for review and decision making. Systems analysts at the National Health Information Center use them for analyzing overall operation, updating EHR, and validating it for consistency with standards and code.

7.6 Exercises

7.6.1 Challenges of Transinstitutional Health Information Systems

Look at the challenges, which transinstitutional health information systems are facing, especially at patient identification and integration. Try to argue from your point of view, why these challenges are greater than the same ones within one hospital.

7.6.2 Strategies for Transinstitutional Electronic Health Records

As outlined, different strategies for maintaining EHRs in transinstitutional health information systems are possible. Describe the advantages and disadvantages of the different strategies with your own words. Which strategy would you prefer? Why?

7.6.3
The Term "Electronic Health Record"

Look at examples Sects. 7.5.3 and 7.5.4 and refer to Sect. 4.4. Do you think the term "electronic health record" is used with the same meaning in each case? Could you suggest using a different term as introduced in this book in order to harmonize these examples?

7.6.4
Transinstitutional Information Systems in other Sectors

In which sectors outside of health care can transinstitutional information systems be found? Where do they play a vital role?

7.7
Summary

Since medical treatment often involves many different actors over a long period of time, relevant medical data should be available regardless to the institution where they have been produced.

Transinstitutional information systems feature all enterprise functions to be performed in the member institutions of the respective health care network.

At the domain layer, a unique patient and a case identifier are needed to support the function *patient admission*. These identifiers have to be valid and available throughout the whole health care network. *Decision making, planning, and organization of patient treatment* can be improved by including experts from different institutions. By sharing resources, such as radiological equipment, health care can be organized more efficiently.

The logical tool layer of a transinstitutional health information system consists of the application components of all involved institutional information systems. The challenges for integration are even more complex in comparison to institutional information systems. Additionally, the problems of encryption and patient identification are reinforced.

Different strategies for organizing transinstitutional EHRs can be identified, which may appear in combination. In the provider-centric strategy, the medical records are kept by the institution that created them and are made available to other organizations on request. In the patient-centric strategy, the patient is in authority of his data and controls the content of and access to his record. In the regional- or national-centric strategy, the EHR is maintained by public services. The strategy of independent health banks is characterized by neutral actors that are responsible for managing the EHR, while not being part of the actual health care system.

At the physical tool layer a transinstitutional health information system depends on a trustworthy and secure communication network.

8 Quality of Health Information Systems

8.1 Introduction

The International Organization for Standardization (ISO) defines quality in general as the ability to meet all the expectations of the purchaser of goods or services, or in other words, as the degree to which a set of inherent characteristics fulfills requirements, where "requirements" means need or expectation. Three major approaches to quality assessment are typically distinguished: Quality of structures, quality of processes, and quality of outcome. In the context of health care, the concept of quality of structures applies to the human, physical, and financial resources that are needed to provide medical care (e.g., educational level of staff, availability of medical equipment). Quality of processes describes the quality of activities carried out by care providers (e.g., adherence to professional standards, appropriateness of care). Finally, quality of outcome describes the effects of patient care, that is, the changes in the health status of the patient (e.g., mortality, morbidity, costs). While quality of structures influences quality of processes, quality of processes in turn influences quality of outcome.

Those concepts can be transferred to health information systems. In this context, quality of structures refers to the availability of technical or human resources needed for information processing (e.g., number and availability of computer systems and other ICT, i.e., the HIS infrastructure). Quality of processes deals with the quality of the information processes that are necessary to meet the user's needs. Quality of outcome describes whether the goals of information management have been reached, or, in a broader sense, to what extent, for example, a hospital information system contributes to the goals of the hospital.

These quality concepts for health information systems can help to identify and solve problems concerning information processing. In other words, quality characteristics may help to describe HIS "diseases" (the problems), the corresponding HIS "diagnoses" (identification of the problems), and adequate HIS "therapies" (solution of the problems).

It may not be so difficult to describe what a bad health information system means. But what are the characteristics and features of a good health information system? In this chapter, we introduce some of the most essential ones.

A. Winter et al., *Health Information Systems*,
DOI: 10.1007/978-1-84996-441-8_8, © Springer-Verlag London Limited 2011

After reading this chapter, you should be able to answer the following questions:

- Which facets of quality have to be considered in HIS?
- What are the characteristics of the quality of structures of HIS?
- What are the characteristics of the quality of processes of HIS?
- What are the characteristics of quality of outcome of HIS?
- What does information management have to balance in order to increase the quality of a HIS?
- How can quality of HIS be evaluated?

8.2 Quality of Structures

In the context of health information systems, the quality of structures refers to the technical or human resources needed for information processing. With respect to the technical resources it comprises quality characteristics of data, quality of computer-based application components, quality of physical data processing systems, and quality of architectures.

After reading this chapter, you should be able to answer the following questions:

- What criteria for quality of data exist?
- What criteria for computer-based application components and physical data processing systems exist?
- What criteria for the overall HIS architecture exist?

8.2.1 Quality of Data

Data that are stored and processed in a health information system should adhere to certain criteria for quality of data, such as

- Integrity (see Sect. 6.5.2): Comprises the mere correctness (e.g., correct diagnosis), object identity (e.g., correct identification of every patient by a unique patient identification number), referential integrity (e.g., each clinical report can uniquely be linked to a patient), and consistency of redundant data (e.g., the name of a patient is not spelled differently in different databases).
- Reliability*:* Data are reliable when they are verifiable. For example, there is no element of uncertainty with regard to the clinical findings because they are signed by a responsible doctor.
- Completeness: Describes whether data are sufficiently complete for a given purpose. For example, administrative data on a patient should be complete to allow patient identification.
- Accuracy: Describes that data should be free from mistakes. For example, patient laboratory findings are free of measurement or transcription errors.
- Relevancy: Degree to which data are of relevance for a given situation. For example, no irrelevant data such as "number of grandchildren's friends" are stored.

- Standardization: Data are uniformly recorded and there are clear rules on what data and how the data are recorded and stored. For example, the "nutritional status" shall be recorded for all inpatients using the value set {cachectic, thin, normal weight, overweight, adipose, others}. A high degree of standardization leads to well-structured data and thus fosters their processability (e.g., specific items from lab results can be extracted and processed to produce a 1-week overview of one parameter) whereas low standardization (e.g., when recording data simply as narrative texts) leads to unstructured and hardly processible data. To support standardization, coding systems such as ICD-10 or LOINC may be used.
- Authenticity: Describes that data have an established authorship. For example, the authorship of a discharge report is clear and indisputable.
- Availability: Describes the degree of availability of data. For example, recent lab results are available at the patient's bedside.
- Confidentiality and security: Clinical data should be kept confidential. For example, the diagnoses of a patient are only accessible by the treating health care professionals.

8.2.2 Quality of Computer-Based Application Components and Their Integration

ISO 25000[1] provides six quality characteristics for software, which can be applied to computer-based application components:

- Functionality: Does an application component have the required functionality? For example, a *RIS* contains functionality required for report writing, it provides correct output when searching for a patient, and it guarantees security of stored data.
- Reliability: Can an application component provide defined services for a defined time under certain conditions? For example, a *RIS* has no down-times and is tolerant with regard to wrong data entry by a user.
- Efficiency: How much resources are needed for an application component? For example, a *RIS* has a good response rate of less than 1 s for most of the functionalities.
- Maintainability: How much effort does it take to modify an application component? For example, an upgrade of the *RIS* software can be done quickly and without endangering overall application component's stability.
- Portability: How easily can a software product be transferred to another environment? For example, a *RIS* software follows established market standards with regard to the used database systems and operating systems.
- Usability: Is the application component easy to use? For more details on software ergonomics, see next paragraph.

[1] ISO. International Standard ISO/IEC 25000. Information technology – Software product evaluation – Quality characteristics and guidelines for their use. Geneva: International Organization for Standardization, International Electrotechnical Commission; 2005. http://www.iso.org

Good usability is very important for software used within health care institutions. Health care professionals spend only a smaller amount of their working time at computers and they often have to use various application components for their work. In addition, staff turnover is very high. Therefore, software products should be easy to learn and to use intuitively. This is addressed by ISO 9241[2], which defines specific quality characteristics for software ergonomics. Part 9241-110 of this standard deals with dialogue principles for user interface design:

- Suitability for the task: Does the user interface support the user in fulfilling her or his tasks effectively and efficiently?
- Suitability for learning: Is the user supported to learn and use the user interface?
- Suitability for individualization: Can the user interface be adapted to the tasks and to the individual skills and needs of the user?
- Conformity with user expectations: Is the user interface consistent and adapted to the characteristics of the user (e.g., his knowledge, skills, and expectations)?
- Self-descriptiveness: Is each step of the user interface understandable for the user by providing direct feedback or explanation?
- Controllability: Can the user, after having initiated the first step, control the flow and speed of tasks?
- Error tolerance: Can the task be completed if obviously wrong input is entered by the user, with either little or no effort to correct it?

There exist further quality criteria for software products that are of relevance for health care:

- Adaptability: Can a software product be easily adapted to the working context? For example, functionality of a *RIS* software can be adapted to the particular workflow in a specific radiology.
- Availability: Is the application component made available at all places where it is needed? This means: Is access integration guaranteed (see Sect. 6.5.3.3)? For example, is the *RIS* available in all treatment rooms of the outpatient unit?
- Sustainability: How sustainable is the overall software product? For example, a *RIS* software is still built on the programming language that is not further supported and developed.
- Maturity: Is the software product free of errors? For example, a *RIS* runs after installation immediately and durably without relevant errors.
- Certification: Is the software product certified? For example, the *PACS* software is certified according to the national law for medical devices.
- Standardized interfaces: Whether software products support different standards for integration (such as HL7) as introduced in Sect. 6.5.4 is another important aspect of

[2]ISO. International Standard ISO 9241. Ergonomics requirements for office work with visual display terminals (VDTs). Geneva: International Organization for Standardization, International Electrotechnical Commission; 2006. http://www.iso.org

quality of structures. Otherwise integration in AC^n architectures is hardly reachable in an economically reasonable way.

Since health care professionals are usually confronted with more than one application component and thus with a multiplicity of software products, presentation integration (see Sect. 6.5.3.4) should be guaranteed as well.

A high quality of structures at the logical tool layer of a HIS is achieved, if data, semantic, access, presentation, and functional integration hold as described in Sect. 6.5.3. Contextual and process integration are part of quality of processes (see Sect. 8.3).

8.2.3 Quality of Physical Data Processing Systems

The quality of physical data processing systems can be described by the following major characteristics:

- Availability: For example, computers are available both in the ward office and at the patient's bedside.
- Appropriateness: For example, the bedside computer does not dominate the physician-patient relationship.
- Mobility: For example, mobile tools like PDA and tablet-PC, which are not restricted to a certain working place, are available.
- Multiple usability: For example, a personal computer or a mobile tool can be used for more than one task.
- Flexibility: For example, the mobile tools used on a ward can be updated with new memory easily.
- Maintainability: For example, costs for purchase and support of tools are low.
- Stability and reliability: For example, a server has no down-times.
- Security: For example, the mobile tools support data safety and data security as well as electrical safety. There exist standards such as ISO27001[3] that focus on these safety aspects.
- Harmlessness: For example, a computer in the operating room is designed not to harm the patient or the clinical user by electric hazards.
- Usability: For example, a mobile tool allows easy data entry by a touch screen.
- Standardization: For example, all computer-based physical tools follow predefined standards for technical interfaces (see Sect. 6.7.2 for details).
- Performance: For example, the network bandwidth allows quick data transmission.
- Up-to-dateness: For example, all client computers used are not older than 3 years.
- Certification: For example, the tools used in the intensive care unit are certified according to the national law for medical devices.

---

[3] ISO. International Standard ISO/IEC 27001. Information Security Management – Specification with Guidance for Use. Geneva: International Organization for Standardization, International Electrotechnical Commission; 2005. http://www.iso.org

8.2.4 Quality of the Overall HIS Architecture

HIS architecture should ensure that the different computer-based and non-computer-based information processing tools can be smoothly and efficiently integrated, in order to provide a maximum quality of information processing.

There are some general characteristics that can be used to describe structural quality of a HIS architecture:

- Transparency: The details of the HIS architecture are described in an up-to-date documentation (e.g., using $3LGM^2$ as modeling language).
- Adaptability: In general, the hospital information system should be sufficiently flexible to adapt to the changing needs of the hospital. For example, it should be easy to add new computer-based application components to the information system, and application components should be easily replaceable by other (more advanced) application components. A star-based architecture (CP^1 architecture) with a communication server (see Sect. 6.5.1.3) supports exchanging or adding of new computer-based application components. Additionally, the available bandwidth of the network infrastructure should be easily extendable to match increasing volume of communication.
- Saturation: An architecture is saturated if as many enterprise functions as possible are supported by computer-based tools, and if there are no or only a small number of non-computer-based tools still in use.
- Functional leanness: As described in detail in Sects. 5.3.2.4 and 8.7.4, functional redundancy is an indication for superfluous application components. The opposite, functional leanness (see Sect. 8.5.4), assures that each function is only supported by one application component.
- Controlled redundancy of data: Usually, redundant data storage should be avoided at the logical tool layer. As has been discussed in Sect. 6.5.1.1 (AC^n, V^n) architectures, that is, "best-of-breed" architectures are quite common for HIS. And since (AC^n, V^n) architectures are always of DB^n style, data redundancy is nearly unavoidable in these architectures. Good architectural quality can only be achieved if all measures are taken to provide consistency of redundant data (see Sect. 6.5.2.3). However, at the physical tool layer, data redundancy is often valuable. For example, data may be stored redundantly in different sites in order to avoid data loss in case of systems failures. Or patient data may be available in the electronic patient record, but also as copy in a microfiche archive or in a paper archive. Also, data may be duplicated on different hard discs in a specific database server (e.g., using redundant array of independent discs [RAID] technology), allowing reconstruction of data when a hard disc fails.

8.2.5 Exercises

8.2.5.1 Quality Criteria in $3LGM^2$ Models

Please look at the quality criteria for the HIS structure presented in Sect. 8.2. Which of those criteria can be represented by a $3LGM^2$ model of a HIS? And which cannot?

8.2.5.2
Quality of Computer-Based Application Components

Look at the list of quality criteria for computer-based application components in Sect. 8.2.2. Which one do you find most important? Explain your choice!

8.2.5.3
Usability of Software Products

In Sect. 8.2.2, we argued that "Good software usability is very important for software used within hospitals." Try to find examples (e.g., from the literature) where bad usability had a negative effect on *patient care*! For literature search, you can use PubMed, http://www.pubmed.org and http://iig.umit.at/efmi/badinformatics.htm.

8.2.5.4
Quality of HIS Architectures

Look at the quality criteria for HIS architectures described in Sect. 8.2.4. Now look at the example of a HIS architecture in Fig. 6.53. Which quality criteria may be fulfilled here, which may not, and which cannot be decided based on the details given in the example?

8.2.6
Summary

Criteria for quality of structures of health information systems comprise quality of data, quality of computer-based application components, quality of physical data processing systems, and quality of HIS architecture.

- Quality of data comprises issues such as referential integrity, correctness, integrity, reliability, completeness, accuracy, relevance, processability, authenticity, standardization, availability, confidentiality, security, and safety.
- Quality of computer-based application components is based on aspects of software quality (such as functionality, reliability, usability, efficiency, portability, adaptability, sustainability, scalability, maturity, and certification) and software ergonomics (such as suitability, conformity, self-descriptiveness, controllability, and error tolerance).
- Quality of physical data processing systems comprises availability, appropriateness, mobility, multiple usability, flexibility, maintainability, stability, security, harmlessness, usability, standardization, performance, up-to-dateness, and certification.
- Quality of architecture comprises transparency, adaptability, saturation, functional leanness, and controlled data redundancy.

8.3 Quality of Processes

In medicine, quality of processes describes the quality of activities carried out by care providers (e.g., adherence to professional standards, appropriateness of care). In the context of health information systems, quality of processes deals with the quality of the information processes that are necessary to meet the user's needs. An information process is a sequence of enterprise functions (see Sect. 5.3.2.1).

Criteria for quality of information processes in HIS comprise single recording and multiple usability of data, controlled transcription of data, leanness of information processing tools, efficiency of information logistics, and patient-centered information processing. All those quality criteria support good process integration, that is, that business processes (see Sect. 3.3.3) are effectively supported by a set of interacting application components (see Sect. 6.5.3.7). After reading this chapter, you should be able to answer the following question:

- What are the characteristics of the quality of processes of HIS?

8.3.1 Single Recording, Multiple Usability of Data

Application components often need the same data. For example, patient administrative data or basic medical data are needed by *RIS* and *LIS*. To avoid duplicate data entry, which is inefficient and prone to error, data should be recorded only once, even when they are stored in different databases. One prerequisite is data integration (see Sect. 6.5.3.1). Multiple usability of data is one of the most important benefits computer support can bring to information systems.

8.3.2 No Transcription of Data

Transcription means the manual transfer of data from one storage device to another storage device, for example, to transfer patient diagnoses from the patient record to an order entry form, or to copy data from a printout into a computer-based application component (Figs. 8.1 and 8.2). Transcription is often combined with a change of the storage media (media crack), for example, transcribing data from a computer-based media to paper (or other way round). Manual transcription is time-consuming and may lead to copy-errors. Therefore, manual transcription has to be avoided.

8.3.3 Leanness of Information Processing Tools

Even if process integration (see Sect. 6.5.3.7) is achieved, the user wants to use as few application components and data processing systems as possible for a given process. Thus

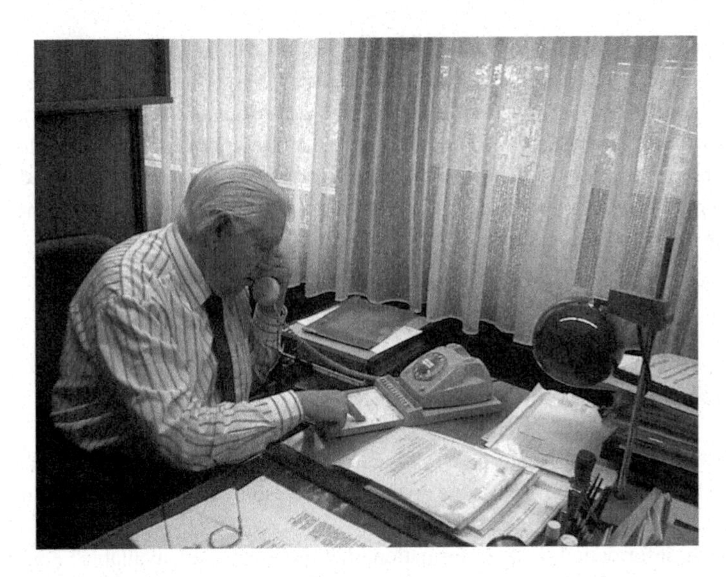

Fig. 8.1 Example of a transcription (1)

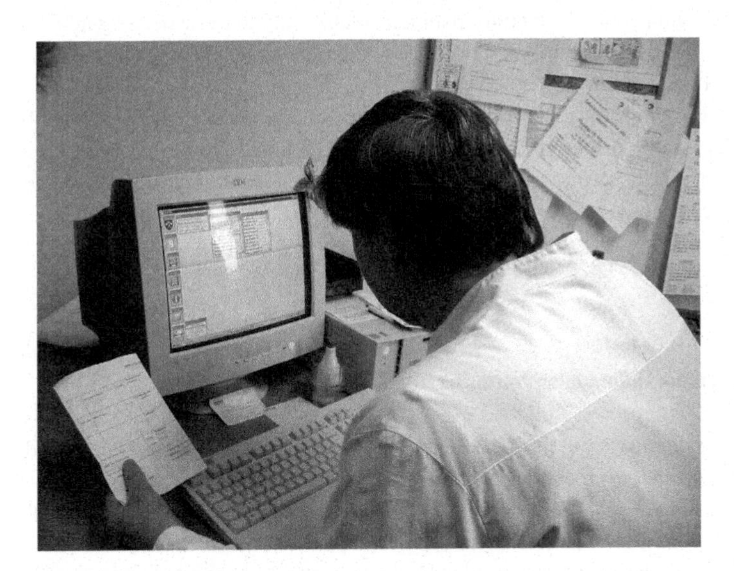

Fig. 8.2 Example of a transcription (2)

for each process, there should be all the tools necessary but as few as possible. For example, let us look at the *execution of nursing procedures*. Maybe a nurse has to use the *nursing management and documentation system*, the *patient administration system*, and the paper-based order entry system. The fewer information processing tools have to be used for one process, the easier it is for the staff. In case different tools have to be used, contextual integration (see Sect. 6.5.3.5) can help to reduce the efforts for the user when he has to change between the tools.

8.3.4 Efficiency of Information Logistics

Information processing should be as efficient as possible. This means that information logistics should be as good as possible given the used resources. Good information logistics comprises the following aspects:

- The right information: Is the information, that the users need, available? For example, is the recent lab result available for the physician?
- At the right time: Is the information available when it is needed (just in time)? For example, are the recent lab results available before the physician's round starts?
- At the right place: Is the information available where it is needed? For example, are the recent lab results available at the patient's bedside?
- To the right people: Is the information available only to those needing it? For example, are the recent lab results only available to the treating health care professionals? Is data protection guaranteed?
- In the right form: Is the information available in a usable format? For example, can lab results also be displayed over a longer period of time? Can information personally be filtered (personal filtering), not overwhelming the health care professional with too much information (information overload)?

8.3.5 Patient-Centered Information Processing

Since *patient care* is highly specialized and distributed, it creates great demand for integrated information processing among health care professionals and among health care institutions (see Sect. 4.3). Information processing, therefore, should center on the patient (not on the institution). This means, for example, that all relevant data about a patient, regardless of what institution produced the data, should be made available to any health care professional in any institution involved in the care of the patient. The availability of an electronic health record system that stores all data about a patient is usually the precondition for real patient-centered information processing.

8.3.6 Exercises

8.3.6.1 Quality of Processes in an Intensive Care Unit

Imagine the following situation in an intensive care unit: Every hour, the responsible nurse reads selected data from a bedside patient monitoring device and enters this information in the *PDMS*. Within the *PDMS*, theses data can be used to generate trends over a longer period of time, and to calculate certain patient-related scores (such as TISS – Therapeutic Intervention Scoring System[4]).

- Which quality criteria described in Sect. 8.3 are not fulfilled?
- Which solution would you suggest to improve quality?

8.3.6.2 Transcription of Data

Look at Figs. 8.1 and 8.2. They show examples of transcription. Answer the following questions:

- In which process may this transcription take place?
- Which data may be transcribed?
- Which tools are involved? Is the transcription associated with a media crack?
- Which negative consequences may this transcription have?
- What can be done to avoid the transcription or to avoid errors?

8.3.6.3 Leanness of Information Processing Tools

Explain how the leanness of information processing tools, as described above, is correlated with the transcription of data and media cracks.

8.3.6.4 Quality of Processes

Have a look at Fig. 8.3, an extract from a simplified UML activity diagram based process model of the process "ordering meals" from the Plötzberg Medical Center and Medical School (PMC). Which of the criteria for quality of processes is not fulfilled? How could the process be changed (e.g., by using other information processing tools) to improve the quality of processes?

---

[4]Therapeutic Intervention Scoring System. http://www.sfar.org/scores2/tiss2.html

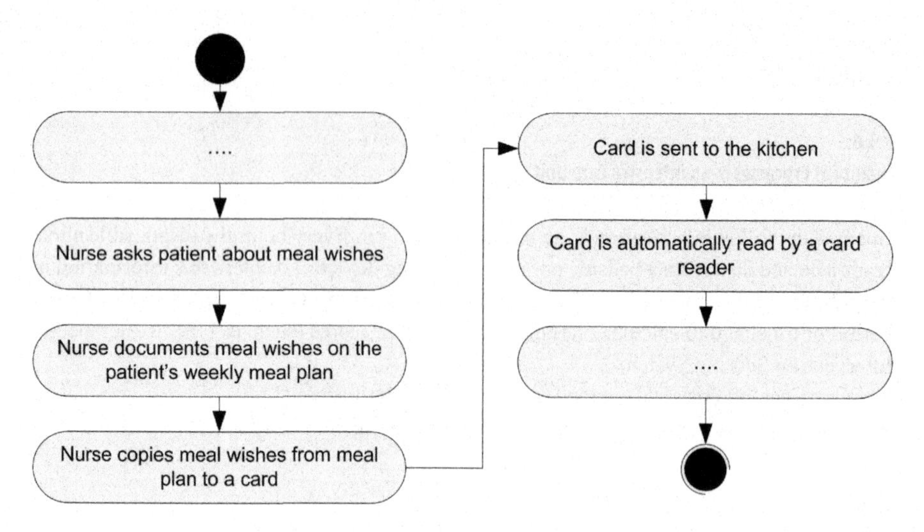

Fig. 8.3 Extract from the business process "meal ordering"

8.3.7 Summary

The criteria for quality of processes of hospital information systems are:

- single recording, multiple usability of data;
- no transcription of data, no media cracks;
- leanness of information processing tools;
- efficiency of information logistics (e.g., correctness and completeness, just-in-time information, availability, personal filtering);
- patient-centered information processing.

8.4 Quality of Outcome

In medicine, quality of outcome describes the effects of patient care, that is, the changes in the health status of the patient (e.g., mortality, morbidity, costs). In the context of health information systems, quality of outcome describes whether the goals of information management have been reached, or, in a broader sense, to what extent the health information system contributes to the goals of the respective institution and to the expectations of different stakeholders.

Quality of outcome thus means whether the health information system finally fulfills the needs of its different user groups and supports efficient and effective patient care. Quality of outcome describes the measurable value of the HIS for the institution and its various stakeholders. Despite good quality of structures and processes, it is not proven that

the hospital information system contributes to the aims of the hospital or the expectations of the stakeholders. Quality of structures and quality of processes is just a prerequisite for quality of outcome.
After reading this chapter, you should be able to answer the following question:
- What are the characteristics of quality of outcome of HIS especially in hospitals?

8.4.1 Fulfillment of Hospital's Goals

For the hospital as an enterprise, the hospital information system should typically contribute to high quality patient care, efficient usage of resources, and fulfillment of legal requirements as general goals of all hospitals.
Additionally, each hospital may have specific goals as defined in an enterprise strategy, such as
- support of clinical research;
- support of medical education;
- offering holistic, interprofessional, patient-oriented care;
- offering high-quality care for a special patient group (offering specialized medical competence centers);
- offering shared-care in close cooperation with certain health care providers;
- attracting patients from other regions;
- being very cost-effective; or
- using up-to-date and expensive technology.

The hospital information system must contribute to the specific strategic goals of the hospital (strategic alignment, see Sect. 9.4.1.1). For example, a HIS may support the hospital goals by offering:
- efficient communication with other health care providers (e.g., quick communication of discharge reports);
- a comprehensive electronic patient record that can be used by all departments and health professionals in the institution;
- mobile tools for all professionals and bedside terminals, or, on the contrary, no IT tools near the patient;
- restricted access to electronic patient records for teaching purposes;
- a personal health record offering patients access to "their" electronic health record;
- data analysis functionality of electronic health record data for clinical research;
- highly standardized, modern, and effective IT tools.

8.4.2 Fulfillment of the Expectations of Different Stakeholders

Distinct stakeholders have specific expectations. The following user needs should be addressed.

8.4.2.1 Patients and Relatives

Patients want to be treated in a both emphatic and effective way, they want to recover quickly, be released from pain, and be able to get home soon. They do not want to be harmed during the diagnosis and treatment process by preventable medication errors. They do not want to be interviewed or examined repeatedly on the same questions. Patients want easy access to their patient record and clear explanations on their diseases. Parents want quick information when the state of the treated child changes. Some parents may even want to use telemonitoring facilities (e.g., via a webcam) to observe their kids at every time (see example 8.7.3). Relatives want to easily find a person within the hospital building. During *discharge*, the patient wants to get a summary of this treatment, and clear advice on what to do next. Overall, patients want that their data are handled in a secure and safe way, ensuring confidentiality and avoiding misusage.

8.4.2.2 Health Care Professionals

Health care professionals want to be supported in their daily work by the IT tools. This means, for example, that documentation tasks are supported by easy-to-use data entry forms, and double documentation and transcription should be avoided. New patient information should be available quickly at the place where the professional needs it (e.g., during the ward round). The health professional does not want to lose time by searching for data, or by dealing with complicated or instable software. Information of earlier stays should be available in an aggregated, well-structured form, and communication with professionals outside the hospital should be well supported. Health professionals want to be able to reuse clinical data for other tasks such as clinical research, clinical education, and administrative tasks (multiple usability). Medical knowledge should be accessible easily wherever needed. IT tools should be user-friendly and robust and show sufficient performance, and paper-based and computer-based tools should work hand-in-hand. If possible, only one computer-based application component should be needed for one business process, without any media crack in between.

8.4.2.3 Administrative Staff

For administrative staff, it is most important that up-to-date and complete administrative information is available. They want automatic tools to guarantee and check the correctness and completeness of administrative data, and automatic interfaces to transfer relevant administrative data to health insurances and other types of organizations. They also want to generate all relevant statistics and reports automatically from available data.

8.4.2.4 Hospital Management

Hospital management needs easy access to complete and up-to-date information on the quality of *patient care* and on its costs. For this, it needs access to all kind of quality and performance data produced in the different parts of the hospital.

8.4.3 Fulfillment of Information Management Laws

In each country, different laws affect health information processing, addressing, for example, organization of health care, financing of health care, and health statistics. Those laws must be taken into account by information management.

An important part of these laws deals with data protection. Health-related patient data are most sensitive and must be protected from unauthorized access. Normally, only those health care professionals involved in the treatment of patients should be able to access patient data, and only those data that are of potential importance for optimal *patient care* should be stored. For example, for a surgical patient, earlier psychiatric stays may not be relevant to the surgeon. The information system should be designed in such a way that data protection (as defined by the national laws) is guaranteed.

For example, in the USA, the Health Insurance Portability and Accountability Act (HIPAA) deals with standards for electronic data interchange, protection of security and confidentiality of electronic health information, and unique identifiers for providers and patients.[5] In Germany, for example, laws on the organization of health care (SGB V[6]), on its financing (KHG,[7] KHRG,[8] BPflV[9]), on data protection (BDSG[10]), on digital signatures (SigG,[11] IuKDG[12]), and on hospital statistics (KHStatV[13]) have to be taken into account in information management.

---

[5]http://www.hipaa.org/
[6]http://sozialgesetzbuch.de/gesetze/05/
[7]http://www.buzer.de/gesetz/6105/index.htm
[8]http://www.buzer.de/gesetz/8675/index.htm
[9]http://www.buzer.de/gesetz/4772/index.htm
[10]http://www.buzer.de/gesetz/3669/index.htm
[11]http://www.buzer.de/gesetz/6596/index.htm
[12]http://www.artikel5.de/gesetze/iukdg.html
[13]http://www.gesetze-im-internet.de/khstatv/BJNR007300990.html

8.4.4 Exercises

8.4.4.1 Expectation of Patients and Relatives

Imagine the last time you (or one of your relatives) was patient in a health care institution. List the aspects where you have been satisfied during your stay there, and which aspects were not satisfactory. In which way does this list contain criteria related to health information systems? Does your list correspond to the criteria discussed in Sect. 8.4.2.1?

8.4.4.2 National Laws for Information Processing

As described above, information processing has to take into account the different laws of the respective country. Find out – for example, using information from the Internet, from publications, or from other lectures – which laws are important for your country with regard to information processing. Briefly describe the content of the laws.

8.4.5 Summary

The criteria for quality of outcome of health information systems are

- fulfillment of the hospital's goals;
- fulfillment of the expectations of different stakeholders;
- fulfillment of the information management laws.

8.5 Balance as a Challenge for Information Management

Besides quality criteria, optimal balance is also a determinant of the quality of a health information system. This is a particular challenge for information management, as it must weigh the different – and possibly contradicting – goals of the hospital. The solution will require the ability of those responsible for information management to carry through with their goals, and the willingness of the affected stakeholders to compromise. Above all, an appropriate organization of *strategic information management* is required (see Chap. 9).

After reading this section, you should be able to answer the following question:

- What does information management have to balance in order to increase the quality of a health information system?

8.5.1
Balance of Homogeneity and Heterogeneity

The collection of information processing tools (both on the logical and on the physical tool layer) should be as homogeneous (i.e., comparable in appearance and usability, for example, using tools from the same vendor) as possible and as heterogeneous as necessary. In general, a homogeneous set of information processing tools makes training and support of users easier and thus leads to reduced costs for the HIS. However, in reality, we usually find a very heterogeneous set of tools at both the logical and the physical tool layer. Why?

In a hospital we need application components at the logical tool layer for the support of the hospital functions. Maximum homogeneity, at least for the computer-supported part of a hospital information system, can easily be reached by a (DB^1, AC^1, V^1) architecture, when just one computer-based application component exists that is implemented through a single software product from a single manufacturer. But usually diverse software products from different manufacturers have to be purchased, which can lead to very heterogeneous (DB^n, AC^n, V^n) architectures. These products might please the various stakeholders of the hospital (which will all have optimal support for their own tasks), but they will make integration, operation, and user support much more difficult. These difficulties are often overlooked by the concerned stakeholders. In this situation, it is the task of information management to ensure and support an appropriate compromise between the hospital's need for economical homogeneous information processing and the needs of the various stakeholders.

At the physical tool layer, heterogeneity is often the consequence of the evolution of the HIS, comprising different generations of computer systems. This could be prevented only if all components are completely exchanged regularly, which is generally not sensible.

Heterogeneity is not always bad. Moreover, heterogeneity is appropriate to a certain degree. But when heterogeneity of information processing tools is not systematically managed, it can lead to the uncontrolled proliferation of tools and to unnecessary costs. The better all stakeholders are involved in *strategic information management* through an appropriate organization, the more this situation can be avoided (see Sect. 9.3).

8.5.2
Balance of Computer-Based and Non-Computer-Based Tools

It is the task of information management to manage information processing in such a way that the goals of the hospital can be reached best. So, for a hospital whose goal is to provide very personal and humane treatment, it might be sensible, for example, to abstain from the use of technology and especially computers for all immediate physician-patient contact. It is possible to write notes on the ward with paper and pen (and even so-called digital pens) rather than using electronic tools, depending on what best supports the hospital's functions. For a hospital whose goal is technological leadership, it might be appropriate to proceed in the opposite direction (see Fig. 8.4).

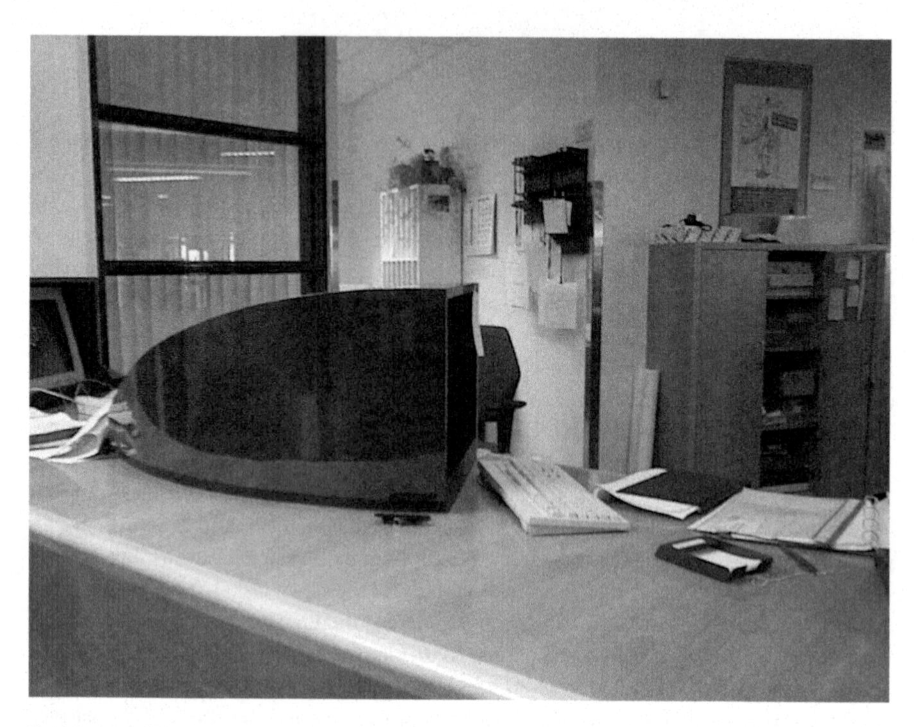

Fig. 8.4 A stylish client at a patient admission unit

That is, the optimum of computer support is not defined by the maximum; rather, it evolves through the various goals of the hospital and its stakeholders as well as through the hospital functions to be supported.

8.5.3 Balance of Data Security and Working Processes

The data saved in a hospital information system are worth protecting. Every patient must be confident that his or her data will not be made available to an unauthorized third party. To ensure this, the appropriate laws of the particular country are to be adhered to. However, hospital information systems are not just purely technical, but rather are socio-technical systems. This means that people are also part of the information system and are therefore also responsible for data security and protection.

A hospital information system should implement strict access control methods to ensure that unauthorized access is impossible. However, this can lead to hindrances in the daily work of the health care professionals. For example, it may occur that a medication cannot be prescribed in an emergency when the attending physician belongs to another hospital department and therefore does not have the right to read the lab result or to order a medication. This can, in an extreme case, even lead to a life-threatening situation. Thus, an access control system that is strict and adapted to predefined tasks and roles in a department can hinder the cooperation between health care professionals and other departments. This would be unfortunate, as it is the job of information management to build the HIS such that cooperation is supported. Consequently, following a thorough risk analysis, it should be weighed whether access control measures in certain situations should be less strict for medical staff, thereby strengthening their own level of responsibility.

Similar risks should be considered in determining how long data should be kept. Health care laws, research needs, and lawsuit requirements should be addressed. So, for example, following the expiration of the storage period, if documents are destroyed, it could be difficult to prove that the hospital carried out a correct medical process in the event of a lawsuit. The resulting consequences would be requests for damage compensation and possibly punishment. However, long-term storage of data may be costly and space-consuming (e.g., archive room, disk storage capacity). Risk management must be carried out with strong support from hospital management.

8.5.4 Balance of Functional Leanness and Functional Redundancy

Functional leanness describes a situation where one hospital function is supported by one and only one application component; the opposite is functional redundancy (see also Sect. 8.7.4), which results in additional costs both for investment and maintenance. But as discussed with controlled data redundancy (compare Sect. 8.2.4), functional redundancy is not always bad. For example, *patient admission* may be supported by application components other than the *patient administration system* to allow easy *patient admission* during night time in a radiology department by using the *RIS*. Even if this conflicts with functional leanness, it may be suitable here to have a more convenient and well-known tool in the diagnostic area and a faster and more sophisticated tool staffing the patient administration unit. Thus, it is the management's task to check carefully where and why there is functional redundancy, because unmanaged functional redundancy may lead to functional oversaturation and unnecessary costs.

As a consequence, these checks may lead to the necessity of declaring an application component to be superfluous. Do not hesitate to remove those components; otherwise the HIS will become logically oversaturated.

8.5.5 Balance of Documentation Quality and Documentation Efforts

Documentation of clinical data is needed for many purposes, such as for information exchange within the health care team, for clinical decision making, for clinical research, for reimbursement issues, for hospital controlling, and for legal statistics. Consequently, many groups inside and outside the hospital profit from a complete, accurate, and timely clinical documentation.

On the other side, high-quality documentation takes time. Physicians and nurses responsible for clinical documentation may feel that the time needed for documentation reduces the time they have for *patient care*. The feeling is especially strong in institutions where documentation is not well supported by existing tools and documentation processes. Insufficient organization of documentation may lead to documentation which is more time-consuming than necessary, to double documentation of the same data, and to transcriptions and media cracks. This all reduces the motivation for documentation and may lead to the feeling that documentation is not helpful but a burden. This in turn may reduce the quality of the documented data. This fact is especially relevant if data items need to be documented by staff that will not use these data for their own purposes. Due to the integrated nature of the processes within a hospital, this is rather common.

Thus, information management carefully has to balance the amount of documentation that is really needed for the various purposes, and the effort that health care professionals have to invest. Well-designed documentation forms, high level of standardization, integrated documentation tools, and a systematic planning of documentation help to reduce effort and to increase the awareness that documentation is an important and indeed useful part of clinical practice.

8.5.6 Exercises

8.5.6.1 Best-of-Breed Versus All-in-One

Imagine you are responsible for the HIS architecture of a newly built hospital. Two alternatives are being discussed: A (DB^1, AC^1) architecture ("all-in-one" solution, see Fig. 6.52 as an example) and an (AC^n, V^n) architecture ("best-of-breed" solution, see Fig. 6.48 as an example). Discuss the strengths and weaknesses of each alternative with focus on the balance of homogeneity and heterogeneity. What would be your choice? Explain your answer.

8.5.7 Summary

Besides quality criteria, which should be fulfilled as well as possible, an optimally balanced situation is also a determinant of the quality of the hospital information system. This is a particular challenge for information management. These criteria comprise:

- Balance of homogeneity and heterogeneity: The collection of information processing tools (at both the logical and the physical tool layer) should be as homogeneous as possible and as heterogeneous as necessary.
- Balance of computer-based and paper-based tools: The optimum of computer support is not defined through the maximum; rather, it evolves through the various goals of the hospital and its stakeholders as well as through the hospital functions to be supported.
- Balance of data security and working processes: The need for data security must be balanced with the need for smooth working processes in a multi-professional and often ad hoc working context in hospitals.

- Balance of functional leanness and functional redundancy: Functional redundancy results in additional costs both for investment and maintenance, but there may be reasons to have redundant functionality.
- Balance of documentation quality and documentation efforts: Many groups profit from a high-quality documentation, but documentation takes time and effort. Well-designed documentation forms, high level of standardization, integrated documentation tools, and a systematic planning of documentation help to increase the motivation for documentation.

As a consequence, it is hardly possible to provide information managers with a simple checklist to find out whether the HIS is good or not. Moreover, HIS quality is a matter of finding optima in a multidimensional space with myriads of restrictions. But this makes information management an extraordinary interesting task.

8.6 Evaluation of Health Information Systems Quality

Evaluation can be defined as the act of measuring or exploring properties of a health information system. The result of an evaluation should give information to support decisions concerning the HIS, such as decisions on replacing or further deploying an application component. This definition highlights the fact that evaluation can comprise both quantitative ("measuring") as well as qualitative ("exploring") aspects, and that evaluation should answer a clear question and thus support information management decisions. Evaluation studies can, for example, help to justify IT investments, to verify that the information system is effective and safe, or to understand problems and to improve the information system.

In this section, we will give an introduction to evaluation methods. After reading, you may want to look at Sect. 9.5 to find details on specific approaches and initiatives dealing with HIS quality, such as COBIT, CCHIT, IHE, and others. After reading this section, you should be able to answer the following questions:

- What are the major phases of an IT evaluation study?
- What are the major IT evaluation methods?

8.6.1 Typical Evaluation Phases

All quality criteria as described in the earlier sections can be evaluated in dedicated evaluation projects. When planning and conducting such an evaluation study, it is necessary – as in any empirical investigation – to follow a systematic, step-wise approach. The following steps are recommended[14]:

[14]Nykänen P, Brender J, et al. GEP-HI – Guidelines for Best Evaluation Practices in Health Informatics: EFMI-WG on Evaluation of Health Information Systems; 2010. Available at http://iig.umit.at/efmi/

Fig. 8.5 The major steps of an evaluation study. Boxes comprise activities; arrows into a box from top are input; arrows out from a box are output. Feedback loops indicate that earlier steps may have to be redone or refined

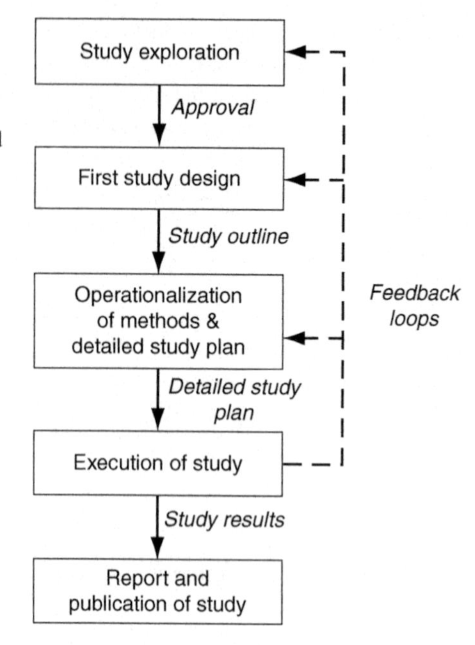

- study exploration;
- first study design;
- operationalization of methods and detailed study plan;
- execution of study;
- report and publication of study.

Figure 8.5 summarizes the described steps of an evaluation study.

8.6.1.1 Study Exploration

The study exploration phase forms the basis for an evaluation study and results in a preliminary outline of the study, which can be characterized by the following questions:

- Who wants the information from the evaluation study? (Identify the major sponsors for the evaluation.)
- What is the strategic objective of the study?
- What is the intended audience?
- What is the organizational and political context for the evaluation studies to take place?
- What are the major stakeholder groups that should be involved in the preparation of the study?
- What is the available budget?
- Is there sufficient political acceptance in the institution to go on?

This phase should end with a written approval by the relevant decision makers before going on.

8.6.1.2
First Study Design

The First Study Design Phase has the purpose of sketching the foundation for study. The following activities have to be done:

- establish the evaluation team;
- formulate in detail the study questions you want to answer and the evaluation criteria you want to access;
- identify any constraints the study may have (e.g., budget, location, time, political aspects);
- select the (quantitative or qualitative) methods you want to apply to answer your study questions;
- describe the organizational context and technical setting your study will take place in;
- outline the time plan for the evaluation study and inform the involved user groups;
- pay attention to any legal or ethical aspects that may occur;
- decide on a strategy for reporting the evaluation results.

At the end of this phase, you should have a written agreement on the study outline.

Please note that different groups may have different evaluation questions in mind. As it is impossible to evaluate all possible criteria, you typically will have to select the most important ones.

8.6.1.3
Operationalization of Methods and Detailed Study Plan

This phase is dealing with the selection of an appropriate design and methods to answer the leading questions (the information need), in accordance with the setting, the resources (available competences, staff, time, money, readiness of the participants to take part, etc.), and the objectives of the study. You will have to decide on study design, outcome measures, on details of the quantitative and qualitative methods (see also next section for more details on evaluation methods), on participants, whether it is a laboratory study or a field study, on study flow, and on project management and risk management aspects. The result of this phase is a detailed study plan that will be followed in the next phase.

Please note that several experimental, quasi-experimental and nonexperimental study designs can be applied to IT evaluation studies. The study design has to be carefully selected depending on the study questions you may have. For quantitative studies that want to prove a hypothesis (e.g., on the effect of an information system), experimental designs (such as randomized controlled trials) are typically seen as having a higher internal validity than quasi-experimental designs (such as before-after trials or time series analysis). For qualitative studies, nonexperimental designs such as case studies are normally chosen, but there also exist approaches of qualitative experiments.

8.6.1.4 Execution of Study

During this phase, the study plan is followed, that is, qualitative and/or quantitative data are gathered and analyzed as planned. Depending on the study design, data will have to be gathered at several locations and/or at several points in time. Special attention should be given to quality of data and to any unintended factors that may influence the findings of the study. Observations will be analyzed and interpreted to answer the original study questions.

8.6.1.5 Report and Publication of Study

The results of the study should be published in a report for the decision makers and stakeholders of the study. In some cases, international scientific publication may also be done. In any case, publication should follow established reporting guidelines such as the STARE-HI guidelines.[15]

8.6.2 Typical Evaluation Methods

8.6.2.1 Quantitative Evaluation Methods

Quantitative methods deal with quantitative data, that is, with numbers. Numbers have the advantage that they can easily be statistically analyzed, aggregated, and compared. The basic idea of quantitative methods is that objects have attributes (such as duration or amount) that can be exactly measured. To get data representative for a predefined population, a sampling is selected and then analyzed.
Typical quantitative evaluation methods comprise:

- time measurements (e.g., time-motion and work sampling);
- event counting;
- quantitative questionnaires.

Time Measurements

The time-motion analysis is based on trained observers that measure the duration of observed events (e.g., tasks) while using a predefined list of event categories. Typically, for time-motion analysis, one observer for one observed actor (e.g., one user) is needed. This disadvantage is resolved by the work sampling analysis. Here, trained observers document

[15]STARE-HI – Statement on Reporting of Evaluation Studies in Health Informatics. http://iig.umit.at/efmi/starehi.htm

which task is just being executed only at predefined (e.g., every 5 min) or randomly selected time intervals. By this, they can observe several actors in parallel. By counting the number of observed tasks in each category, the overall distribution and thus the duration of each task can be calculated. However, to get precise numbers, a relatively large number of observations have to be done here. Please note that both approaches (time-motion and work sampling) are typically conducted by external trained observers, but can principally also be conducted by the actors (e.g., users) themselves – this, however, may endanger the quality of the data.

Event Counting

Event counting comprises observations of clinical situations or processes or analysis of available data (e.g., log files), counting the number of events that occur in a given time period. This can, for example, be counting of medication errors (based on an analysis of patient records), counting the number of clicks when using certain software, counting the number of physician-patient interactions or counting the number of patients entering a department. As for any measurement, special attention should be given to train the observers and to use standardized observation protocols to achieve interobserver reliability.

Quantitative Questionnaires

Questionnaires that use standardized, closed questions lead to quantitative results. For questionnaires addressing subjective opinions and feelings, the five-point Likert scale is typically used ("strongly agree" – "agree" – "neither/nor" – "disagree" – "strongly disagree"). The quality of data achieved by questionnaires depends on a thorough formulation of questions and answers and an intensive pretest of the questionnaire. The available literature should thus be consulted before planning a questionnaire to ensure objectivity, reliability, and validity of results. If possible, available and validated questionnaires should be reused.

8.6.2.2 Qualitative Evaluation Methods

Qualitative methods deal with qualitative data, that is, with text and any other non-number data. Qualitative data can describe individual situations and contexts in detail.

Typical qualitative evaluation methods comprise:

- qualitative interviews;
- qualitative observations;
- qualitative content analysis.

Qualitative Interviews

This comprises all forms of semi- or unstructured interviews that use open questions, thus generating free-text as results. This allows the respondent to answer freely, and it allows interaction between interviewer and respondent. The interview can be conducted with one or more respondent at the same time. Group interviews support interaction between respondents, but should only be done in groups without hierarchical dependencies. In any case, a pretested interview instruction is needed that describes how the interviewer should conduct the interview and document the results. Answers are typically recorded by an audio recorder and later transcribed in verbal or aggregated protocols. The analysis of the data can be done by, for example, qualitative content analysis (see below).

Qualitative Observations

This comprises open, less-standardized, nonquantitative observations of processes or events. In contrary to quantitative observations, the aim is not to count and measure, but to get insight into a situation. The observations are typically documented in a field diary and/or on predefined observation protocols. Qualitative observations generate text (such as observer notes) that can be analyzed by qualitative content analysis. Please note that for qualitative observation, there should be a certain familiarity of the observer with the observed field (e.g., with the situation in the clinical department).

Qualitative Content Analysis

Text obtained from qualitative interviews or observations can be analyzed by a methodological, planned approach based on categories. Here, the material is stepwise analyzed and coded into several available categories. The categories can either be defined beforehand (deductive approach), they can be developed while reading and analyzing the text (inductive approach), or they can be defined beforehand and refined while analyzing the text (mixed approach). The coding of text into categories should be reproducible; it must therefore be clearly documented and explained by so-called anchor examples. Typically, the text material is read and coded more than once to make sure that nothing is overlooked, and that the categories are homogeneous and all filled with text examples. Based on the categories and the text passages that are related to them, the text can then be further analyzed to identify larger patterns and to answer the study questions.

8.6.2.3
Special Evaluation Studies

The quantitative and qualitative evaluation methods described above form the basis for special types of evaluation studies. The following list presents some examples.

- User survey: Quantitative analysis of user satisfaction with an application component.
- Delphi survey: Consensus method for the prediction of the future. A panel of experts is surveyed on a given topic in several iterative rounds. The result of each round is presented to each expert in anonymized form; the experts are then invited to modify their judgment in the next round.
- SWOT analysis: Quantitative and/or qualitative analysis of the most significant strengths (positive features), weaknesses (negative features), opportunities (potential strengths), and threats (potential weaknesses) that characterize an information system component.
- Effectiveness study: Quantitative analysis of the effects of an information system component.
- Cost-effectiveness analysis: An economic analysis to compare the costs and consequences of an information system component. It does not require that all important effects and benefits are expressed in monetary terms.
- Cost–benefit analysis: An economic analysis that converts effects of an information system component into the same monetary terms as the costs and compares them.
- Utility analysis: An economic analysis that compares costs and consequences of an information system component, taking personal preferences into account by including weighting factors for each criterion.
- Return-on-investment (ROI) study: An economic analysis that describes how much an investment on an information system component paid back in a fixed period of time.
- Usability study: Assessment of the user friendliness of an IT component with special focus on the interaction between an IT component and its users.

8.6.3 Exercises

8.6.3.1 Selection of Evaluation Criteria

It seems quite clear that you cannot evaluate all possible evaluation criteria as defined in this chapter in one evaluation study. Imagine that you were asked to "evaluate the new *RIS* system in the Department of Radiology." How would you proceed to come to a subset of criteria? Which stakeholder groups would you involve in decision making? What would be your role during this process?

8.6.3.2 Planning of an Evaluation Study

Your task is now to prepare the *RIS* evaluation study mentioned before. You decided to focus on the cost-benefit ratio of this application component. Define an adequate evaluation plan. What would be the detailed questions? What measuring methods would be used? What would be an adequate study design? Discuss the different possibilities.

8.6.3.3
The Baby CareLink Study

Please look at example 8.7.3. Which method is used to assess quality of care? Can you think of other methods to assess the quality of care in a neonatal intensive care unit?

8.6.4
Summary

Evaluation studies should follow a well-defined structured approach comprising: study exploration, first study design, operationalization of methods and detailed study plan, execution of study, and report and publication of study. Special emphasis has to be put on the clear formulation of the evaluation criteria that are investigated.

There are quantitative and qualitative evaluation methods. Typical quantitative methods comprise time measurement, event counting, and user surveys. Typical qualitative methods comprise qualitative interviews, qualitative observations, and qualitative data analysis. Special evaluation studies comprise user surveys, Delphi surveys, SWOT analysis, several economic analyses, and usability studies. The challenge is to select the adequate evaluation method for each evaluation criterion.

8.7
Summarizing Examples

The following examples present various attempts to describe quality criteria for HIS.

8.7.1
The Baldrige Health Care Information Management Criteria

This (shortened) example is taken from the Malcolm Baldrige National Quality Award Program.[16] This award is annually given to US organizations that are judged to be outstanding in seven areas: leadership; strategic planning; customer and market focus; measurement, analysis, and knowledge management; workforce focus; process management, and results.

"Describe how your institution ensures the quality and availability of needed data, information, software, and hardware for your workforce, suppliers, partners, collaborators, and customers.

(a) Data, Information and Knowledge Management
   1. How do you ensure the following properties of your organizational data information and knowledge? Accuracy; integrity and reliability; timeliness; security and confidentiality

[16] National Institute of Standards and Technology, Baldrige National Quality Program. http://www.baldrige.nist.gov/

2. How do you make needed data and information available to your workforce, suppliers, partners, collaborators, and customers?

(b) Management of information resources and technology
   1. How do you ensure that hardware and software are reliable, secure, and user friendly?
   2. In the event of an emergency, how do you ensure the continued availability of hardware and software systems and the continued availability of data and information?
   3. How do you keep your software and hardware systems current with business needs and directions?"

8.7.2 Information Management Standards of the Joint Commission

The Joint Commission[17] is an independent, not-for-profit organization. It evaluates and accredits more than 16,000 health care institutions in the USA, for example, hospitals, health care networks, ambulatory care units, long-term-care facilities, and laboratories. Accreditation means to certify that an institution meets predefined quality standards. Joint Commission standards are nationally recognized as those that are conducive to providing a high standard of *patient care*. External evaluation is done at regular time intervals (e.g., 3 years).

The Joint Commission has defined standards that must be fulfilled to achieve accreditation. Those standards comprise, for example, aspects of *patient care*, data security, and staff management. Among others, the Joint Commission also defines the following major information management standards:

1. The hospital plans and designs information management processes to meet internal and external information needs that are appropriate for the hospital's size and complexity.
2. Confidentiality, security, and integrity of data and information are maintained.
3. Uniform data definitions and data capture methods are used whenever possible.
4. Decision makers and other appropriate staff members are educated and trained in the principles of information management.
5. Transmission of data and information is timely and accurate, and the formats for disseminating data and information are standardized.
6. Adequate data integration and data interpretation capabilities are provided.
7. The hospital defines, captures, analyzes, transforms, transmits, and reports patient-specific data and information related to care processes and outcomes.
8. The hospital collects and analyzes aggregate data to support patient care and operations.
9. The hospital provides systems, resources, and services to meet its needs for knowledge-based information in patient care, education, research, and management.
10. Comparative performance data and information are defined, collected, analyzed, transmitted, reported, and used consistently with national and state guidelines for data set parity and connectivity.

[17]http://www.jointcommission.org

The information management standards are further divided into several subsections. For example, the subsections of information management standard number 7 comprise among others the following criteria:

- The institution initiates and maintains a medical record for every individual assessed or treated.
- The medical records contain sufficient information to identify the patient, support the diagnosis, justify the treatment, and document the course and results accurately.
- At *discharge* from inpatient care, a clinical resume concisely summarizes the reason for hospitalization, the significant findings, the procedures performed and treatment rendered, the patient's condition on *discharge*, and any specific instructions given to the patient and/or family, as pertinent.
- All significant clinical information pertaining to a patient is entered into the medical record as soon as possible after its occurrence.
- All entries in medical records are dated and authenticated, and a method is established to identify the authors of entries.

8.7.3 The Baby CareLink Study[18]

Baby CareLink is a telemedicine program that incorporates videoconferencing and World Wide Web technologies to enhance interactions among families, staff, and community providers during the treatment of very low birth weight (VLBW) infants. The videoconferencing module allows virtual visits and distance learning from a family's home during an infant's hospitalization as well as virtual house calls and remote monitoring after *discharge*. Baby CareLink's WWW site contains information on issues that confront these families. It also allows sharing of patient-based data and communications among authorized hospital and community users.

In a randomized trial of Baby CareLink comprising 30 control and 25 study patients, a standardized 80-item survey using a five-point-Likert scale was administered to the participating families after *discharge*, to assess their satisfaction with the quality of care. It could be shown that families in the CareLink group were significantly more satisfied and reported significantly fewer problems with the quality of care. The duration of hospitalization was similar in the two groups, but all infants in the CareLink group were discharged directly to home, whereas 20% of control infants were transferred to community hospitals before ultimately being discharged to home. Overall, CareLink significantly improved family satisfaction with inpatient VLBW care and lowered costs associated with hospital-to-hospital transfer.

8.7.4 In-Depth Approach: The Functional Redundancy Rate

The easier quality criteria for HIS are computable, the more frequent they will be used. A prerequisite of computability, however, is the formal description of criteria.

---

[18]This example is based on Gray JE, Safran C, Davis RB, et al. Baby CareLink: Using the Internet and telemedicine to improve care for high-risk infants. Pediatrics. 2000;106(6):1318–1324.

As we experienced in the previous sections, the metamodel 3LGM² (recall Sect. 5.3) is helpful for describing architectures of HIS. We will now show a little bit more in detail how 3LGM²-based models can be used to automatically compute a particular quality criterion, which is the functional redundancy rate (FRR). On that basis we want to support information managers to find answers to the following question:

- How many application components in my HIS can be shut down without loss of functionality?

Functional redundancy deals with the adequate relationship between enterprise functions and application components to support these tasks. We can model this support relationship, that is, a part of the interlayer relationships mentioned in Sect. 5.3.2.4, by a matrix *SUP*.

Let $\underline{EF} := \{EF_1, ..., EF_p\}, P > 0$ be a set of enterprise functions, and $\underline{AC} := \{AC_1, ..., AC_n\}$, $N > 0$ a set of application components.

The two-dimensional matrix *SUP* describing the relationship between enterprise functions and application components is defined as $SUP := (sup_{p,n})_{p=1...P, n=1...N}$ with

$$sup_{p,n} = \begin{cases} 1 \; if \; function \; ef_p \; is \; supported \; by \; application \; component \; ac_n \\ 0 \; else \end{cases}$$

Let us look at the following example: Suppose a set of enterprise functions $\underline{EF}$:={*A,B,C,D,E,F,G*}, where the letters represent enterprise functions as follows: *A* for *medical admission*, *B* for *administrative admission (inpatients)*, *C* for *administrative admission (outpatients)*, *D* for *execution of radiology diagnostics*, *E* for *decision making*, *F* for *visitor and information service*, and *G* for *medical and nursing care planning*. Additionally, suppose a set of application components $\underline{AC}$:={*1,2,3,4,5,6,7,8,9*}, where the numbers represent application components as follows: (*1*) for *medical documentation system*, (*2*) for *patient administration system*, (*3*) for *cardiovascular information system*, (*4*) for *RIS*, (*5*) for *decision support system*, (*6*) for *pharmacy information system*, (*7*) for *pathology information system*, (*8*) for *dialysis information system*, and (*9*) for *teleradiology system*.

Table 8.1 contains the matrix *SUP* describing the interlayer relationships between these functions and application components, whereas Fig. 8.6 illustrates these relationships.

Table 8.1 The matrix SUP for EF and AC. The matrix is illustrated in Fig. 8.6

		Application components n=1,…, 9								
		1	2	3	4	5	6	7	8	9
Enterprise functions p=1, …, n	A	1	0	0	0	0	0	0	0	0
	B	0	1	0	0	0	0	0	0	0
	C	1	1	1	1	0	0	0	0	0
	D	0	0	0	1	0	0	0	0	0
	E	0	0	0	0	1	0	1	0	0
	F	0	0	0	0	0	1	0	0	0
	G	0	0	0	0	1	0	1	1	1

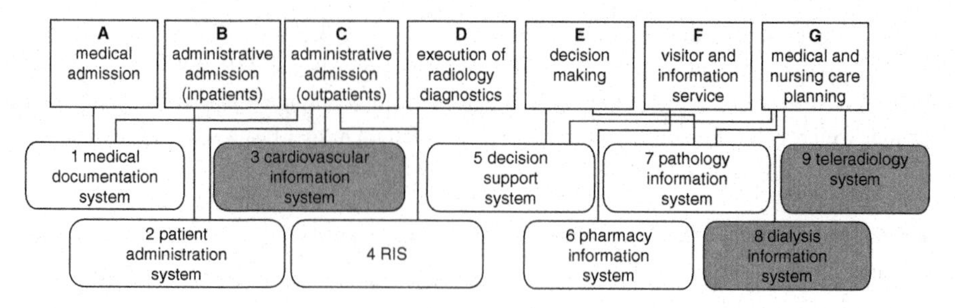

Fig. 8.6 Matrix SUP: rectangles denote enterprise functions, rounded rectangles denote application components, and connecting lines illustrate a "1" in the respective position of the matrix, that is, that a certain enterprise function is supported by a certain application component. For example, enterprise function E *decision making* can be supported by application component 5 *decision support system* or 7 *pathology information system* alternatively

In order to reduce complexity of the HIS it is interesting to know which application components could be omitted without loss of functionality, that is, without hindering the execution of any enterprise function. Before we define a measure for functional redundancy we want to explain, how we can detect redundant support of enterprise functions by application components.

For every enterprise function $ef_p \in \underline{EF}$ we can easily calculate $isup_p := \sum_{n=1}^{N} sup_{p,n}$. Every $isup_p$ denotes the number of application components actually supporting the individual enterprise function ef_p; we call it its individual degree of support by application components. Every $isup_p > 1$ may be an indicator that some application components are dispensable, with $isup_p - 1$ indicating the number of possibly superfluous components. However, this number needs a careful investigation because some of the apparently superfluous application components may be necessary for other enterprise functions. Obviously, measuring functional redundancy in a way, which is supportive for information management, needs a measure, which takes these interrelationships into account.

Continuing part 1 of our example we can easily calculate $isup_p$ as shown in Table 8.2.

Table 8.2 $isup_p$

p	ef_p	$isup_p$
1	A	1
2	B	1
3	C	4
4	D	1
5	E	2
6	F	1
7	G	4

The value of $isup_3=4$ indicates that perhaps there are three superfluous application components supporting C (*administrative admission* (*outpatients*)). But detailed analysis shows that the application components *1* (*medical documentation system*), *2* (*patient administration system*), and *4* (*RIS*) cannot be omitted, because they are needed for the functions A (*medical admission*), B (*administrative admission* (*inpatients*)), and D (*execution of radiology diagnostics*). However, application component *3 (cardiovascular information system*) seems to be a good candidate for being removed from this information system because function C as the only function it supports is also supported by application components *1*, *2*, and *4*. A measure of redundancy should, therefore, correctly indicate that considering the enterprise function C (*administrative admission* (*outpatients*)) only one application component could be omitted (namely, *cardiovascular information system*).

How can an algorithm automatically check, whether particular application components can be omitted or not, given $\underline{EF}$, $\underline{AC}$ and SUP?

The challenge is to calculate a minimal subset $\underline{AC}^{min} \subseteq \underline{AC}$ of application components, which guarantees that all functions are supported and that there are no superfluous application components in use. Each set $\underline{AC}^{min}$ we call a "minimal functionally nonredundant set of application components." In general, there is more than one such set $\underline{AC}^{min}$ for a given information system, that is, there is more than one way to cut down functional redundancy.

Let us describe any subset $\underline{AC}' \subseteq \underline{AC}$ of application components being actually in use by a vector $\overrightarrow{USE}$, indicating whether application components are member of the subset $\underline{AC}'$ or not: $\overrightarrow{USE} := (use_n)_{n=1...N}$ with

$$use_n = \begin{cases} 1\ if\ ac_n \in \underline{AC}' \\ 0\ else \end{cases}$$

Hence, $\underline{AC}^{min}$ can be described by $\overrightarrow{USE}^{min} := (use_n^{min})_{n=1...N}$ and $use_n^{min} \in \{0,1\}$. Given what application components are in use, that is, given the respective vector USE, we can calculate the individual degree of support for all enterprise functions as well as:

$\overrightarrow{ISUP}^T = SUP * \overrightarrow{USE}$ with $\overrightarrow{ISUP} = \left(isup_p\right)_{p=1...P}$.

As stated above, we want that, despite of some application components being not in use, every function is supported by at least one application component. We introduce a vector $\vec{e}$ of length P containing only "1": $\vec{e} = \left(e_p\right)_{p=1...P}$ with $e_p := 1, p = 1...P$.

Now we can state the first postulation (P1): For every vector $\overrightarrow{USE}$, which is as a candidate for being considered as a possible reduced set of application components, the following constraint holds: $SUP * \overrightarrow{USE} \geq \vec{e}^T$.

Second, we want to have as few application components in use as possible. We introduce a vector $\vec{c}$ of length N containing only "–1": $\vec{c} = \left(c_n\right)_{n=1...N}$ with $c_n := -1, n = 1...N$.

This leads to the second postulation (P1): $\vec{c}^T * \overrightarrow{USE} \rightarrow max$.

Since *SUP* is a matrix of zeroes and ones, we have a pure 0-1 linear programming problem. This particular problem here is well known in literature as the "set covering problem." Corresponding to our statement that there will be more than one "minimal functionally nonredundant set of application components" there are also different solutions for the set covering problem.

The simplest algorithm for computing these solutions, known as "brute-force," checks all combinations of application components for postulations (P1) and (P2). Of course this would need too much computing resources for realistic information systems with several tenths of application components. Moreover, set covering is an NP-complete problem generally, which, roughly, means that the complexity of any algorithm will be in the order of an exponential function of N. Fortunately, for usual models of a HIS certain assumptions can be made, which can be used to define a heuristic algorithm. The 3LGM² tool (see footnote 8 in Chap. 5) provides such an algorithm, which actually computes solutions for this particular set covering problem even in large HIS models very fast.

The solution is a set $\underline{USE}^{\min}$ of all vectors $\overrightarrow{USE_k}^{\min} := \left(use_{k,n}^{\min}\right)_{n=1...N}$, for which (P1) and (P2) hold. The set is defined as $\underline{USE}^{\min} := \left\{\overrightarrow{USE_1}^{\min},...,\overrightarrow{USE_K}^{\min}\right\}$.

This corresponds with the set $\underline{AC}^{\min} := \left\{\underline{AC}_1^{\min},...,\underline{AC}_K^{\min}\right\}$ of minimal functionally nonredundant sets of application components $\underline{AC}_k^{\min}$. In the sense of the set covering problem we could say every $\underline{AC}_k^{\min}$ covers $\underline{EF}$. Because of (P2), all those sets $\underline{AC}_k^{\min}$ are of the same cardinality $M := \left|\underline{AC}_k^{\min}\right|$.

We can now define *Functional Redundancy Rate* (*FRR*) as $FRR := \frac{N-M}{N}$.

FRR can be interpreted as the percentage of application components, which could be removed from the information system without loss of functionality.

Since the given information system in our example is very small, we can immediately identify two minimal functionally nonredundant configurations without using complicated algorithms, but by merely looking accurately at Fig. 8.6:

$\underline{AC}_1^{\min} = \{1,2,4,5,6\}$ and $\underline{AC}_2^{\min} = \{1,2,4,6,7\}$, which correspond to the vectors $\overrightarrow{USE_1}^{\min} = (1,1,0,1,1,1,0,0,0)$ and $\overrightarrow{USE_2}^{\min} = (1,1,0,1,0,1,1,0,0)$.

For $\overrightarrow{USE_1}^{\min}$ as one of the two minimal solutions in our example holds: $SUP * \overrightarrow{USE_1}^{\min} = \left(\overrightarrow{ISUP_1}^{\min}\right)^T = (1,1,3,1,1,1,1)$ (see Table 8.3).

Thus, (P1) holds for $\overrightarrow{ISUP_1}^{\min}$. In the same way (P1) can be shown to hold for $\overrightarrow{ISUP_2}^{\min}$ as well.

FRR is only dependent on *N* and on *M*, being the number of application components and the cardinality of all minimal functionally nonredundant sets of application components, respectively. With $N=9$ and $M=5$, we get: $FRR = \frac{9-5}{9} = 0{,}44$.

Hence, 44% of the application components in our example could be removed.

Table 8.3 Vector $\overrightarrow{ISUP}^{min}$

p	ef_p	$isup_p$
1	A	1
2	B	1
3	C	3
4	D	1
5	E	1
6	F	1
7	G	1

8.8 Summarizing Exercises

8.8.1 Evaluation Criteria

Look at the quality criteria for structures, for processes, and for outcomes as described in this chapter. Please select three criteria that you personally find most important. Please discuss your choice.

8.8.2 Joint Commission Information Management Standards

Please look at the ten major Joint Commission Information Management Standards presented in Sect. 8.7.2. Analyze how they correspond to the quality criteria for structures, for processes, and for outcomes as described in this chapter. To which quality criteria can they be matched?

8.9 Summary

Three major approaches to quality assessment are typically distinguished: quality of structures, quality of processes, and quality of outcome. Quality characteristics may help to describe "HIS diseases," find "HIS diagnoses," and derive adequate "HIS therapies."

In the context of hospital information systems, quality of structures refers to the availability of resources needed for information processing. It comprises quality of data, quality of computer-based application components, quality of physical data processing systems, and quality of HIS architecture.

Quality of processes deals with the quality of the information processes, which are necessary to meet the user's needs. It comprises single recording and multiple usability of data, no transcription of data, leanness of information processing tools, efficiency of information logistics, and patient-centered information processing.

Quality of outcome describes whether the goals of information management have been reached, or, in a broader sense, to what extent the hospital information system contributes to the goals of the hospital and to the expectations of different stakeholders, and the fulfillment of information management laws.

It is a particular challenge for information management to take into account those criteria where only an adequate balance is a determinant of the quality of a hospital information system. This comprises the balance of homogeneity and heterogeneity, the balance of computer-based and paper-based tools, the balance of data security and working processes, the balance of functional leanness and functional redundancy, and the balance of documentation quality and documentation efforts.

Evaluation studies should follow a well-defined, structured approach, comprising: study exploration; first study design; operationalization of methods and detailed study plan; execution of study; and report and publication of study.

Evaluation methods that can be used comprise quantitative methods such as time measurement, event counting, and user surveys, and qualitative methods such as qualitative interviews, qualitative observations, and qualitative data analysis.

Strategic Information Management in Hospitals

9

9.1 Introduction

Until now we have discussed how health information systems look like and how their quality can be described and measured. We will now examine how high quality health information systems can be achieved and how high quality can be maintained, especially in hospitals.

High quality HIS can only by achieved and HIS failures can only be prevented if the HIS are systematically planned, monitored and directed. We summarize this triad by the term 'information management'.

In this chapter, we will first differentiate information management with regard to different scopes. Hence we introduce definitions for *strategic, tactical* and *operational information management*. But this chapter, like the entire book, will focus on *strategic information management*. Systematic information management as a whole requires clear organizational structures. Implementing these is one of the first tasks of *strategic information management*. After discussing appropriate organizational structures for information management in hospitals we will explain what planning, monitoring and directing means especially in a strategic context.

After reading this section, you should be able to answer the following questions:

- What does information management mean and how can *strategic, tactical* and *operational information management* be differentiated?
- What organizational structures are appropriate for information management in hospitals?
- What are the tasks and methods for strategic HIS planning?
- What are the tasks and methods for strategic HIS monitoring?
- What are the tasks and methods for strategic HIS directing?
- How can experts for information management in hospitals be gained?

A. Winter et al., *Health Information Systems*,
DOI: 10.1007/978-1-84996-441-8_9,

9.2 Strategic, Tactical and Operational Information Management

In this section, we present in more detail the tasks of information management in hospitals. After reading this section, you should be able to answer the following questions:

- What does information management in general and in hospitals encompass?
- What are the three main scopes of information management?
- What are the tasks of *strategic, tactical*, and *operational information management* in hospitals?
- What is meant by IT service management and how is it related to information management?

9.2.1 Information Management

The concept 'management' can stand for an institution or for an enterprise function (see Sect. 6.3.3.8 and footnote 3 in Chap. 6). As an institution, management comprises all organizational units of an enterprise that make decisions about planning, monitoring, and directing all activities of subordinate units. As an enterprise function, management comprises all leadership activities that determine the enterprise's goals, structures, and activities.

We can distinguish between (general) management dealing with the enterprise as a whole and management dealing with distinguishable units of the enterprise. The management of the business unit information processing is called information management. In general, information management should contribute to fulfill strategic enterprise goals. Information management in an enterprise manages its information system and thus deals with the following objects:

- enterprise functions and entity types,
- application components, and
- physical data processing systems.

Information management

- plans the information system of an enterprise and its architecture,
- directs its establishment and its operation, and
- monitors its development and operation with respect to the planned objectives.

Different management scopes have different perceptions and interests. Hence, it is helpful to divide information management with regard to its scope into *strategic, tactical*, and *operational management*, which all comprise as main tasks planning, directing, and monitoring.

- *Strategic information management* deals with the enterprise's information processing as a whole and establishes strategies and principles for the evolution of the information system. An important result of strategic management activities is a strategic information management plan.

- *Tactical information management* deals with particular enterprise functions or application components that are introduced, removed, or changed. Usually these activities are done in the form of *projects*. Such *tactical information management projects* are initiated by *strategic information management*. Thus, *strategic information management* is a vital necessity for *tactical information management*. The result of *tactical information management projects* is the enterprise information system.
- *Operational information management* is responsible for operating the components of the information system. It cares for its smooth operation in accordance with the strategic information management plan. Additionally, *operational information management* plans, directs and monitors permanent services for the users of the information system.

This separation is essential because each of these information management scopes has different perspectives, and therefore uses different methods and tools. For example, *strategic information management* focuses on strategic information management plans (compare Sect. 9.4.3). Tactical management needs, for example, methods for project management, user requirements analysis, and software development or customizing. Operational management requires methods and tools for topics that range from intra-enterprise marketing of services to service desk and network management.

Figure 9.1 presents the relationships among *strategic, tactical*, and *operational information management*. Within *strategic information management* a strategic information management plan has to be created as result of planning activities. This depends clearly on strategic goals of the enterprise, which are given by the strategic enterprise management. Since the strategic information management plan contains a list of projects to be performed in the coming years (compare Sect. 9.4.3), strategic directing means to initiate these projects as tasks of *tactical information management*. Strategic monitoring collects different information regarding the state of the information system, its operation, users' opinions and directives of the strategic enterprise management. Within each project of *tactical information management* the course of the project has to be planned (project plan) and the project will be directed according to this plan. The results are components (application components and/or physical data processing systems) of the information system. Again, monitoring is needed in collecting information of the information system's state and deriving consequences for the respective projects but also for strategic decisions. When a project ends, the results have to be operated and thus we enter the scope of *operational information management*.

Management comprises only those tasks that are nonexecutive. Therefore, operational tasks (such as operating a computer server) are not part of management's tasks. However, those operational tasks have to be planned, directed, and monitored. This is carried out by *operational information management*.

Figure 9.2 presents a three-dimensional classification of information management activities. It shows the three objects of information management (functions, application components, and physical data processing systems), the three tasks (planning, directing, monitoring), and the three scopes (strategic, tactical, operational).

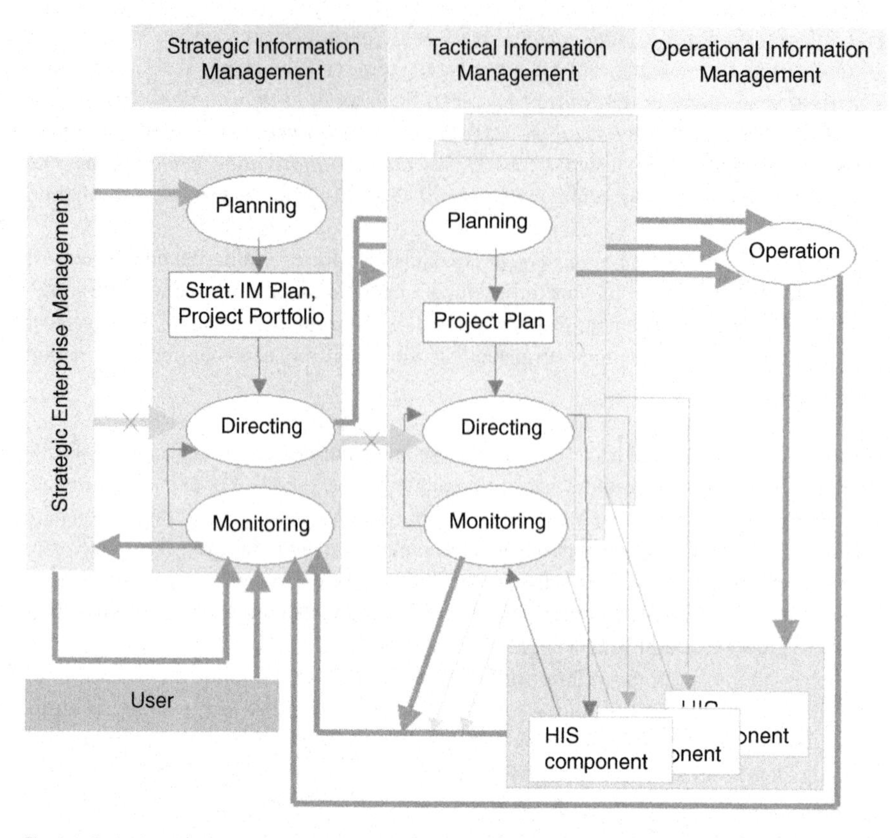

Fig. 9.1 Relationship between planning, directing, and monitoring during *strategic, tactical*, and *operational information management.* For explanation see paragraph before

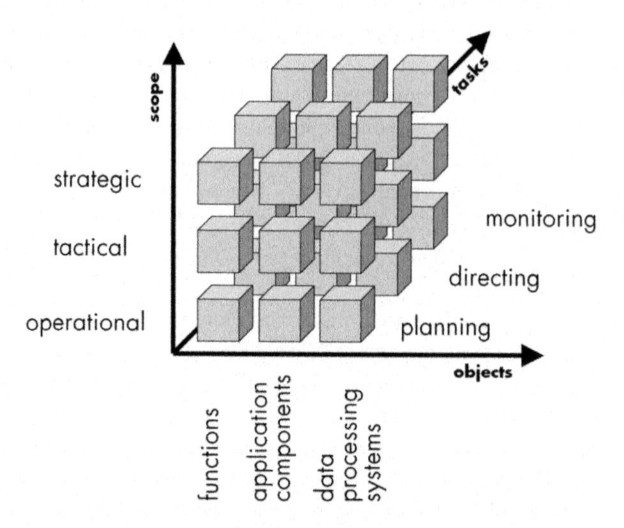

Fig. 9.2 Three-dimensional classification of information management activities

9.2.2 Information Management in Hospitals

We can now apply the defined management concepts to the enterprise "hospital". Information management in hospitals is the management of hospital information systems; hence we can use "HIS management" as a synonym. The tasks of information management in hospitals are:

- planning the hospital information system and its architecture;
- directing its establishment and its operation;
- monitoring its development and operation with respect to the planned objectives.

Information management in hospitals is performed in an environment full of influencing factors. For example, decisions made by the hospital's management directly influence information management (e.g., a decision to cooperate in a health care network). New legal regulations have an effect on information management (e.g., a law enforcing the introduction of a new billing system based on patient grouping). Patients and users of the hospital information system with their values, attitudes, comments, demands, and fears also influence information management. On the other side, information management itself may affect, for example, the management of the enterprise (e.g., information management may propose to introduce a hospital-wide, multiprofessional *electronic patient record system*; this must in turn lead to strategic activities such as process reorganization).

Figure 9.3 presents this relationship between HIS management and HIS operation, and the influencing factors.

We now look at the activities of *strategic, tactical*, and *operational information management* in hospitals.

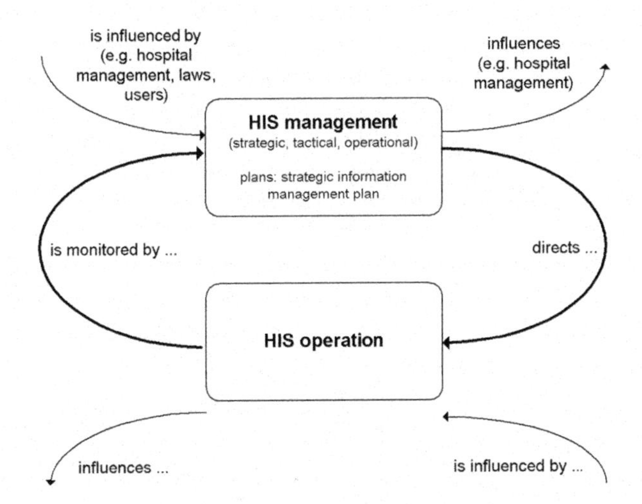

Fig. 9.3 *Strategic, tactical*, and *operational information management* in hospitals, HIS operation, and their relationships

9.2.3 Strategic Information Management

Strategic information management deals with the hospital's information processing as a whole. It depends strictly on the hospital's business strategy and strategic goals and has to translate these into an appropriate information strategy. The planning activities of *strategic information management* result in a specific strategic information management plan. This plan includes the direction and strategy of information management and gives directives for the construction and development of the hospital information system by describing its intended architecture. A proposal for the structure and content of strategic information management plans is presented in Sect. 9.4.3. The strategic information management plan is the basis for strategic project portfolios. They contain concrete projects, which implement the objectives of the strategy, and shall be revised regularly. For example, the strategic information management plan might contain the introduction of a *clinical information system* on all wards within the next 2 years to provide health care professionals with the right information, in the right place, at the right time. The strategic project portfolios could then contain individual projects, for example, on *decision making, planning and organization of patient treatment*, *order entry*, and *medical admission*.

Directing as part of *strategic information management* means to transform the strategic information management plan into action, that is, to systematically manipulate the hospital information system to make it conform to the strategic plan. The system's manipulation is usually done by the initiation of projects of the strategic project portfolio. The projects deal with the construction or further development and maintenance of components of the hospital information system. Planning, directing, and monitoring these projects are the tasks of *tactical information management*. Operational management will then be responsible for the proper operation of the components. An example of strategic directing would be to initiate a project for the introduction of a *provider/physician order entry system*.

Monitoring as part of *strategic information management* means continuously auditing HIS quality as defined by means of its strategic information management plan's directives and goals. Auditing should determine whether the hospital information system is able to fulfill its tasks efficiently, that is, whether it can contribute significantly to the hospital's goals (Sect. 8.4.1), meet the stakeholders' expectations (Sect. 8.4.2) and fulfill the laws (Sect. 8.4.3).

The management's task is to install "sensors" to audit the information system's quality (compare Sect. 8). Management has to receive information from the current projects, from operational management, from users, and from the various stakeholders. Additional information can be gained through evaluation projects (see Sect. 8.6).

Monitoring results are used as input for the directing tasks of information management, which could for example initiate further projects. Monitoring results will also give feedback to update the strategic information management plan, which could for example lead to further activities of strategic management.

Strategic information management and its strategic information management plan are the vital requirements for *tactical* and *operational information management* in a hospital.

9.2.4 Tactical Information Management

Tactical information management deals with particular enterprise functions or application components. It aims to introduce, remove, change, or maintain components of the hospital information system. Such a component could be a *provider/physician order entry system*. Related activities are usually performed within projects. These projects have to be initiated as part of an information strategy, which is formulated in the project portfolio of a strategic information management plan as drawn up by the *strategic information management*. The result of all tactical information management projects is the HIS itself.

The organization of the operation and maintenance of information processing tools is part of *operational information management*. However, if problems occur during the operation of HIS components (e.g., frequent user complaints about a *medical documentation system*), appropriate projects may be executed by *tactical information management* (e.g., introducing a better version of the *medical documentation system*). Typically, those tactical information management projects comprise a planning phase, a running phase (which could contain, for example, system analysis, evaluation, selection, specification, or introduction), and a finishing phase (see Fig. 9.4).

Planning in *tactical information management* means planning projects and all the resources needed for them. Even though tactical information management projects are based on the strategic plan, they need a specific tactical project plan. This plan has to describe the project's subject and motivation, the problems to be solved, the goals to be achieved, the tasks to be performed, and the activities to be undertaken to reach the goals.

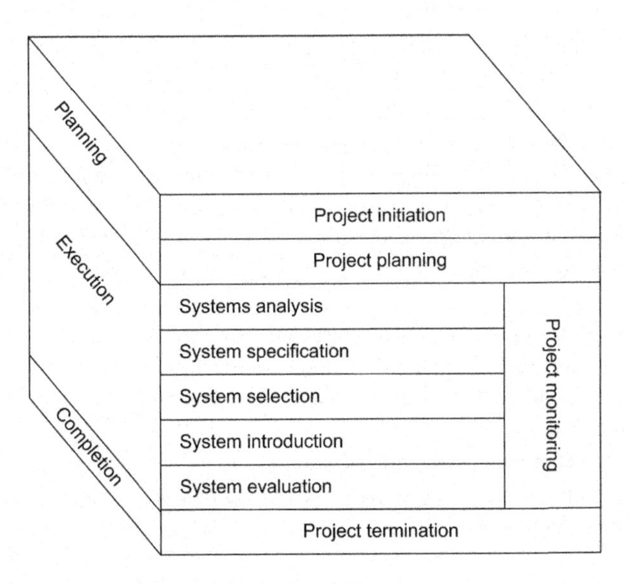

Fig. 9.4 Typical phases of *tactical information management projects*

Directing in tactical management means the execution of such tactical information management projects in hospitals, based on a project plan. Therefore, it includes typical tasks of project management such as resource allocation and coordination, motivation and training of the staff, etc.

Monitoring means continually checking whether the initiated projects are running as planned and whether they will produce the expected results. Monitoring results influence project planning, as a project's plan may be updated or changed according to the results of the project's monitoring in a given situation.

9.2.5 Operational Information Management

Operational information management is responsible for operating the components of the hospital information system. It has to care for its operation in accordance with the strategic information management plan.

Planning in *operational information management* means planning organizational structures, procedures, and all resources such as finances, staff, rooms, or buildings that are necessary to ensure the faultless operation of all components of the hospital information system. For example, *operational information management* may require the installation of a service desk and a service support system that enables the quick transmission of users' error notes to the responsible services. Such systems but also respective staff resources need to be available for a longer period of time. Therefore, they should be allocated as part of a strategic information management plan. Moreover, planning in this context concerns the allocation of personnel resources on a day-to-day basis (e.g., planning of shifts for staff responsible for user support or network management).

Directing means the sum of all management activities that are necessary to ensure proper responses to operating problems of components of the hospital information system, that is, to provide backup facilities, to operate a service desk, to maintain servers, and to keep task forces available for repairing network components, servers, personal computers, printers, etc. Directing in this context deals with engaging the resources planned by the strategic information management plan in such a way that faultless operation of the hospital information system is ensured. *Operational information management* does not mean to exchange a server, but to organize the necessary services and resources.

Monitoring deals with caring for the verification of the proper working and effectiveness of components of the hospital information system. For example, a network monitoring system may regularly be used to monitor the availability and correct working of network components (compare Fig. 9.5).

To guarantee the continuous operation of the most important components of a HIS, it is helpful to draw up a concept for *operational information management*. Such a concept should clarify the following:

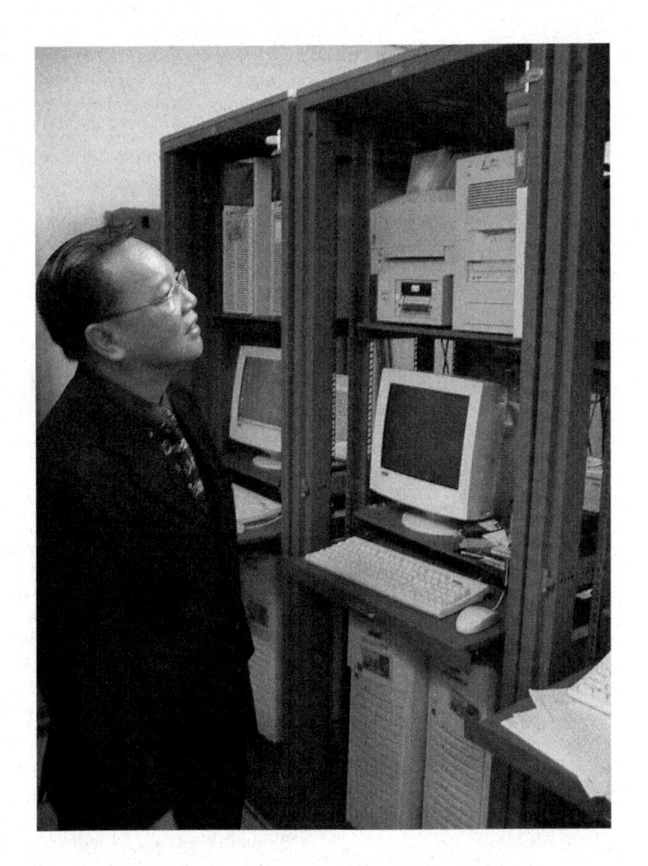

Fig. 9.5 Monitoring of the server of a hospital information system

- Which components have to be supported?
- What tasks comprise operational support?
- Who is responsible for the operational support?
- What should be the intensity of operational support?

Typically, three levels of operational support can be distinguished. First-level support is the first address for all user groups with any kind of problem. It may consist, for example, of a central 24-h-hotline (service desk) that is responsible for the management of user accounts and first trouble shooting, or of decentralized information processing staff. When the first-level support cannot solve the problems, it hands them over to the second-level support, specially trained informatics staff in the central information management department who are usually responsible for the operation of the specific application components. The third-level support, finally, addresses the most severe problems that cannot be solved by the second-level support. It can consist, for example, of specialists from the software vendor (Fig. 9.6).

Table 9.1 presents objects, responsibilities, tasks, and the intensity that should be defined as part of the operational management concept for the computer-based part of a HIS. As an example, a concept for operational management in a hospital could clarify

Table 9.1 Dimensions to be considered for *operational information management* of the computer-based part of hospital information systems

Dimension	Facets
Objects	Decentralized application components (e.g., in departments)
	Central application components (e.g., *patient administration system*)
	Workstations
	Decentralized servers
	Central servers
	Networks
	Backbone
Responsibility	Local (in departments)
	Central (in departments for information processing)
	Vendors
Task	First-level support (incident taking, incident analysis, problem solving if necessary, user training)
	Second-level support (training courses, regular operation, data protection)
	Third-level support (software development, problem solving, contact with vendors)
Intensity	Availability (e.g., 24 h/day, 7 days/week)
	Presence (e.g., locally, by pager, by hotline)
	Timeliness (e.g., answering time < 2 h)

- that central servers and networks are supported by the central information management department, which offers first- and second-level support 24 h a day. A service desk guarantees response time in less than 1 h. Third-level support (see Table 9.1) is provided for certain application components by the vendors of the respective application software products.
- that clients (e.g., personal computers) are supported by the local technical staff in each department. They offer first- and second-level support during the day. They are available by pager.

9.2.6 Relationship Between IT Service Management and Information Management

IT service management (ITSM) is information management centered on the customer's perspective of IT's contribution to the business, in contrast to technology-centered approaches. It comprises all measures and methods that are necessary to support the business processes.

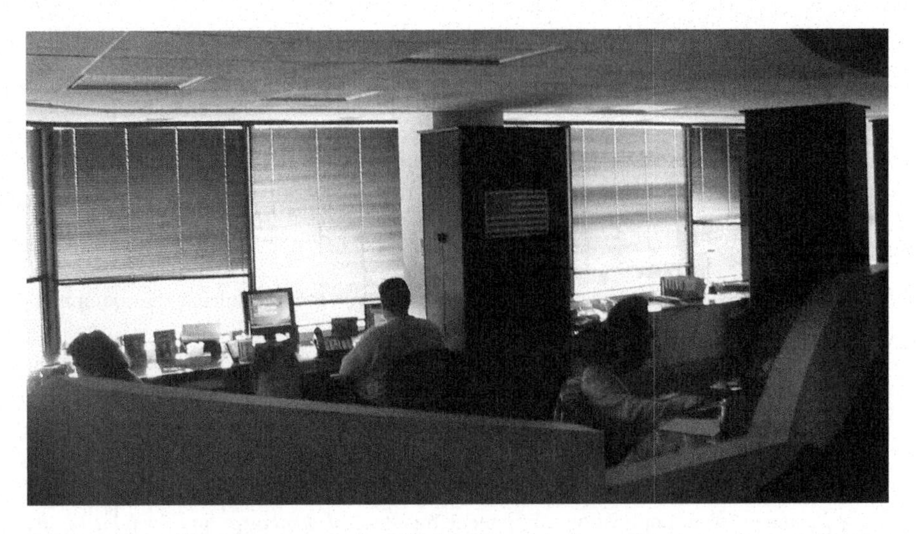

Fig. 9.6 An immediate support center for third-level support of a vendor

Independent of how an institution defines the term "service," there must be an added value for the customer. If, for example, the nurse does not have to call the laboratory for a quick test result but has it immediately available on her portable, it gives her an added value because she can concentrate on her core functions. So, IT Service Management has the task to design, provide, deliver and improve such customer-centered services. The IT Infrastructure Library (ITIL) is the de-facto standard framework for IT Service management. ITIL was developed for the British Government in order to define best practices for all governmental computing centers. In its version 3, the phases of ITIL are described in five core publications:

- service strategy,
- service design,
- service transition,
- service operation,
- continual service improvement.

These publications comprise 26 processes which range from strategic alignment of the IT to continual improvement of processes. Among others, ITIL V3 defines a Service Lifecycle consisting of a circle of service design, service transition and service operation. Service operation usually influences new service designs – and the circle moves on.

Many hospitals use ITIL for selected information management tasks, but have not already implemented the whole lifecycle. Typical ITIL processes that can often be found implemented in hospitals are in the phase of service operation the incident management process and the problem management process, the service desk, and in the phase of service transition the change management and the service asset and configuration management.

ITIL conformant information management processes may be part of *strategic, tactical*, and *operational information management* as best practice.

9.2.7
Example

9.2.7.1
Typical Projects of Tactical Information Management

Typical *tactical information management projects* in the Plötzberg Medical Center comprise:

- analysis of the structure and processes of *order entry* in order to select a new computer-based application component to support this function;
- further development of a *medical documentation system* in order to support new legal demands on diagnoses-related patient grouping and billing;
- introduction of an *operation management system* for *execution of diagnostic, therapeutic and nursing procedures* and *medical discharge and medical report writing* in an operation theater;
- replacement of an application component for *medical discharge and medical report writing* in outpatient units;
- design, implementation, and introduction of an application component to support *medical and nursing care planning;*
- assessment of the user acceptance of a new application component for an intensive care unit.

9.2.8
Exercises

9.2.8.1
Influences on HIS Operation

Look at Fig. 9.3 and find examples of factors influencing HIS operation.

9.2.8.2
Typical Projects of Tactical Information Management

Look at Fig. 9.4 which shows typical phases of information management projects. Match the typical tactical information management projects from example 9.2.7.1 to those typical project phases.

9.2.8.3
Diagnostics and Therapy of HIS

Planning, monitoring, and directing of hospital information systems to a certain extent can be compared to health and the diagnostics and therapy of diseases. Discuss similarities and differences.

9.2.9 Summary

Information management in hospitals is a complex task. To reduce complexity, we distinguish between *strategic, tactical*, and *operational information management*. Each of these information management scopes has different perspectives and uses other methods and tools.

The tasks of information management are:
- planning of a hospital information system and its architecture;
- directing its establishment and its operation;
- monitoring its development and operation with respect to the planned objectives.

IT Service Management comprises tasks of all scopes of information management but emphasizes that information management should be regarded as a service offered by the information management department to a customer in or outside the hospital.

9.3 Organizational Structures of Information Management

Organizational structures for information management in hospitals differ greatly among hospitals. In general, each hospital should have an adequate organization for *strategic, tactical*, and *operational information management*, depending on its size, its internal organization, and its needs.

Organizational structures can be defined at the overall hospital level (e.g., a chief information officer (CIO), a central information management department), and at the departmental level (e.g., specific information management staff for a certain department, a certain outpatient unit).

9.3.1 Chief Information Officer

It is generally useful to centralize responsibilities for information management in one role. This role is usually called chief information officer (CIO); but the role is also often called vice president (or director) of information systems (or information services, information management, information and communication technology, information resources) or chief of information services.

The CIO bears the overall responsibility for the *strategic, tactical*, and *operational* management of the information system and the budgetary responsibility, and has the authority for all employees concerned with information management. The specific position of the CIO demands dedicated professional skills. Of course health/medical informatics competencies are required. But additionally more general executive and managerial competencies, and business and economic competencies are necessary as well.

Depending on the size of the hospital, the role and the tasks of a CIO may be performed by one dedicated person (e.g., a full-time health/medical informatics specialist) or by a high-ranking member of the hospital's board (e.g., the chief executive officer, CEO). The CIO may be supported by an information management board. Such a board can often be found in larger hospitals (Fig. 9.7). Members should include one representative from the hospital's board of directors, representatives from the main departments and user groups, and the director of the information management department (see Sect. 9.3.2) if this director is not the CIO simultaneously. If no dedicated CIO position exists, the president of this board can be regarded as the CIO of the hospital.

The CIO should report directly to the CEO or the hospital's board of directors and, therefore, should be ranked rather high in the hospital's organizational hierarchy, optimally as a member of the top management team of the hospital. The CIO's role should be a strategic one that comprises the following tasks of *strategic information management*:

- make or prepare all relevant strategic decisions on the HIS, especially with respect to infrastructure, architecture, and information management organization;
- align the hospital's business plan with the strategic information management plan;
- establish and promote the strategic information management plan;
- initiate and control projects for *tactical information management*;
- initiate HIS evaluation studies and adequate HIS monitoring activities;
- identify and solve serious information management problems;
- report to the CEO or the hospital's board of directors.

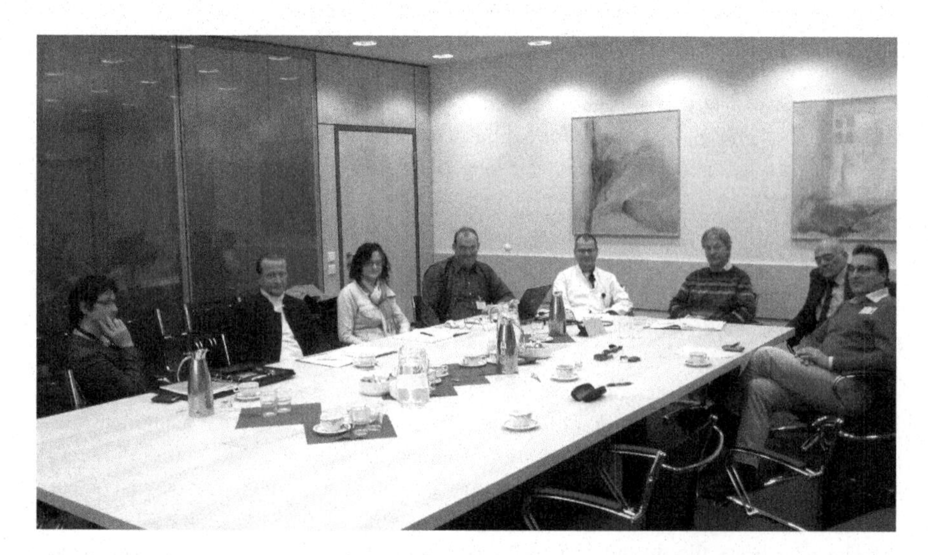

Fig. 9.7 An information management board meeting at a university hospital. Participants in this meeting are (from the left): the director of procurement, the chair of the staff council, the assistant of the information management department's director, the director of the information management department, a senior physician as chair of the board, a medical informatics professor as vice-chair of the board, a director of a medical research department as representative of the medical faculty and medical school, the director of nursing. The director of finance and vice-director of administration took the photo

The CIO's membership in the top management team should provide the possibility to influence the hospital's strategies using information technology as a strategic resource. Therefore, business knowledge and the ability to effectively communicate with other business managers, for example the chief financial officer (CFO) or the chief operating officer (COO), is important for a CIO. Nevertheless, reality often differs greatly from this image. Whether the role of the CIO is a strategic one or a more tactical or even operational one depends on internal hospital factors such as the CIO's top management membership, the internal communication networks among top executives and the CIO, the top management's strategic knowledge about ICT, the hospital's strategic vision of ICT, and on the personal skills of the CIO.

9.3.2 Information Management Department

There is usually one central information management department (often called the department for medical informatics, hospital computing center, or ICT department). This unit takes care at least of the *tactical* and *operational information management* of those parts of the HIS with hospital-wide relevance (e.g., the *enterprise resource planning system*, the *clinical information system*, and the *computer network*). In larger hospitals, there may be subdivisions with respect to tasks (e.g., different units for desktop management, user support, clinical systems, or networking).

If the information management department also cares of *strategic information management*, the head of this department is typically the CIO.

With regard to the responsibilities for *tactical* and *operational information management*, it is sometimes not useful and often not feasible to totally centralize these services. Especially in larger hospitals, they are performed in cooperation between central units and the decentralized staff. This staff may be dedicated medical informaticians or especially skilled users. These local information managers have responsibilities for *tactical* and *operational information management* with regard to their department, but in accordance with the central information management department. For example, they may (with support from the central unit) introduce a hospital-wide application component in their department, and operate it. On the other hand, they will also take care of additional information needs of their departments, for example by introducing a dedicated departmental system. However, this should be done only in accordance with the strategic information management plan.

9.3.3 Example

9.3.3.1 Organizational Structures for Information Management

Figure 9.8 presents the overall organization of information management at the Plötzberg Medical Center and Medical School (PMC).

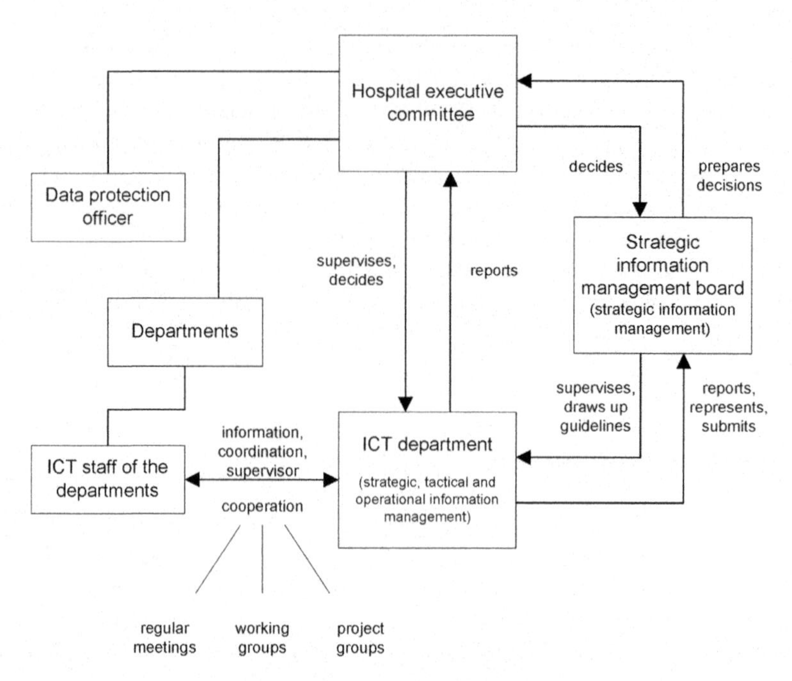

Fig. 9.8 Organization of information management at the Plötzberg Medical Center and Medical School (PMC)

9.3.4 Exercises

9.3.4.1 Information Systems Managers as Architects

Information systems managers can be partly compared to architects. Read the following statement, and discuss similarities and differences between information system architects and building architects:

> We're architects.... We have designed numerous buildings, used by many people.... We know about users. We know well their complaints: buildings that get in the way of the things they want to do.... We also know well users' joy of relaxing, working, learning, buying, manufacturing, and worshipping in buildings which were designed with love and tender care as well as function in mind.... We're committed to the belief that buildings help people to do their jobs or impede them and that good buildings bring joy as well as efficiency.[1]

[1]Caudill WW et al. Architecture and You. New York: Whitney Library of Design; 1978. p. 6.

9.3.4.2
Organizational Structures for Information Management in a Hospital

Look at a real hospital you know and at its information system.
- Which organizational units are involved in information management?
- Which boards and persons are involved in information management?
- Who is responsible for *strategic information management*?
- Who is responsible for *tactical information management*?
- Who is responsible for *operational information management*?
- Who is the CIO, and what is his or her responsibility?

9.3.4.3
Centralization of Organizational Structures

Discuss the pros and cons for centralization and decentralization of *strategic, tactical*, and *operational information management.* Find concrete examples for your arguments.

9.3.4.4
Organizational Structures for Information Management at PMC

Look at the description of the organizational structures for information management at the Plötzberg Medical Center and Medical School (PMC) in Fig. 9.8. Discuss the advantages and disadvantages of this organizational structure and discuss alternatives.

9.3.5
Summary

Each hospital should have an adequate organization for *strategic, tactical* and *operational information management.*

In general, a chief information officer (CIO) is responsible for information management. The CIO's most important tasks should be the strategic alignment of business plans and the strategic information management plan. She or he is responsible for all scopes of information management in the hospital.

There is typically one central department for information management. Usually the CIO directs this department. In addition, there may also be decentralized information management staff, located at the individual departments of the hospital. But this staff has to be coordinated by the CIO as well.

9.4 Strategic Planning

We will now focus on *strategic information management.* Strategic planning is the first step of a systematic *strategic information management* process and leads to a strategic information management plan as basis. It comprises planning of the HIS architecture and of the organization of information management.

After reading this section, you should be able to answer the following questions:
- What are the typical tasks for strategic HIS planning?
- What are the typical methods for strategic HIS planning?
- What is the goal and typical structure of a strategic information management plan?

9.4.1 Tasks

The most important tasks of strategic HIS planning are strategic alignment of business plans and strategic information management plans, long-term HIS planning, and short-term HIS planning.

9.4.1.1 Aligning Business Plans and Information Management Plans

The basis for *strategic information management* in a hospital are the strategic goals as defined in the hospital's business plan. Advances in ICT may influence these strategic business goals. Therefore, it is one main task of *strategic information management* to align business plans and strategic information management plans. Hospitals aim to provide efficient, high-quality health care. However, this mission may be further refined by goals as in Sect. 8.4.1, for example.

Different hospitals may choose different subsets of these goals, which would result in different information management strategies and different architectures of HIS. If hospital chosen goals are conflicting, *strategic information management* must try to solve these conflicts and establish a clear order of priorities, in accordance with the enterprise's business plan.

It is obvious that the CIO as person in charge for *strategic information management* needs knowledge about the enterprise strategy and the enterprise business plan. But also, the hospital's management needs knowledge about the potential of information processing with regard to formulation, realization, and evaluation of the hospital's strategy. *Strategic information management* must be able to offer this information to hospital management in adequate and understandable form. Methods for strategic alignment are presented in the methods section, below.

9.4.1.2
Long-Term HIS Planning

Strategic planning of HIS distinguishes between long-term and short-term HIS planning.

The strategic information management plan contains the results of long-term planning of HIS. It describes the hospital's goals, the information management goals, the current HIS state, the future HIS state, and the steps to transform the current HIS into the planned HIS. *Strategic information management* must create and regularly update this plan. The strategic plan must take into account quality criteria for HIS structures, processes, and outcome. It must be guaranteed that the strategic information management plan is the basis for all other information management activities. HIS planning is an ongoing process, and there is no use in trying to solve all problems at the same time. Solely a stepwise approach, based on different levels of priorities, is possible and useful. The strategic information management plan, therefore, must contain a general priority list of most important projects to be done in the coming years.

The long-term strategic information management plan is usually valid for a longer period of time (e.g., 3–5 years). However, requirements (e.g., due to legal changes or new user requests) and resources (staff, money) may change quicker than the strategic information management plan; or strategic monitoring (see Sect. 9.5) results may require an adjustment.

The detailed structure of strategic information management plans is described later on.

9.4.1.3
Short-Term HIS Planning

Major task of short-term HIS planning is to establish an (annual) project list with recent projects, priorities, and upcoming planned projects. This project list, also called the project portfolio, has to be approved by the hospital management, which decides which projects to execute and how to organize necessary resources. The project portfolio has to match the (more general) priority lists described in the strategic information management plan. However, its annual update reflects detailed prioritization and changes in the environment.

Because of the temporal limited validity of the strategic information management plan, HIS planning is a permanent task of *strategic information management* in hospitals.

9.4.2 Methods

9.4.2.1 Strategic Alignment

The role of information management varies between two extremes. At one extreme, information management may be seen as a purely supporting function; that is, the hospital strategy determines the information management planning activities. This is called "organizational pull." At the other extreme, information management is seen as the strategic resource, from which the hospital gains competitive advantage. The application of technological advances mainly determines the further development of the hospital and its position on the health care market. This is called "technology push." Strategic alignment describes the process that balances and coordinates the hospital goals and the information management strategies to get the best result for the hospital.

Several models exist for strategic alignment. The component alignment model (CAM) of Martin et al. considers seven components – the external environment, emerging information technologies, organizational infrastructure, mission, ICT infrastructure, business strategy and ICT strategy – that should be continually assessed with respect to their mutual alignment. Tan's critical success factor (CSF) approach is a top-down approach that first identifies factors critical to the hospital's success or failure. Strategic information management planning is then derived with regard to these factors.

Successful strategic alignment requires that hospital top management as well as information managers have a basic knowledge of each other's competence and share the same conception of the role of information management.

9.4.2.2 Portfolio Management

An important instrument for information management strategic planning is portfolio management. Originally coming from the field of finance to acquire a well-balanced securities portfolio, today the term portfolio management is used to refer to multiple strategic management problems.

Portfolio management concerning information management categorizes certain components of an information system, like application components or physical data processing systems, but also projects, using certain criteria to assess the value of these components for the enterprise and to balance risks and returns. The assumption is that there are different management issues and priorities for each class.

Project portfolio management categorizes projects, looking, for example, at project objectives, costs, time lines, resources, risks, and other critical factors. McFarlan proposes eight distinct project categories along the dimensions of project size, experience with the technology, and project structure. Each category carries a different degree of risk, and thus he recommends different project management tools to use. Today, project portfolio management is primarily used to plan and control IT investments.

The portfolio proposed by the Gartner Group distinguishes three categories according to the contribution of an application component to the hospital's performance. Utility applications are application components that are essential for the hospital's operation, but have no influence on the success of a hospital, and, therefore, are independent of the hospital's strategic goals. A good example is the *patient administration system*. Enhancement applications are application components that improve the hospital's performance, and, therefore, contribute to the hospital's success (e.g., computer-based *nursing management and documentation system*). Frontier applications are application components that influence the hospital's position in the health care market, for example, the enforced use of telemedicine. Information management planning should aim at a well-balanced application portfolio – on the one hand, to efficiently support essential hospital functions, and on the other hand, not to miss future technological innovations.

9.4.3 The Strategic Information Management Plan

An important aim of strategic HIS planning is to establish the strategic information management plan. The previous sections made clear that without a strategic information management plan, neither tactical nor operational management would work appropriately. A strategic information management plan is an important precondition for systematic directing and monitoring the hospital information system.

The strategic information management plan should be written by the CIO and approved by the hospital management. Without proper strategic planning, it would be a matter of chance if a hospital information system fulfilled strategic information goals. But considerable efforts have to be made for creating strategic plans.

In this section, the goals and structure of strategic information management plans are presented in more detail. Figure 9.9 presents an overall view on strategic information management planning.

9.4.3.1 Purpose of Strategic Information Management Plans

Different stakeholders[2] are involved in the creation, updating, approval, and use of strategic plans. Such stakeholders may include:

- top management;
- employees, e.g., physicians, nurses, administrative staff;
- clinical, administrative, service departments;
- information management department;
- funding institutions;
- consultants;
- hardware and software vendors.

[2]The term stakeholder is used to refer to anyone who has direct or indirect influence on or interest in a component of an information system.

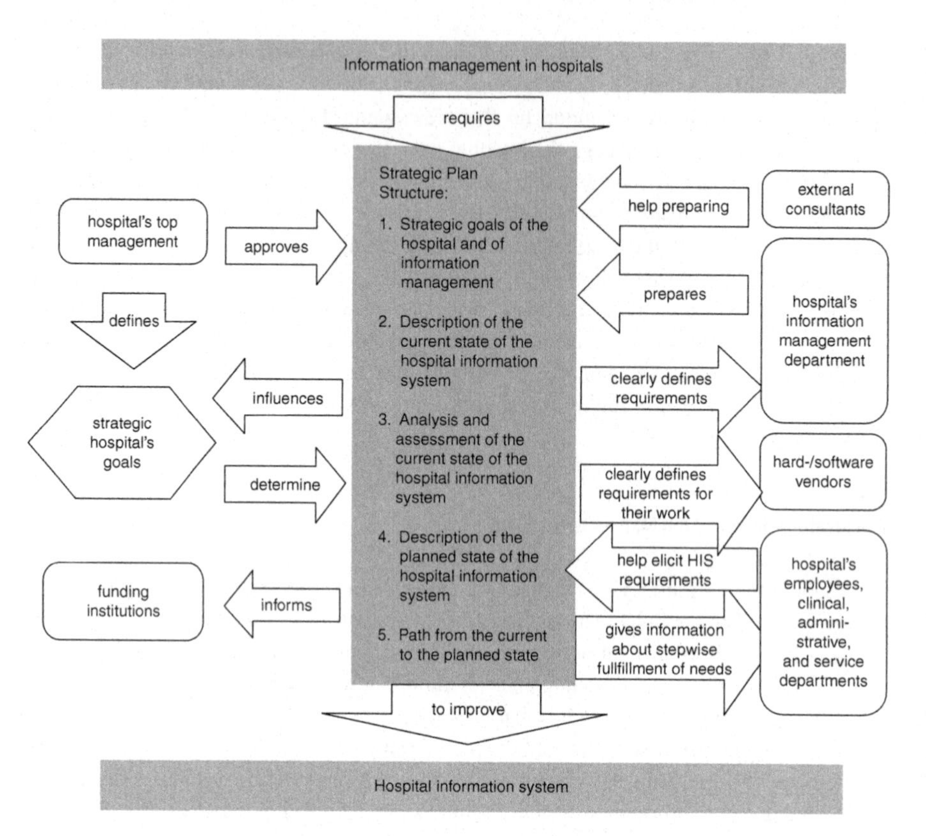

Fig. 9.9 Strategic information management planning of hospitals. A strategic information management plan gives directives for the construction and development of a hospital information system. It describes the recent and the intended hospital information system's architecture. (Details are explained in the following sections)

These stakeholders may have different expectations of a strategic plan and are involved in different life-cycle phases for strategic plans:

- creation, i.e., writing a first plan;
- approval, i.e., making some kind of contract among the stakeholders;
- deployment, i.e., asserting that the plan is put into practice;
- use, i.e., the involved stakeholders refer to the plan when needed;
- updating when a new version is required (because of new requirements, new available technologies, failure to achieve individual tasks, or just leaving the time frame of the plan). After the first version, the creation and update phases merge into a cyclic, evolutionary development of the plan.

The CIO and the information management department usually create and maintain proposals for the strategic information management plan. They are interested in clearly defined requirements for their work, which is greatly concerned with *tactical information management* issues. Top management is interested in the seamless and cost-effective operation of the hospital. Top management approves the plans (probably together with the funding institutions). Representatives of the employees should be involved in eliciting the requirements, since they will use the resulting information systems. The current strategic plans will be used by the information management departments and the vendors of HIS components when constructing or maintaining components of hospital information systems. External consultants may help to create plans, but also be engaged in negotiations for the approval of the plans.

The most essential purpose is to improve a hospital information system so that it can better contribute to the hospital's goals. This purpose should determine the structure of strategic plans; that is, it should show a path from the current situation to an improved situation, in which the hospital's goals are achieved as far as possible and reasonable.

9.4.3.2
Structure of Strategic Information Management Plans

A strategic information management plan should encompass the hospital's business strategy or strategic goals, the resulting information management goals, the current state of the hospital information system, and an analysis of how well the current information system fits the goals. The planned architecture should be derived as a conclusion of this analysis.

The strategic plan also has to deal with the resources needed to realize the planned architecture, and has to include rules for the operation of the resulting hospital information system and a description of appropriate organizational structures. Examples of resources are money, personnel, soft- and hardware, rooms for servers and (paper-based) archives, and rooms for training. The resources should fit the architecture and vice versa.
The general structure of strategic information management plans in hospitals can be summarized as follows:

- strategic goals of the hospital and of information management,
- description of the current state of the hospital information system,
- analysis and assessment of the current state of the hospital information system,
- description of the planned state of the hospital information system, and
- path from the current to the planned state.

This is only a basic structure that may be adapted to the specific requirements of individual hospitals. Particularly, a short management summary and appendices describing the organizational structure, personnel resources, the building structure, etc. are likely to complement a strategic plan.

Strategic Goals of the Hospital and of Information Management

Based on a description of the hospital's strategic goals (e.g., presented in a mission statement), the *strategic information management* goals should be derived using the method of strategic alignment (see Sect. 9.4.2.1). Despite the imperative to individually derive information management goals from the hospital's strategic goals predefined catalogs of goals may be helpful. One of these catalogs is provided by the information management standards of the Joint Commission in the USA (see Sect. 8.7.2).

Of course there will be goal conflicts eventually. They need to be taken into account and resolved.

Description of the Current State of the Hospital Information System

Before any planning commences, the hospital information system's current state should be described. This may require some discipline, because some stakeholders may be more interested in the planned (new) state than in the current (obsolete) state.

The description, i.e., a model of the current state is the basis for identifying those functions of the hospital that are well supported, for example, by information and communication technology, and those functions that are not (yet) well supported. Thus, application components as well as existing information and communication technology have to be described, including how they contribute to the support of the hospital's functions.

Hence the metamodel $3LGM^2$ (see Sect. 5.3) and related software is very helpful for this task.

Analysis and Assessment of the Current State of the Hospital Information System

The model of the current state has to be analyzed with respect to the achievement of information management strategies. Note that missing computer support for a certain function may not be assessed in all cases as being poor support for that function. For example, missing computers in patient rooms and consequently paper-based documentation of clinical findings may be conforming more to a goal of being a humane hospital than the use of computers and hand-held digital devices in this area.

Description of the Planned State of the Hospital Information System

Based on the analysis of the current state, a new state should be modeled that achieves the goals better than the current state does, provided that the current state does not already achieve the hospital's goals. Note that besides technical aspects, organizational aspects also have to be discussed. The model of the planned state can thus be completed by the description of the planned organizational structure of information management. In many cases, this is an opportunity to introduce a CIO or to clarify his or her role.

Migration Path from the Current to the Planned State

This section should describe a step-by-step path from the current to the planned state. In the strategic information management plan every such step is a project. Every project description should include assigned resources, that is, personnel, estimated investment costs as well as future operating costs, etc., and concrete deadlines for partial results. The resulting path of projects could also assign priorities to individual projects as well as dependencies between projects.

This migration path is the basis for annual project portfolio preparation.

9.4.4 Example

9.4.4.1 Structure of a Strategic Information Management Plan

Table 9.2 presents the structure of the strategic information management plan for 2010–2015 of the Plötzberg Medical Center and Medical School (PMC).

9.4.5 Exercises

9.4.5.1 Life Cycle of a Strategic Information Management Plan

Why is a strategic information management plan usually valid for 3–5 years? Could there be situations where a shorter or longer period may be useful? Explain your answer.

9.4.5.2 Deviation from a Strategic Information Management Plan

A strategic information management plan should serve as a guideline for information management. Could there be situations where information management is allowed to deviate from the strategic information management plan after it has been approved? Explain your answer.

9.4.5.3 Strategic Information Management and Strategic Hospital Management

We have discussed the strategic alignment of business plans and information management plans. Could you imagine situations where this alignment is difficult? Find examples where the hospital's goals and the information management goals may conflict. Discuss reasons and possible solutions.

Table 9.2 Structure of the strategic information management plan (2010–2015) of the Plötzberg Medical Center and Medical School (PMC)

1. Intention of this strategic information management plan
2. Plötzberg Medical Center and Medical School (PMC) 2.1 Mission statement 2.2 Strategic goals 2.3 Environment analysis 2.4 Organizational structure 2.5 Hospital indicators 2.6 Hospital layout
3. Current state of the information system 3.1 Goals of information management 3.2 Organization of information management 3.3 Guidelines and standards for information processing 3.4 Functionality 3.5 Application components 3.6 Physical data processing systems
4. Assessment of the current state of the information system 4.1 Goals attained 4.2 Weak points and strengths of the information systems 4.3 Required activities
5. Future state of the information system 5.1 Visions and perspectives 5.2 Planned functionality 5.3 Planned application components 5.4 Planned physical data processing systems 5.5 Planned organization of information management
6. Planned activities until 2015 6.1 Overview 6.2 Task planning 6.3 Time planning 6.4 Cost planning
7. Conclusion

9.4.5.4
Establishing a Strategic Information Management Plan

Imagine you are the CIO of a hospital in which almost no computer-based tools are used. One of the hospital's goals is to support health care professionals in their daily tasks by offering up-to-date patient information at their work-place.

Which main goals for information management would you define based on this information? Which hospital functions should be supported by new computer-based information processing tools?

9.4.6
Summary

Strategic information management deals with the hospital's information processing as a whole. It comprises planning of the HIS architecture and of the organization of information management.

Tasks of strategic HIS planning include strategic alignment of business plans and information management plans, long-term HIS planning, and short-term HIS planning. Strategic alignment describes a process to balance and coordinate hospital goals and information management strategies to get the best result for the hospital. The long-term planning of HIS is defined in the strategic information management plan. Short-term strategic HIS planning establishes an (annual) project portfolio.

A strategic information management plan is an important precondition for systematic monitoring and directing of the hospital information system. A strategic information management plan should encompass the hospital's business strategy or strategic goals, the resulting information management strategies, the current state of the hospital information system, and an analysis of how well the current information system fits the strategies. The planned architecture should be derived as a conclusion of this analysis. Finally, the path from the current to the planned state should be described.

The strategic information management plan should be written by the CIO and adopted by the hospital management.

9.5
Strategic Monitoring

After having planned the HIS strategically, one may expect the HIS will operate well in most of its functions, with most of its information processing tools, and in many parts of its operating organization. However, in many cases problems may occur. If we consider the quality criteria as discussed in Chapter 8 problems like the following may arise: Confidentiality of data may not be assured in some circumstances; transmission of reports may not be timely; adequate data integration capabilities may not be provided and thus consistency of redundant data may not be assured in a number of application components;

since there is no data warehouse, the hospital may not be able to collect and analyze aggregated data to support *patient care* and operations; the needs for knowledge-based information in *patient care* may hardly be met, since easy access to current medical journals is not provided. But there may be additional problems to be taken into account at a strategic level such as, for example, users may be increasingly dissatisfied with an application component, technical or motivational problems may lead to a decrease in documentation quality; increased documentation time may limit the time available for direct patient care; there may be unplanned high efforts for support and training; or the number of medical errors may rise due to software errors or unusable software.

Besides low software quality, also badly organized projects in *tactical information management* or errors in *strategic information management* may lead to the described problems.

Problems may get visible very slowly, for example, when a formerly "good" HIS component is not updated to match the overall technical progress, leading to more and more inacceptable performance and functionality; or, when more and more new application components have to be integrated into a spaghetti-styled architecture. But problems may also arise very suddenly, for example when a server suddenly crashes, and no replacement is available; or, when due to a software error, a wrong finding is presented to a patient, a physician takes a wrong decision, and the patient is harmed.

After reading this section, you should be able to answer the following questions:

- What are the typical tasks of strategic HIS monitoring?
- What are the typical methods of strategic HIS monitoring?

9.5.1 Tasks

As explained in Sect. 9.2.3, strategic monitoring means to continuously audit HIS quality, to make sure it corresponds to the quality defined in its strategic information plan. The management's task is to install "sensors" to audit the information system's quality. In general, strategic management has to make sure that it regularly receives and analyzes HIS quality information (permanent monitoring). In addition, information can be gained through dedicated evaluation projects (ad-hoc monitoring).

Typically, both permanent monitoring activities as well as ad-hoc monitoring activities are combined for strategic HIS monitoring. Both represent sub-types of an evaluation study. Thus, both activities should be planned and executed as described in details in Sect. 8.6, comprising the activities of study exploration, first study design, operationalization of methods and detailed study plan, execution of the study, and report and publication of the study.

9.5.1.1 Permanent Monitoring Activities

A hospital information system is too complex to allow monitoring all its components with regard to all quality criteria as defined in Chapter 8. However, it is useful to define subsets of criteria that should then be monitored on a regular (daily, weekly, monthly, yearly) basis.

Quantitative measurements for regular monitoring of the achievement of strategic goals are also called key performance indicators. These indicators could comprise, for example:

- functional coverage of the application components (e.g., level of saturation of the overall HIS architecture, see Sect. 8.2.2, or percentage of documents primarily created in computer-based form);
- user satisfaction (e.g., by regular user surveys);
- standardization of the HIS architecture (e.g., percentage of interfaces using standards such as HL7);
- homogeneity of the HIS architecture (e.g., number of different application components);
- availability of the application components (e.g., down times per year);
- performance of the application components (e.g., response time);
- costs for information management (e.g., overall costs, costs in relation to number of users or number of workstations);
- quality of IT training (e.g., IT training hours per user);
- quality of IT support (e.g., number of hotline calls that are successfully solved within 2 h);
- quality of *tactical information management* (e.g., percentage of successfully completed IT projects).

To allow monitoring on a regular base, these key performance indicators should be collected in quantitative and as far as possible in automated form. Reports should be presented to the information management board.

Besides monitoring those indicators, further permanent monitoring tasks may comprise patient satisfaction surveys, medical error reports, or the local press containing comments on the hospital's HIS. In addition, national legislation (e.g., new data protection law) and standardization initiatives (e.g., new version of HL7) should be monitored as both may affect the HIS.

Sudden changes in monitored numbers can indicate problems (e.g., malfunctioning of a component), which could then initiate more detailed analysis and corrections that are then to be initiated by strategic directing.

Permanent monitoring activities can be used locally, but they can also be used to compare HIS quality with other organizations or with established standards in the form of a so-called benchmarking. Details on HIS benchmarking are explained later in Sect. 9.5.3.1.

9.5.1.2 Ad Hoc Monitoring Activities

Ad-hoc monitoring activities may be initiated when larger changes of a component are planned, or when sudden larger problems of HIS components have been observed. Ad-hoc activities help to analyze a certain situation in detail, in order to better understand reasons and consequences of an observed or expected problem. The execution of those ad-hoc activities entails systems evaluation studies which are planned and conducted by *tactical information management*.

Evaluation studies can focus on structure quality, process quality and quality of outcome of a HIS component (see Sects. 8.2–8.4). For example, during the introduction of a *nursing documentation and management system*, the effects on nursing care could be analyzed by a sub-set of the following evaluation questions:

- How accurate and complete is nursing documentation after introduction of a computer-based nursing documentation system?
- How are nurses satisfied with the new component?
- Is the offered functionality sufficient to support all steps of the nursing care process?
- Is there any redundant functionality with other components?
- Did the introduction of the component affect the time that is available for direct patient care?
- Does the quality of nursing care change?
- Did the level of data integration with regard to nursing data improve after the introduction of the component?
- How is the consistency of nursing data, comparing the new component and the remaining paper-based patient chart?
- What did the purchase and introduction of the component cost?
- What do support and training of the component cost?
- Are there any unexpected negative effects on nursing care?

Typically, quantitative and qualitative methods (see Sect. 8.6 for details) can be combined to answer study questions. Strategic HIS monitoring collects and reports the results, to directly give feedback to strategic HIS planning.

9.5.1.3
Certification of HIS

Certification in general means to confirm that an object or organization has certain characteristics. HIS certification in general describes a process where an accredited body confirms that the HIS fulfills certain pre-defined quality characteristics. While approaches to assess the overall HIS quality are rare, there exist established certification systems for individual software products (e.g., software for a *medical documentation system*) such as CCHIT and EuroRec (for details on different approaches, see Sect. 9.5.3). Depending on the certification approach, security, functionality or interoperability of the application component are assessed.

Many vendors try to obtain these certificates, as they hope to get an competitive advantage. In fact, when buying software for a new application component, more and more hospitals check for the availability of these certificates. In general, certification increases transparency of different products and fosters buyers' knowledge about products, as certification organizations often compile information about the different products and technologies. Increased transparency and knowledge in turn have a positive impact on the buyers' willingness to invest in new technology. Even when a HIS certification does not guarantee that a HIS is good with regard to all and every criteria, certification may contribute to an increased quality of HIS in general.

9.5.2 Methods

Details on planning and execution of evaluation studies as well as on general evaluation methods have already been presented in Sect. 8.6. They form the basis for ad-hoc studies. We will now concentrate on HIS benchmarking, as an approach for permanent monitoring activities, as well as on HIS certification approaches.

9.5.2.1 HIS Benchmarking

Benchmarking in general describes a process in which organizations evaluate various aspects of their performance and compare it to a given standard or to the best organizations ("best-practice"). Typically, benchmarking comprises quantitative evaluation criteria such as costs, quality of structures, quality of processes, or quality of outcome. In strategic hospital management, benchmarking is seen as an important approach to assess a hospital's performance. Benchmarking is often seen part of a continuous quality improvement process, in which organizations measure and then steadily improve their performance.

If a hospital wants to establish permanent monitoring activities on its HIS in the form of a best-practice-benchmark, it needs to select standardized and clearly defined evaluation criteria. Often, regional groups of hospitals join together on an ad-hoc basis to define and compare their HIS benchmarking criteria. Besides, there are also international standards for HIS benchmarking. For example, the criteria defined by COBIT (compare the example 9.5.3.2) or criteria derived from ITIL (Sect. 9.2.6) are used to benchmark especially the quality of information management.

9.5.2.2 HIS Certification

Several approaches for the certification of hospitals and their HIS exist. For example, ISO 9001 standard[3] assesses the hospital's compliance with certain quality management standards. An ISO 9001 certificate states that an organization follows certain formalized business processes, that it monitors the outcome of its processes, and that it facilitates their continuous improvement; ISO 9001 focuses on the quality of processes. Another example is the Joint Commission's certification program; details of which have already been presented in Sect. 8.7.2. So-called excellence programs, such as the EFQM Excellence Model[4] in Europe or the Malcolm Baldrige National Quality Award in the U.S. (for details, see Sect. 8.7.1) also strive for quality improvement. They use a scoring system that makes it possible to compare the performance of organizations to one another, and to continually observe improvement in

---

[3]International Organization for Standardization. ISO 9001 standards on quality management, http://www.iso.org

[4]European Federation for Quality Management (EFQM) http://ww1.efqm.org

quality of structures, quality of processes, or quality of outcome. Most of these certification or excellence programs also comprise aspects on the quality of a HIS. For example, the Baldrige program (see Sect. 8.7.1) and the Joint Commission standards (see Sect. 8.7.2) offer specific health care information management criteria, to different extents.

There also exist certification approaches specific for hospital information systems. In the USA, the Certification Commission for Healthcare Information Technology (CCHIT)[5] is developing quality criteria and a certification process for Electronic Health Records. In Europe, the EuroRec Institute[6] is developing a repository of certification criteria to support quality certification for Electronic Health Records. Finally, the IHE initiative[7] tries to achieve interoperability between different clinical information systems based on existing standards such as HL7 and DICOM. IHE offers a standardized interoperability testing of clinical application components of different vendors in so-called Connectathons that take place in different parts of the world each year.

9.5.3 Examples

9.5.3.1 A HIS Benchmarking Report

The CIO of the Plötzberg Medical Center and Medical School (PMC) bi-annually reports to the hospital's management about the amount, quality, and costs of information processing of Plötzberg's hospital information system. For this report, the CIO uses HIS benchmarking criteria that have been agreed to by a regional group of hospitals' CIOs (see Table 9.3). Each year, the hospitals exchange and discuss their reports as part of a best-practice-benchmark.

9.5.3.2 COBIT

CobiT[8] is developed by the IT Governance Institute. It provides a common language for executives to communicate goals, objectives and expected results of IT systems and IT projects. COBIT is built on a process model that defines 34 IT-related processes within four domains: plan and organize; acquire and implement; deliver and support; monitor and

[5]Certification Commission for Healthcare Information Technology, http://www.cchit.org
[6]EuroRec, http://www.eurorec.org
[7]IHE International, http://www.ihe.net
[8]http://www.isaca.org/cobit

Table 9.3 Extract from the PMC HIS benchmarking report 2010 (KPI = key performance indicator)

KPIs for the organization	
Number of staff	5,500
Number of beds	1,100
Number of inpatient cases	40,000
Mean duration of stay	8.1 days
KPIs for HIS costs	
Overall IT costs	€5 million
IT investment costs	€0.8 million
IT costs per inpatient case	€125
IT costs in relation to hospital budget	1.7%
KPIs for HIS management	
Number of HIS staff	45.5
Number of HIS users	4,800
Number of workstations	1,350
Hospital staff per workstation	4.1
Number of IT problem tickets	15,500
Percentage of solved tickets	97.5%
Availability of the overall HIS systems	97.5%
Number of IT projects finalized	13
Percentage of successful IT projects	76%
KPIs for HIS functionality	
Percentage of all documents available electronically	45%
Percentage of all diagnosis coded electronically	77%
Functionality index[9] of patient administration system	52%
Functionality index of medical documentation system	87%
Functionality index of …	…
KPIs for HIS architecture	
Number of computer-based application components	84
Percentage of standard interfaces between applications	87%
Functional redundancy rate[10]	0.44

[9]A functionality index describes how many of the related hospital functions are already supported by a computer-based application system.
[10]For details, see Sect. 8.7.4.

evaluate. For each of these 34 processes, among others, information is provided on how the specific process goals can be measured, what the key activities and major deliverables are, and who is responsible for them. The following list presents an overview of the four domains and selected, simplified key metrics (key performance indicators) for each of them.

Plan and Organize

This domain covers strategy and tactics, and concerns the identification of the way IT can best contribute to the achievement of the business objectives. Selected key metrics:

- percentage of strategic IT objectives that are aligned to the strategic hospital plan;
- percentage of redundant or duplicated data elements within the IT architecture;
- number of business processes that are not yet supported by IT;
- percentage of stakeholders that are satisfied with IT quality;
- percentage of IT projects that are on time and within budget.

Acquire and Implement

IT solutions need to be identified, developed or acquired, implemented and integrated into the business process as well as maintained. Selected key metrics:

- percentage of users that are satisfied with the functionality of the new IT system;
- number of IT problems that lead to non-operation periods;
- percentages of IT systems that do not conform to the defined technical standards;
- percentage of IT systems where adequate user training is provided.

Deliver and Support

This domain is concerned with the actual delivery of required IT services, including management of security and continuity, service support for users, and management of data and operational facilities. Selected key metrics:

- percentage of stakeholders that are satisfied with IT support;
- number of user complaints with regard to an IT service;
- percentage of satisfactory response times of an IT system;
- number of lost hours due to unplanned IT downtimes.

Monitor and Evaluate

All IT processes need to be regularly assessed over time for their quality and compliance with control requirements. Selected key metrics:

- frequency of reporting from IT management to enterprise management;
- satisfaction of management with IT performance reporting;
- number of independent IT reviews.

9.5.3.3 CCHIT Functional Quality Criteria

CCHIT is a not-for-profit organization and offers certification for inpatient EHRs, ambulatory EHRs and other application components.[11] The certification primarily covers functionality, security, and interoperability, and is hierarchically structured in criteria and sub-criteria. Table 9.4 shows some examples of functional criteria.[12] Vendors are provided with a certification handbook and test-scripts for self-evaluation. The actual certification is then carried out by CCHIT auditors. The CCHIT certificate is typically valid for 3 years.

Table 9.4 Examples of CCHIT functional criteria for medication ordering

	Criteria
10.01	The system shall provide the ability to define a set of items to be ordered as a group
10.04	The system shall provide the ability to allow the clinician to order medication doses in mg/kg/min, μg/kg, and μg/kg/min
10.06	The system shall provide end-users with the ability to browse or search for a drug by therapeutic class when ordering a medication
10.14	The system shall provide the ability to modify medication orders including dosing information without having to discontinue the order
10.26	The system shall provide the ability to compute drug doses, based on appropriate dosage ranges, using the patient's body surface area and ideal body weight
12.01	The system shall provide the ability to check for potential interactions between medications to be prescribed/ordered and current medications and alert the user at the time of medication prescribing/ordering if potential interactions exist

[11]Certification Commission for Health Information Technology, http://www.cchit.org

[12]Taken from Inpatient EHR Criteria at http://www.cchit.org/sites/all/files/certifications/2011Inpatient_4.zip

9.5.4 Exercises

9.5.4.1 An Information Processing Monitoring Report

Look at the HIS benchmarking report in example 9.5.3.1. Figure out some numbers for a hospital you know. It may help to look at the strategic information management plan of this hospital.

9.5.4.2 COBIT

Please look at the examples of COBIT key metrics presented in Sect. 9.5.3.2. Analyze how they correspond to the quality criteria for structures, for processes, and for outcomes as described in Chapter 8. To which quality criteria can they be matched?

9.5.4.3 Most Relevant Key Performance Indicators

In case you had to select the five most relevant indicators for HIS quality for your hospital: Which would you select? You can look at examples in Sect. 8.7 and in Sect. 9.5.3 to get ideas. How would you proceed to get regular information on your five most relevant indicators?

9.5.4.4 Organizing User Feedback

You are asked to organize regular user feedback facilities for the *medical documentation system* of your hospital. How would you proceed? How would you gather user feedback? Which user groups would you take into account? Which types of data (quantitative and/or qualitative) would you collect? Which technical means would you use? Discuss different possibilities.

9.5.5 Summary

The task of strategic HIS monitoring is to continually audit the quality of the hospital information system at strategic level. Monitoring can be done on a permanent base, but also as dedicated ad-hoc monitoring activities.

Permanent monitoring activities comprise the definition of a subset of quantitative key performance indicators that are to be automatically monitored on a regular (daily, weekly, monthly, yearly) basis. Permanent monitoring is supported by national and international certification, accreditation or excellence activities. Ad hoc monitoring activities are organized as regular evaluation studies.

9.6 Strategic Directing

Strategic directing of HIS is a consequence of planning and monitoring hospital functions, HIS architectures, and information management organizations.
After reading this section, you should be able to answer the following questions:
- What are the typical tasks of strategic HIS directing?
- What are the typical methods of strategic HIS directing?

9.6.1 Tasks

Strategic directing of information systems mainly transforms the strategic information management plan into projects. These projects are taken from the strategic project portfolio or the migration path as established in the strategic information management plan. The decision to initiate projects is part of strategic information planning; the execution of this decision is part of strategic information directing.

Planning, running, and (successfully) finishing projects are tasks of *tactical information management*. However, strategic directing must initiate them and prepare an adequate framework for them. In detail, the following main tasks can be identified:
- initiation of projects;
- general resource allocation;
- general time allocation;
- general controlling of the project progress;
- adoption of the project's results.

9.6.2 Methods

For a project of important strategic relevance (e.g., introduction of a hospital-wide *clinical information system*), a project management board will typically be established.
Such a project management board supports the project manager by providing an interface between the project manager, future user groups, vendors involved in the project, and strategic information management authorities like CIO and information management board. Its tasks are:
- controlling the project with respect to allocated resources, allocated time and the planned results,
- settling disputes and solving conflicts which may arise between project management, vendors, involved hospital departments and strategic management authorities.

Typically, the project management board comprises representatives from strategic information management authorities, from hospital management and from the hospital departments and vendors involved. The project manager reports to this board and should be part of it.

9.6.3 Example

9.6.3.1 Project Management Boards at PMC

Currently, two project management boards are established at Plötzberg Medical Center and Medical School (PMC):

1. Project management board for the *clinical information system*. Head of the board is the CIO. Members are representatives from the hospital board of managers (vice president for nursing, vice president for administration), representatives from the main user groups (senior physician from the surgery department, senior physician from the internal medicine department), a representative of the software vendor, as well as the project manager.
2. Project management board for the introduction of a new computer-based intensive care *patient data management system*. Head is the manager of the quality assurance department. Members are the manager of the information management department, representatives from main user groups (senior physician and head nurse from the surgery department), and the project manager.

9.6.4 Exercise

9.6.4.1 A Project Management Board at PMC

At the Plötzberg Medical Center and Medical School (PMC), a project is going to be initiated to introduce a hospital-wide *nursing documentation system*. This application component comprises functionality of comprehensive nursing data management as well as supporting communication with other health care professionals.

Due to the high significance of nursing documentation, a project management board will be installed. Who should the members of this board be? Explain your answer.

9.6.5 Summary

Strategic directing of information systems mainly consists of transforming the strategic information management plan into projects. It is at least as important as strategic planning and strategic monitoring, but often, from a methodological point of view, an immediate consequence of them.

For projects of important strategic relevance (e.g., introduction of a hospital-wide *electronic patient record system*), a project management board typically is established. This project management board serves as an interface between *strategic* and *tactical information management*.

9.7
Last But Not Least: Education!

For *strategic information management* in hospitals, well-educated specialists in health informatics/medical informatics are needed. They should have appropriate knowledge and skills to systematically manage such information systems, in order to appropriately and responsibly apply information and communication technology to the complex information processing environment of hospitals – and beyond (see, e.g., the next chapter).

Curricular national frameworks for educating such specialists are very important. In this book and with respect to this importance, we want to refer to the recently updated recommendations of the International Medical Informatics Association (IMIA) on education.[13] These recommendations are designed to help in establishing courses, course tracks or complete programs in biomedical and health informatics and to further develop existing educational activities in the various nations. They also provide examples of how education has been established within nations.

The IMIA recommendations by the way clearly and explicitly mention the relevance of educating knowledge and skills in health information systems and its architectures and strategies (see also the citations at the beginning of this book).

As education is not in the scope of this book, we only want to refer to the need to educate. The exclamation mark at the end of this section heading should help to highlight the outstanding importance of education for professional and high-quality information management.

9.8
Summarizing Examples

9.8.1
Deficiencies in Information Management

The following letter was written by the head of the Department of Internal Medicine of the Plötzberg Medical Center and Medical School (PMC) to the chief executive officer. He complains about failures in information management.

> Dear colleague,
>
> I am sitting here again, having organized the duties for Good Friday and the whole Easter weekend in a way that *patient care* as far as the physicians are concerned is guaranteed. I can also be sure that nursing is well organized for these days, so I want to use the holidays to catch up with my work in the clinic. On the other hand, I have to realize that the network

[13]Mantas J et al.; IMIA Recommendations on Education Task Force. Recommendations of the International Medical Informatics Association (IMIA) on Education in Biomedical and Health Informatics. Methods Inf Med. 2010;49:105–120. Accessible, e.g., at www.IMIA.org

of our clinic is down yet again and that consequently, starting from the door-keeper's office to every ward and every lab, there isn't any kind of data processing or EDP support. The door-keeper sends visitors coming to see their relatives to the wards by trusting their luck. At the wards, essential information is missing and scientific work is delayed by the cutting off of all internal and external scientific networks.

With this letter I want to express my protest once again and complain about the fact that the way information processing is managed in our hospital is completely unacceptable. I do not know what still has to happen so that we can finally get an emergency service for nights and for holidays. This is why I want to ask you to immediately make sure in the board of the PMC and in the Committee for Information Processing that such a technical standby service is installed for the maintenance of the network and for breakdowns in the same way that we provide on-call services for all important clinical processes.

In summary, I want to express my deep disappointment about the whole situation. Nowadays, information processing has gained such an important standing in daily patient care that we can really put patients at risk if we do not immediately – and with this I mean at once – find a remedy for this problem.

Yours sincerely,
in a very annoyed mood
Prof. Dr. K.
Director of the Dept. of Internal Medicine

9.8.2 Computer Network Failures[14]

The computer system of Plötzberg Medical Center and Medical School (PMC) crashed repeatedly over 3½ days last week, periodically blocking access to patient records, prescriptions, laboratory reports, and other information, and forcing the hospital to revert to the paper-based systems of what one executive called "the hospital of the 1970s."

Hospital executives said yesterday that patient safety was never jeopardized. But scores of employees worked overtime printing records, double-checking doses, physically running messages from the labs to the wards and back – even rushing to buy copier paper on the credit card of the chief operating officer (COO), Dr. E. The crisis, which lasted from Wednesday afternoon until Sunday, took the hospital by surprise. Its electronic network was named the nation's best in health care last year by the magazine Information Week, and its chief information officer (CIO), Dr. H., is an authority on medical computing.

As hospitals are urged to convert their record keeping to computers as part of the battle against errors, hospital and public health officials are calling the incident a wake-up call for hospitals across the country, whose computer systems may not be able to keep up with their growing work load. At PMC, the systems handle 40 terabytes of information daily – or 40 times the information in the Library of Congress.

[14]This example is based on a report in Boston Globe, November 19, 2002, page B1.

"Imagine if you built a house and you put in an extension cord to it, and then you hook up a lawnmower, and then you hook up a barbecue. Eventually the breaker is going to blow," the CIO, Dr. H., said. "I as CIO feel a moral obligation to share the lessons we have learned over the last few days with every other CIO in the country. Have you got systems in place to deal with a problem like this? And if you have infrastructures that are at risk, have you done due diligence to really look at your hospital and make changes?"

Although computer systems have allowed hospitals to work with more speed and flexibility, executives said, last week's events showed how frightening it can be when they fail. "Any time you're taking care of very sick patients, when everything isn't as you're used to it, you get a little nervous," said the COO, Dr. E.

The crisis began when a researcher installed software to analyze data, and a large amount of information started flowing over the network. Doctors noticed intermittent problems with e-mail and data entry. But at 4 p.m. on Wednesday, most of the systems – from e-mail to accessing patient records to entering laboratory data – slowed or stopped and stayed down for 2 h.

The hospital called in a special forces team of specialists from the manufacturer that provides and maintains its computer networks. But the crashes kept happening every 4–6 h, so rather than go back and forth between paper and computer systems, the hospital decided to switch to all-paper.

The emergency room shut down for most of Friday, and the hospital decided to refuse all transfers except in life-threatening emergencies. Some lab tests that normally take 45 min to complete took closer to 2 h, so doctors reverted to lower-tech methods of diagnosis. "There was a sense of old-fashioned medicine," said Dr. S., an intensive-care physician.

In response to the incident, the manufacturer plans to warn hospitals to update their systems, the CIO said. He also plans to talk about the subject with the systems managers of the state's hospitals on Thursday, at a previously planned meeting of the regional Health Data Consortium.

All hospitals were required to put in disaster plans. PMC had such a plan in place, but because systems evolve so quickly, it was already outdated. The hospital has not calculated how much the computer setbacks will cost. The COO said there may be some delay in receiving payments from insurers because billing relies on the computer network.

9.8.3 Information Management Responsibilities[15]

The senior executives (chief executive officers, chief operating officers, or chief information officers) at ten health care organizations conducted audits to evaluate the effectiveness of information management in their own organizations. The organizations ranged from rural hospitals to university affiliated teaching hospitals, with bed size ranging from 60 to 1,232.

[15]This example is based on Austin KD, Hornberger JE, Shmerling JE, Managing information resources: a study of ten healthcare organizations, J Healthc Manag 45(4);2000:229–238; discussion 238–239.

The audits evaluated how well the following seven information technology management responsibilities were carried out: (1) strategic information systems planning; (2) employment of a user focus in system development; (3) recruiting of competent IT personnel; (4) information systems integration; (5) protection of information security and confidentiality; (6) employment of effective project management in system development; and (7) postimplementation evaluation of information systems.

The audit results suggest that most of these responsibilities are being met to a considerable extent by a majority of the organizations studied. However, substantial variation across organizations was noted. Executives participating in the study were able to define areas in which the management of information resources in their organizations was in need of attention. The audit process encourages senior management to provide the leadership required to ensure that information technology is used to maximum advantage.

9.8.4 Safely Implementing Health Information and Converging Technologies

From the Sentinel Event Alert from the Joint Commission, Issue 42, December 11, 2008[16]:

> "As health information technology (HIT) and "converging technologies" – the interrelationship between *medical devices* and HIT – are increasingly adopted by healthcare institutions, users must be mindful of the safety risks and preventable adverse events that these implementations can create or perpetuate....
>
> There is a dearth of data on the incidence of adverse events directly caused by HIT overall. The United States Pharmacopeia MEDMARX database includes 176,409 medication error records for 2006.... Of those medication error records, 43,372, or approximately 25 percent, involved some aspect of computer technology as at least one cause of the error....
>
> Inadequate technology planning can result in poor product selection, a solution that does not adapt well to the local clinical environment, or insufficient testing or training. Inadequacies include failing to include front-line clinicians in the planning process, to consider best practices, to consider the costs and resources needed for ongoing maintenance, or to consult product safety reviews or alerts or the previous experience of others. Implementing new clinical information systems can expose latent problems or flawed processes with existing manual systems; these problems should be identified and resolved before implementing the new system. Technology-related adverse events also happen when healthcare providers and leaders do not carefully consider the impact technology can have on care processes, workflow and safety.
>
> If not carefully planned and integrated into workflow processes, new technology systems can create new work, complicate workflow, or slow the speed at which clinicians carry out clinical documentation and ordering processes. Learning to use new technologies takes time and attention, sometimes placing strain on demanding schedules. The resulting change to clinical practices and workflows can trigger uncertainty, resentment or other emotions that can affect the worker's ability to carry out complex physical and cognitive tasks. Additionally, safety is compromised when healthcare information systems are not integrated or updated consistently. Systems not properly integrated are prone to data

[16]http://www.jointcommission.org/SentinelEvents/SentinelEventAlert/sea_42.htm

fragmentation because new data must be entered into more than one system. Multiple networks can result in poor interoperability and increased costs. If data are not updated in the various systems, records become outdated, incomplete or inconsistent."

9.8.5 Increased Mortality After Implementation of a Computerized Physician Order Entry System[17]

The Department of Critical Care Medicine of the University of Pittsburgh School of Medicine, Pennsylvania, USA, implemented a commercially sold computerized *physician order entry system* (*CPOE*) in an effort to reduce medical errors and mortality. The researchers had the hypothesis that *CPOE* implementation results in reduced mortality among children who are transported for specialized care. During an 18-month period, demographic, clinical, and mortality data were collected of all children who were admitted via interfacility transport to the hospital. During this period, a commercially sold *CPOE* program was implemented hospital-wide. The data were retrospectively analyzed comparing pre-CPOE and post-CPOE period. The researchers found that, using univariate analysis, mortality rate significantly increased from 2.80% (39 of 1394) before *CPOE* implementation to 6.57% (36 of 548) after CPOE implementation. The authors argue that they found an unexpected increase in mortality coincident with *CPOE* implementation. Reasons they discuss comprise increased time needed for documenting orders which interferes with the time-criticial treatment of very ill patients, interruptions of communication processes between physicians and nurses by the *CPOE*, and delayed administration of time-sensitive medication.

9.9 Summarizing Exercises

9.9.1 Management of Other Information Systems

Are there any differences between management of hospital information systems and management of information systems in other industries? Explain your answer.

9.9.2 Beginning and End of Information Management

When does hospital information management start, and when does it end? Directing and monitoring are ongoing tasks of information management. Is this true for planning as well?

[17]cf.: Han YY, Carcillo JA, Venkataraman ST, Clark RS, Watson RS, Nguyen TC, Bayir H, Orr RA. Unexpected increased mortality after implementation of a commercially sold computerized physician order entry system. Pediatrics. 2005 Dec;16(6):1506–1512.

9.9.3
Cultivating Hospital Information Systems

Look at the following description of the duties of a forest's owner (taken from respective German law) and discuss the similarities and differences of cultivating a forest and of information management in a hospital:

The duties of a forest's owner are:
- to cultivate the forest according to its purpose,
- lastingly...
- carefully...
- systematically... and
- competently...,
- using recognized forest-managerial methods...

9.9.4
Hospital Information System Failure

Look at example 9.8.2. What are the reasons given for this hospital information system failure? What has been the impact of this failure on clinical workflow and *patient care*? Analyze the problems and suggest appropriate activities to prevent the described problems in the future.

9.9.5
Increased Mortality

Please look at example 9.8.3 and try to explain how the *CPOE* could have contributed to an increase in mortality rates. Please look also at example 9.8.4 to solve this question.

9.9.6
Relevance of Examples

Note that the examples given in Sect. 9.8 are partly taken from the first edition of this textbook and are therefore rather old. What do you think about the relevance of these examples for information management nowadays? (How) do you think, technology and organization of information management have changed?

9.9.7
Problems of Operational Information Management

Look at the following problems, derived from the report of the assessment of the *operational information management* at Plötzberg Medical Center and Medical School (PMC). How would you proceed to solve these problems?

- The ICT Department (see example 9.3.3.1) is distributed over several areas that are some miles away from the hospital's building. This causes long delays, loss of information, and delayed response times in case of local problems.
- The costs of information management and information processing are unclear. For example, the total costs of the introduction of an electronic mailing system for all staff of the hospital are not exactly known.
- In the case of emergencies (e.g., fire) in the computing center, there may be extensive data losses and a longer unavailability of important application components.

9.10 Summary

High quality HIS can only by achieved and HIS failures can only be prevented if HIS are systematically planned, monitored and directed.

The tasks of information management in hospitals are planning, directing, and monitoring of HIS. It can be distinguished into *strategic, tactical*, and *operational information management. Strategic information management* deals with the hospital's information processing as a whole. *Tactical information management* deals with particular enterprise functions or application components. *Operational information management* is responsible for operating the components of the hospital information system.

Each hospital should have an adequate organization for *strategic, tactical*, and *operational information management*. In general, a chief information officer (CIO) should be responsible for information management and a central information management department. If there is decentralized information management staff, located at the individual departments of the hospital, this staff has to be controlled by the CIO.

Consequently high quality HIS need not only adequate financial investments but also considerable financial and human resources for their *strategic, tactical*, and *operational information management*.

Strategic HIS planning deals with planning of HIS architecture and the organization of information management. Tasks of strategic HIS planning are the strategic alignment of business plans and information management plans, the long-term HIS planning, and the short-term HIS planning. The main methods are the strategic alignment of hospital goals and information management goals, adequate portfolio management, and the establishment of a strategic information management plan.

Strategic HIS monitoring aims to continually audit the quality of the hospital information system. It comprises permanent monitoring activities as well as ad hoc monitoring activities such as dedicated evaluation studies.

Strategic HIS directing mainly consists of transforming the strategic information management plan into projects.

Summarizing, some quality criteria for an efficient information management can be defined, such as:

- systematic *strategic information management* with a strategic information management plan as the basis;

- systematic *tactical information management*, with clear management of the projects;
- systematic *operational information management*, with an appropriate support strategy to guarantee the continuous and faultless operation of the information processing tools;
- clear decision structures, roles, and responsibilities for *strategic, tactical*, and *operational information management*;
- sufficient and ongoing training of the users;
- motivation and competence of IT staff, which is essential for the efficient functioning of the information systems and for a high acceptance by the users.

Strategic Information Management in Health Care Networks

10

10.1 Introduction

In Chap. 7, we discussed specific architectural aspects that have to be considered in a transinstitutional health information system, which is the information system of a health care network. We will now examine how *strategic information management* works in such networks.

Similar to information system architectures, principles of *strategic information management* in health care networks turn out to be similar to *strategic information management* in hospitals. But since such a network is a group of legally separated health care institutions, the managerial authority in health care networks can hardly be centralized in one organizational unit. Thus, we are faced with polycentric or decentralized organizations, resulting in the following challenges:

- While members of health care networks remain legally autonomous, the mutual dependency rises with increasing importance of the network.
- While members of health care networks have to cooperate in order to provide high-quality and efficient care, they may compete in other sectors.
- While trust between health care network members is an important factor for the success of the network, the economic risk rises with increasing dependency on cooperation partners.
- While members of health care networks have to specialize in their core competencies on the one hand, they need to align their transinstitutional care processes on the other hand.

A consequence of these characteristics is that in health care networks each member follows its own strategy on the one hand but the network has to fulfill its goal on the other hand. Typically no single person in charge, i.e., a CIO (see Sect. 9.3.1), exists in health care networks. Hence, the typical (ideal) organizational structure of *strategic information management* as presented in Sect. 9.3 cannot always be applied.

In this chapter, we can forbear from repeating the principles of strategic planning, monitoring, and directing health information systems. But we have to supplement Sect. 9.3 by examining additional organizational aspects of *strategic information management* when legally separated institutions cooperate in networks.

A. Winter et al., *Health Information Systems*,
DOI: 10.1007/978-1-84996-441-8_10, © Springer-Verlag London Limited 2011

In contrast to single institutions with hierarchical structures, such as hospitals, the interests of many legally autonomous actors have to be coordinated in health care networks. After reading this chapter you should be able to answer the following questions:

- What are health care networks?
- How can health care networks be described?
- What organizational structures are appropriate for information management in health care networks?

10.2 Description of Health Care Networks

In order to understand the challenges and possible information management mechanisms, we need to be able to describe health care networks systematically. The attributes in Table 10.1 can be used.

10.3 Organizational Structures of Information Management in Health Care Networks

Information management in health care networks is the sum of all planning, directing, and monitoring activities with regard to the transinstitutional information system of the respective network (see Sect. 9.2). In contrast to information management in hospitals, a multiplicity of strategic interests exist in health care networks that may interfere with each other and have to be coordinated with respect to the strategic goals of the network as a whole. This coordination requires adequate organizational structures, which can be characterized by two dimensions: centrality of information management and intensity of information management.

10.3.1 Centrality of Information Management in Health Care Networks

Centrality of information management describes how the competencies of information management are shared among the network members. A high degree of centralization means that few or only one network member is authorized to make decisions.

Regarding centrality, a continuum with two extremes can be identified: the complete centralized information management and the complete decentralized information management. Most of the real world examples are featuring characteristics of both extremes and can therefore be termed hybrid management mechanisms.

In case of complete centralized information management, one member of a health care network provides a *strategic information management* plan for the network and is in charge of implementing the strategy. This is often the case when one member is a large

Table 10.1 Attributes for the description of health care networks

Attribute	Description
Structural attributes of health care networks:	
Range	Geographic extension of the network, e.g., local, regional, national, international
Size	Number of the network members
Configuration	Describes to what extent different types of institutions (hospitals, private practices, etc.) are part of the network
Stability	Describes the extent of member fluctuation
Network management system, i.e., managerial characteristics of a network:	
Legal form	Legal foundation or corporate form of the health care network
Financing form	Describes the mechanism, how the network is maintained financially
Openness	Describes the conditions for becoming a network member
Centrality of network management	Describes, how the authority to make decisions is allocated among the network members
Attributes of the network care system:	
Comprised groups of patient	Describes which groups of patients are treated within the network. These groups can be based on medical, demographic, or administrative characteristics
Coordination of care process	Describes the mechanism that leads the patient through the network, e.g., medical guidelines, "gatekeeping," i.e., the care process is coordinated by one institution, or the care process is coordinated by the patient
Temporal attributes of the health care network:	
Life span	Describes the planned period of time in which the network exists
Development stage	Describes the development stage of a network, e.g., planning stage, operative stage, or dissolution stage

institution, such as a hospital and the other members are small, such as physicians in private practices. Normally, the central member can provide many more resources for information management. The interests of the members regarding the information management strategy for the network are not coordinated systematically.

Complete decentralized information management is characterized by mutual coordination of interests among the network members. The information management strategy is developed in a standardized process that is open to all members.

Both mechanisms possess advantages and disadvantages. The efficiency of decision making is higher in the centralized information management. In contrast, coordinating the interests of all network members in the decentralized mechanism can be a time- and resource-consuming process. On the other hand, mutually agreed decisions have a better chance to be accepted by all network members.

10.3.2 Intensity of Information Management in Health Care Networks

Intensity of information management describes the degree to which the decisions of information management in health care networks are obligatory for the network members. Remember that the membership in a health care network is voluntary.

In case of high intensity, the information management decisions have to be implemented by the network members. This can be based on contracts and may be mandatory for the network membership.

Low intensity means that the network members are not bound to implement the strategy of the network information management. Here, the decisions can be understood as guidelines or recommendations.

Again, advantages and disadvantages can be identified. A higher degree of information management intensity leads to increased reliability for the network members. If the implementation of a certain communication standard or the purchase of a certain application component is mandatory for all network members, the chance of improving efficiency and quality of transinstitutional information processing increases. In case of low intensity, the individual member cannot rely on the decisions of the other members.

On the other hand, a high degree of intensity leads to external dependencies that institutions normally are trying to avoid. By investing in application components, communication interfaces, or infrastructure that supports the collaboration within the network, the economic risk increases, since the investments may be useless once the network membership has ended or the network dissolves. This is called "lock-in effect".

10.4 Types of Health Care Networks

It turns out that the organizational structure of information management reflects the type of collaboration in a network. Therefore health care networks can be characterized with regard to their information management centrality and intensity. We can identify the following different types of health care networks (see Fig. 10.1):

- Loosely coupled networks show a low degree of centrality and intensity. They are typically regional bordered, homogeneously configured, and are based on social structures.

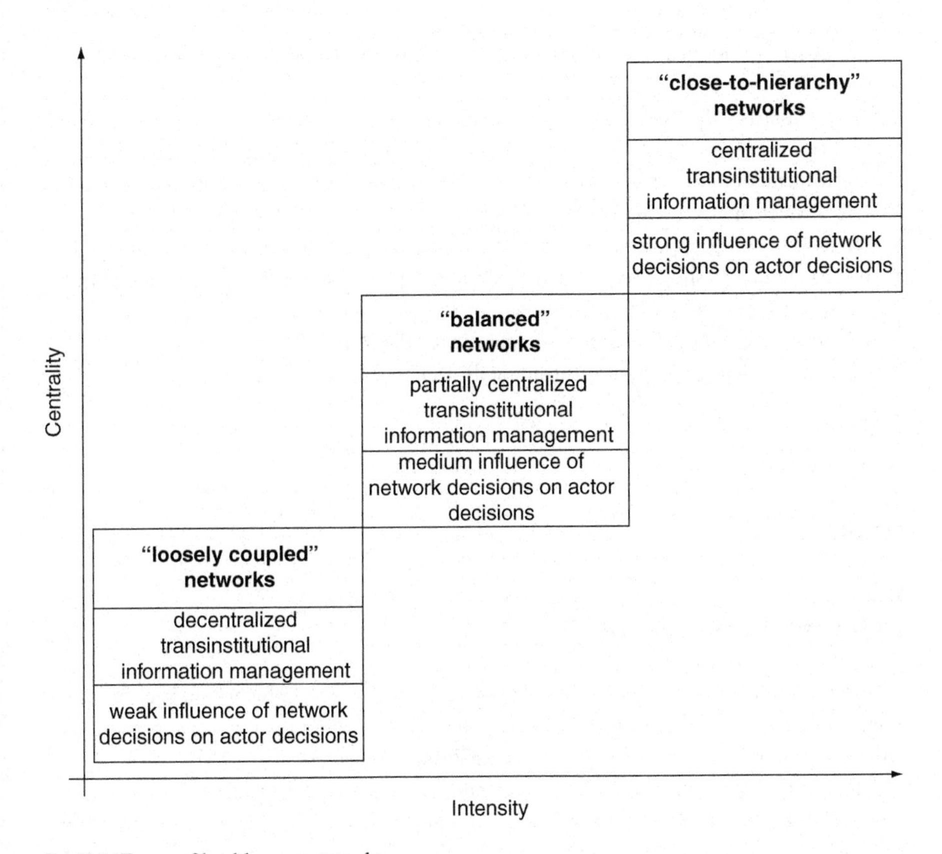

Fig. 10.1 Types of health care networks

- Hierarchy-like networks still fulfill the definition of health care networks, but decision making in information management is highly centralized and the decisions made are compulsory. Typically, these networks are configured heterogeneous and are dominated by one large institution, such as a hospital.
- Balanced networks show medium degrees of centrality and intensity.

10.5 Example

10.5.1 Regional Health Information Organizations

One of the major approaches to reduce costs and increase efficiency in the US health care system is focusing on so-called Regional Health Information Organizations (RHIOs). It has been initiated by the US Department of Health and Human Services in 2004. RHIOs are state-wide, local, or rural health care networks with a strong emphasis on the use of computer-based application components in order to support transinstitutional care processes.

The ultimate goal is to crosslink all RHIOs aiming at establishing a Nationwide Health Information Network (NHIN). This process is in the lead of the National Coordinator for Health Information Technology, a CIO with nationwide competencies. Typically, RHIOs have to answer the following strategical questions:

- What are the appropriate architectures to achieve transinstitutional integration?
- Which standards should be implemented in order to ensure efficient transinstitutional information processing and data protection?
- Which business models ensure sustainability of the RHIO?
- How can all stakeholders profit from the RHIO?

10.6 Exercise

10.6.1 The Plötzberg Health Care Network

In order to improve quality and efficiency of care for patients with chronic back pain, the Plötzberg Medical Center wants to share medical data with regional general practitioners and experts in private practices as well as rehabilitation centers.

The CIO of Plötzberg Medical Center and his experienced team decide to install a portal-based solution to share information from the hospitals EHRs with cooperation partners. A few weeks later, the application component has been introduced and is ready for routine operation. In order to inform the doctors in private practices and rehabilitation centers, a press conference is held. A few more weeks later, though, the CIO notices that the portal is used only by two practitioners on an irregular basis.

Try to help the CIO of the Plötzberg Medical Center by answering the following questions:

- How high is the degree of centrality in the Plötzberg Health Care Network?
- How high is the degree of intensity in the Plötzberg Health Care Network?
- What could be the reasons for the low acceptance of the introduced portal?
- What could be the approaches to raise the acceptance?

10.7 Summary

In contrast to information management in single institutions, such as a hospital, information management in health care networks has to cope with additional problems that result from the non-hierarchical organization of networks. Autonomy and dependency, cooperation and competition, trust and risk between the members are coexisting in networks.

In order to understand health care networks, we need to be able to describe them systematically. Important attributes are the network structure, the network management system, the network care system, as well as temporal attributes of the health care network.

Transinstitutional information management in health care networks can furthermore be characterized by the degree of centrality, i.e., the allocation of managerial authority and the degree of intensity, i.e., the degree to which the decisions of information management in health care networks are obligatory for the network members. Based on centrality and intensity we can differentiate loosely coupled, balanced, and hierarchy-like networks.

11 Final Remarks

Health information systems in general and hospital information systems in particular are sometimes compared to large tankers crossing the oceans. Like tankers, these information systems need careful and long-term planning (planning its course), they need continual monitoring to ensure their course is still followed (staying on course), and they react only very slowly to directing (steering) activities.

Well-educated specialists in health informatics/medical informatics (who are comparable to tanker captains and officers), with the knowledge and skills to systematically manage and operate such information systems, are therefore needed to appropriately and responsibly apply information and communication technology to the complex information processing environment of health care settings.

For better understanding the role of "HIS tanker captains and officers", another analogy in the context of hospital information systems, may be helpful. As mentioned, these information systems have to evolve in parallel and in correspondence to the strategic requirements of a hospital as a whole. The situation of the CIO in a hospital might be regarded as comparable to the environment of the well-known engineer Scotty of "Starship Enterprise," who is always struggling to control the intricate complexities of his warp drive engines in order to fulfill the whims of his captain in a usually insufficient timeframe.

This book discussed health information systems, their architectures and the strategies for information management. A specific focus was laid on hospital information systems. As reader of this book, you should now be able to answer the following questions:

- Why is systematic information processing in health care institutions important?
- What do health information systems look like?
- What are appropriate models and architectures for health information systems?
- How can we assess the quality of health information systems?
- How can we strategically manage health information systems?

And as a summary you may also have found the answer to the question "How can good health information systems be made and maintained?" For us the answer is clear: "By systematic information management!"

This book should be regarded as an introduction to this complex subject. For a deeper understanding, you will need additional knowledge and, foremost, practice in this field.

A. Winter et al., *Health Information Systems*,
DOI: 10.1007/978-1-84996-441-8_11, © Springer-Verlag London Limited 2011

And now a last exercise: Five medical informatics VIPs volunteered to pose in some of the figures used in this book: Prof. Marion Ball (United States), Prof. K.C. Lun (Singapore), Prof. Jochen Moehr (Canada), Prof. Paul Schmücker, and Prof. Gustav Wagner (both Germany). Did you recognize them? Good luck in finding them!

Thesaurus

3LGM²

Abbreviation for →three-layer graph-based →metamodel.

Access integration

Condition of an →information system where the →application components needed for the completion of a certain task can be used where they are needed.

Synonymous term: Zugangsintegration (German)

Activity

Instantiation of an →enterprise function. Different from →enterprise functions, activities have a definite beginning and end.

Synonymous term: Aktivität (German)

Administrative admission

Subfunction of patient admission. Comprises →patient identification and documentation of main administrative →data during the admission of a patient to an institution. Includes assignment of a →patient identification number and of a visit number (case identifier).

Synonymous term: Administrative Aufnahme (German)

A. Winter et al., *Health Information Systems*,
DOI: 10.1007/978-1-84996-441-8_BM1,

ADT

Admission, discharge, and transfer of a patient, as part of →patient administration.

Application component

wAn application component is a set of actually usable rules, which control data processing of certain →physical data processing systems. Rules are considered to be actually usable, if they are implemented such that they are ready to support certain →enterprise functions in a certain enterprise or support communication between application components.

If the rules are implemented as executable software, the application component is called →computer-based application component. Otherwise it is called →non-computer-based application component or organizational system.

Synonymous term: Anwendungsbaustein (German)

Architectural style

Combines →architectures of information systems that are equivalent with regard to certain characteristics. On the →logical tool layer, these characteristics comprise number of databases (DB^1 versus DB^n), number of →application components (AC^1 versus AC^n), number of →software products and vendors (V^1 versus V^n), and communication patterns (star versus spaghetti architecture and CP^1 versus CP^n, respectively). On the physical tool layer, we can, for example, distinguish the →mainframe architecture (1-tier architecture or T^1) and the →client-server architectural style (2-tier architecture or T^2, 3-tier architecture or T^3).

Synonymous term: Architekturstil (German)

Architecture of an information system

Fundamental organization of an →information system, represented by its →components, their relationships to each other and to the environment, and by the principles guiding its design and evolution. Architectures can be summarized into certain →architectural styles.

Synonymous term: Architektur eines Informationssystems (German)

Archiving

Long-time storing (e.g., for 10 or 30 years, depending on legal regulations) of documents and records, especially of →patient records, after discharge of a patient.

Synonymous term: Archivierung (German)

Asynchronous communication

Form of communication where the →application component sending a →message will continue its tasks without interruption even when awaiting a response →message from the communication partner.

Synonymous term: Asynchrone Kommunikation (German)

Benchmarking

Describes a process in which organizations evaluate various aspects of their performance and compare it to given standard or to the best organizations ("best-practice"). Typically, benchmarking comprises quantitative evaluation criteria (→key performance indicators). Method of strategic →monitoring of →hospital information systems.

Business process

Sequence of →enterprise (sub-)functions together with the conditions under which they are invoked, in order to achieve an enterprise goal. Enterprise functions have a definitive beginning and end. While →enterprise functions concentrate on the "what," business processes focus on the "how" of →activities.

Synonymous term: Geschäftsprozess (German)

Business process model

→Model focusing on the dynamic view of →information processing. Concepts typically offered are →activities and their chronological and logical order. Often, other concepts can be added, such as the role or →organizational unit that performs an →activity, or the →information processing tools that are used. Because of the number of different perspectives, various business process →metamodels exist, such as simple process chains, event-driven process chains, activity diagrams, and Petri nets.

Synonymous term: Geschäftsprozessmodell (German)

Certification

Assessment of the compliance with certain predefined →quality characteristics. For example, ISO 9001 standard assesses the hospital's compliance with certain →quality management standards, and the Joint Commission assesses the quality of processes related to patient care, hospital management, and information management. CCHIT and EuroRec certify functionality, security, and interoperability of →electronic health records.

Synonymous term: Zertifizierung (German)

Chief executive officer (CEO)

Responsible for setting and carrying out the strategic plans and policies of an enterprise.

Synonymous term: Geschäftsführer, Vorstandsvorsitzender (German)

Chief financial officer (CFO)

Responsible for financial planning and record keeping of an enterprise.

Synonymous term: Leiter der Finanzabteilung, Finanzvorstand (German)

Chief information officer (CIO)

Responsible for the →strategic, →tactical, and →operational information management and the related budgets in an enterprise. The CIO usually has the authority for all employees concerned with →information management. The specific position of the CIO demands dedicated professional skills.

Synonymous term: Leiter des Informationsmanagements (German)

CIO

Abbreviation for →chief information officer.

Client-server architecture

→Architectural style at the →physical tool layer, comprising various servers and clients, interconnected by a network. The server offers services that can be accessed by the workstations as clients.

Synonymous term: Client-Server-Architektur (German)

Clinical context object workgroup (CCOW)

Develops standards for the synchronization of independent →application components running on one workstation, in order to support →contextual integration.

Clinical documentation

→Documentation in clinical environment. Recording all clinically relevant patient →data that arise during patient care as completely, correctly, and quickly as possible. This supports the coordination of patient treatment between all involved →health care professionals, and also the legal justification of the actions taken. Structured documentation of data is a precondition for data aggregation and statistics, computerized decision support, and retrieval of data. Is supported by →medical documentation systems and →nursing management and documentation systems.

Is not considered as →enterprise function but takes place every time an →enterprise function is executed, new →information is generated, and respective →data are stored.

Synonymous term: Klinische Dokumentation (German)

Clinical document architecture (CDA)

→HL7 document format that describes persistent records of medical →information, encoded in XML.

Clinical information system

→Application component supporting a larger number of hospital functions by closely integrating other →application components such as a →medical documentation system, a →nursing management and documentation system, an →outpatient management system, and a →provider order entry system. Provides harmonized, integrated view on patient data and is thus often also called →electronic patient record system.

Synonymous term: Klinisches Informationssystem, klinisches Arbeitsplatzsystem (German)

COBIT (Control Objectives for Information and Related Technology)

Provides a common language to communicate goals, objectives, and expected results of →application systems and related →projects. COBIT defines 34 IT-related →business processes. For each of them, information on how the specific process goals can be measured, what the key activities and major deliverables are, and who is responsible for them is provided.

Communication interface

Used by →application components for communication among themselves. Can either send or receive →data about →entity types. Part of a →communication link.

Synonymous term: Kommunikationsschnittstelle (German)

Communication link

Communicates →data about a certain →entity type. Connects a →communication interface of one →application component with a →communication interface of another →application component.

Synonymous term: Kommunikationsverbindung (German)

Communication server

→Application component supporting →asynchronous communication between →application components. Stands at the center of the →logical tool layer of a →hospital information system.

Synonymous term: Kommunikationsserver (German)

Communication standard

Describes how messages of a certain data format are communicated when an event occurs. Within →health information systems, well-known examples are →HL7 and →DICOM.

Synonymous term: Kommunikationsstandard (German)

Component of an information system

Typical components of →information systems are →enterprise functions, →business processes, →application components, and →physical data processing systems.

Synonymous term: Komponente eines Informationssystems (German)

Computer-based application component

An →application component where the controlling rules for data processing are implemented as executable software.

Synonymous term: rechnerbasierter Anwendungsbaustein (German)

Computer-based information system

An →information system that comprises (among others) computer-based →information processing tools.

Computer system

A computer-based →physical data processing tool, for example, a terminal, server, or personal computer. Computer systems can be physically connected via data wires, leading to physical networks.

Consistency of data

Situation where redundant copies of →data representing the same →information about one particular object are identical. Consistency of data is an important condition for →integrity within →health information systems.

Synonymous term: Datenkonsistenz (German)

Contextual integration

Condition of an →information system in which the context (e.g., patient identification) is preserved when the user switches between →application components. The general aim is that a task that has already been executed once for a certain purpose does not need to be repeated again to achieve the same purpose. This type of →integration is also referred to as visual integration.

Synonymous term: Kontextintegration (German)

Controlled redundancy

Systematic management of redundantly stored →data within →health information systems. Usually, redundant data storage should be avoided. However, there are situations in which redundant data storage is unavoidable or even desirable. In particular, it must be clear which application component is →master application component for a given →entity type.

Synonymous term: Kontrollierte Redundanz (German)

Controlling

Gathering and aggregating financial and other →data about the hospital's operation in order to control and optimize them. This covers, for example, staff controlling, process controlling, material controlling, and financial controlling.

Cost–benefit analysis

An economic analysis to compare the costs and consequences of a →component of an information system. It converts effects of an →information system component into the same monetary terms as the costs.

Synonymous term: Kosten-Nutzen-Analyse (German)

Cost-effectiveness analysis

An economic analysis to compare the costs and consequences of a →component of an information system. It does not require that all important effects be expressed in monetary terms.

Synonymous term: Kostenwirksamkeitsanalyse (German)

Data

Reinterpretable representation of →information or →knowledge in a formalized manner suitable for communication, interpretation, or processing by humans or machines. Formalization may take the form of discrete characters or of continuous signals (e.g., sound signals). For information to be reinterpretable, there have to be agreements on how →data represent →information.

Synonymous term: Daten (German)

Data integration

Condition of an →information system in which each →data item needs to be recorded, changed, deleted, or otherwise edited just once, even if it is used or stored in several →application components. This means that data that have been recorded are available wherever they are needed, without having to be reentered. Data integration is a prerequisite for →multiple usability of data.

Synonymous term: Datenintegration (German)

Data model

→Model describing the →data processed and stored in an →information system. Concepts typically offered are entity types and their relationships. A typical →metamodel for data modeling is offered by the class diagrams in the Unified Modeling Language (UML).

Synonymous term: Datenmodell (German)

Data transmission connection

Connection of →physical data processing systems, e.g., by communication network or courier service. Uses transmitting media such as signal-based media (cable) or non-signal-based media (e.g., paper).

Synonymous term: Datenübertragungsverbindung (German)

Data warehouse system

→Application component that contains →data which have been extracted from other →application systems, in order to support either hospital management or clinical research.

DICOM (Digital Imaging and Communications in Medicine)

Important →communication standard in health care, used for the transfer of medical images and related →information. DICOM not only defines a →message format, but also couples this closely with exchange formats.

Directing

Executing a plan. Directing in →strategic information management means to transform a →strategic information management plan into →projects. Directing in →tactical information management means the execution of →projects, based on a project plan. Directing in →operational information management means the sum of all management activities that are necessary to ensure proper reactions to operating problems of →components of a →hospital information system.

Synonymous term: Steuerung (German)

Document archiving system

→Application component that supports long-term →archiving of patient-related and other →data and documents based on sustainable standardized data formats, documents formats, and interfaces.

Documentation

Recording of →data. Is not considered as →enterprise function but takes place every time an →enterprise function is executed, new →information is generated, and respective →data are stored.

Synonymous term: Dokumentation (German)

Domain layer

In the →3LGM², the domain layer describes what kinds of →activities in a health care institution are enabled by its →information system and what kind of →data should be stored and processed, independent of its implementation. Consequently, the domain layer describes →enterprise functions and →entity types.

Synonymous term: Fachliche Ebene (German)

Electronic health record (EHR)

Collection of health-related →data relating to one subject of care, i.e., the patient, that is stored in the →computer-supported part of a →health information system. Primarily, EHRs are used to provide →information about a patient whenever and wherever needed. EHRs can be differentiated into provider-centric EHR (→electronic patient records) and patient-centered EHRs that are independent of institutional boundaries.

Synonymous term: Elektronische Gesundheitsakte (EGA) (German)

Electronic patient record (EPR)

→Electronic health record that only contains patient →information that was recorded in one institution, e.g., in a hospital (provider-centric EHR). Here, potentially relevant →information on the patient that was recorded in other institutions may not be available.

Synonymous term: Elektronische Patientenakte (EPA) (German)

Enterprise function

The class of all activities interpreting the same set of →entity types and updating the same set of →entity types is called an information processing enterprise function (for short: enterprise function). An enterprise function is a directive in an institution on how to interpret →data about →entity types and then update data about →entity types as a consequence of this interpretation. The goal of data interpretation and updates is part of or contributes to (sub) goals of the institution. A function has no definitive beginning or end.

Similar to an →activity, an enterprise function is said to interpret →entity types and update →entity types.

Synonymous term: Unternehmensaufgabe (German)

Enterprise resource planning system (ERP system)

→Application component that supports the management of all resources of an organization, including →controlling, financial accounting, facility management, human resources management, →quality management, and supply and disposal management.

Entity type

Is a representation of an object class and of the →data describing the objects of this class, if these →data are stored or could/should be stored in the →information system.

Synonymous term: Objekttyp (German)

Evaluation

Act of measuring or exploring properties of a →health information system. The result of an evaluation should give information to support decisions concerning the →health information system. Evaluation studies are typically conducted as →projects of →tactical information management. Evaluation studies support →monitoring of →hospital information systems.

Federated database system

Integrated system of autonomous (component) database systems. The point of →integration is to logically bring the database schemata of the component database systems to a single database schema, the federated database schema, in order to attain →data integration even when there are redundant data in distributed →health information systems.

Synonymous term: Föderiertes Datenbanksystem (German)

First-level support

User support unit serving as first contact for all user groups with any kinds of →information processing problems. It may consist, for example, of a central 24-h-hotline (service desk) that is responsible for the management of user accounts and first troubleshooting, or of decentralized information processing staff. When the first-level support cannot solve the problems, it hands them over to the →second-level support.

Functional integration

Condition of an →information system where features needed in several →application components are implemented only once and can be invoked by other →application components.

Synonymous term: Funktionsintegration (German)

Functional leanness

Condition of an →information system where an →enterprise function is supported by one and only one →application component. The opposite is →functional redundancy.

Synonymous term: Funktionale Schlankheit (German)

Functional model

→Model representing what is to be done in an institution (e.g., a hospital). Concepts typically offered comprise the →enterprise functions that are supported by the →application components of a →health information system. Functional models describe what is to be done.

Synonymous term: Aufgaben-Modell (German)

Functional redundancy

Condition of an →information system where an →enterprise function is supported by more than one →application component. The opposite is →functional leanness.

Synonymous term: Funktionale Redundanz (German)

Health care network

A group of two or more legally separated health care institutions that have temporarily and voluntarily joined together to achieve a common purpose. The →information system of a health care network is called a →transinstitutional health information system.

Synonymous term: Gesundheitsversorgungsnetzwerk (German)

Health care professional

Staff member directly contributing to patient care, such as a physician or nurse.

Synonymous term: Klinisches Personal (German)

Health information system

→Information system dealing with processing →data, →information, and →knowledge in health care environments. They have a computer-based part and a non-computer-based part. Health information systems can be differentiated into institutional information systems (such as →hospital information systems) and →transinstitutional health information systems.

Synonymous term: Informationssystem des Gesundheitswesens (German)

Health Level Seven (HL7)

Important →communication standard in health care supporting the transfer of patient- and case-based messages, excluding image data. HL7 describes the events and structure of →messages that are exchanged between →application components.

HIS

Abbreviation for →health information system.

Hospital administration

→Hospital function that supports the organization of patient care and guarantees the financial survival and the economic success of the hospital. Subfunctions are →patient administration, →archiving of patient information, →quality management, cost and financial accounting, →controlling, facility management, and →information management;

Synonymous term: Krankenhausverwaltung (German)

Hospital function

→Enterprise function of a hospital.

Synonymous term: Krankenhausaufgabe (German)

Hospital information system

Socio-technical →subsystem of a hospital that comprises all →information processing as well as the associated human or technical actors in their respective information processing roles. The aim of a hospital information system is to sufficiently enable the adequate execution of →hospital functions for patient care.

Synonymous term: Krankenhausinformationssystem (KIS) (German)

Information

Specific determination about entities such as facts, events, things, persons, processes, ideas, or concepts.

Information and knowledge logistics

To make available the right →information and →knowledge at the right time, at the right place, to the right people, in the right form, so that people can make the right decisions.

Synonymous term: Informations- und Wissenslogistik (German)

Information management

Management activities that deal with the →information system of an organization, e.g., a hospital. The goal of information management is systematic →information processing that contributes to the enterprise's strategic goals. The general tasks of information management are →planning the →information system and its →architecture, →directing its establishment and its operation, and →monitoring its development and operation. Information management encompasses the management of all →components of an →information system: management of →information, of →application components, and of →physical data processing systems. With respect to its scope, information management can be divided into →strategic, →tactical, and →operational information management.

Synonymous term: Informationsmanagement (German)

Information management board

Responsible for →strategic information management in a hospital. Members should include representatives from the hospital's board of directors, representatives from the main departments and user groups, and the director of the information management department. If no dedicated →CIO position exists, the president of this board can be regarded as the CIO of the hospital.

Synonymous term: Ausschuss für das Informationsmanagement (German)

Information management department

This unit takes care of at least the tactical and →operational information management of those parts of the HIS with hospital-wide relevance (e.g., the →enterprise resource planning system, the →clinical information system, and the computer network). If the department for →information management also takes care of →strategic information management, the head of this department is typically the →CIO.

Synonymous term: Abteilung Informationsmanagement, IT-Abteilung (German)

Information process

Logical and chronological sequence of →enterprise functions which interpret or update →data about →entities. Different from →business processes, information processes do not contain the conditions under which →enterprise functions are performed.

Synonymous term: Informationprozeß (German)

Information processing

In the context of →hospital information systems, it refers to the processing of →data together with their related →information, and →knowledge.

Synonymous term: Informationsverarbeitung (German)

Information processing tool

An →application component or a →physical data processing system. Can be either computer-based or non-computer-based (e.g., paper-based).

Synonymous term: Werkzeug der Informationsverarbeitung (German)

Information system

Socio-technical →subsystem of an institution that comprises all →information processing as well as the associated human or technical actors in their respective information processing roles. An information system can be divided into →sub-information systems.

Synonymous term: Informationssystem (German)

Information system model

→Model that comprises several models such as a →functional model, →technical model, →organizational model, →data model, and →business process model. Beyond this, information system models consider the dependencies of these →models. An example of a →metamodel for creating information system models is the →3LGM².

Synonymous term: Informationssystemmodell (German)

Infrastructure of an information system

Types, number, and availability of →information processing tools used in a given enterprise.

Synonymous term: Infrastruktur eines Informationssystems (German)

Integrated health care delivery system

One form of a health care network where health care institutions join together to consolidate their roles, resources, and operations in order to deliver a coordinated range of services and to enhance effectiveness and efficiency of patient care.

Synonymous term: Integriertes Gesundheitsversorgungssystem (German)

Integrating the health care enterprise (IHE)

Organization that aims at improving the →interoperability of →application components in healthcare, using existing standards such as →HL7 and→DICOM.

Integration

A union of parts making a whole, which – as opposed to its parts – displays a new quality. We speak of integrated health information system if we want to express that it is a union that represents more than just a set of independent →components. To achieve this integration, the →components need to be →interoperable. We expect positive consequences for the quality of →information processing by integration. Different types of integration on the →logical tool layer are →data integration, →semantic integration, →access integration, →presentation integration, →contextual integration, and →process integration. On the →physical tool layer, →physical integration is important.

Integration technology

Technologies used to achieve →integration within distributed →health information systems, including →federated database systems, →transaction management, and →middleware (e. g. →communication servers, →remote function calls, →SOA).

Integrity

The correctness of →data stored in a →health information system. Important aspects of integrity are →object identity, →referential integrity, and →consistency of data.

Synonymous term: Integrität (German)

Interlayer relationship

Dependencies among →components of different layers in the →$3LGM^2$. Relationships exist between concepts at the →domain layer and the →logical tool layer and between concepts at the logical tool layer and the →physical tool layer.

Synonymous term: Interebenen-Beziehung (German)

Interoperability

Ability of two or more →components to exchange →information and to use the information that has been exchanged. A →component that is called interoperable may, for example, support certain →communication standards or certain →integration technologies.

SynonymWous term: Interoperabilität (German)

IT service management

→Information management that is centered on the customer's perspective of the contribution of a →HIS to a business, in contrast to more technology-centered approaches. The IT Infrastructure Library (ITIL) is the de-facto standard framework for IT service management.

Key performance indicator

Quantitative measures for regularly →monitoring the achievement of strategic goals of an enterprise. Can be used for →benchmarking of →health information systems.

Synonymous term: Kennzahl (German)

Knowledge

General →information about concepts in a certain (scientific or professional) domain (e.g., about diseases or therapeutic methods).

Synonymous term: Wissen (German)

Laboratory information system (LIS)

→Application component supporting the management of analysis in a laboratory: the receipt of the order and the sample, the distribution of the sample and the order to the different analysis tools, the collection of the results, the validation of results, the communication of the findings back to the ordering department, as well as general →quality management procedures.

Synonymous term: Labor-Informationssystem (German)

Leanness of information processing tools

For a given task, from the point of view of the user, there should be as many different →information processing tools as necessary, but as few as possible.

Synonymous term: Schlankheit der informationsverarbeitende Werkzeuge (German)

Logical tool

→Application component.

Synonymous term: Logisches Werkzeug (German)

Logical tool layer

In the →3LGM², the logical tool layer describes the set of →application components used in a health care institution to support its enterprise functions. On this layer, →application components communicate representations of →entity types as →messages via →communication links and store them as→data.

Synonymous term: Logische Werkzeugebene (German)

Mainframe architecture

→Architectural style at the →physical tool layer, consisting of one or multiple (networked) mainframe systems to which various terminals are attached.

Synonymous term: Großrechner-basierte Architektur (German)

Management

Management can stand for an institution or an →enterprise function. As an institution, management comprises all organizational units of an enterprise that make decisions about planning, monitoring, and directing all activities of subordinate units. As an enterprise function, management comprises all leadership activities that determine the enterprise's goals, structures, and behaviors.

Management of information systems

Management of information systems is a synonym to →information management.

Synonymous term: Management von Informationssystemen, Informationsmangement (German)

Master application component

→Application component that contains the original →data about a given →entity type. In case of redundant data storage, other →application components may hold copies of these data, but these →data can only be inserted, deleted, or changed in this master application component; data →integrity in the other →application components has to be maintained by communicating new copies of the original →data to the other →application components.

Synonymous term: Führendes Anwendungssystem (German)

Master Patient Index

→Application component providing a correct →patient identification number even in →transinstitutional information systems with several →patient administration systems.

Manually or semiautomatically found relationships of →patient identification numbers from different institutions are saved in one network MPI and are made available to all member institutions.

Media crack

Change of the storage media during the →transcription of data.

Synonymous term: Medienbruch (German)

Medical documentation system

→Application component supporting specific →documentation tasks (e.g., patient history, planning of care, progress notes, report writing). Typically, it contains specialized modules for different medical fields.

Synonymous term: Medizinisches Dokumentationssystem (German)

Message

Set of →data that are arranged as a unit in order to be communicated between →application components.

Synonymous term: Nachricht (German)

Message type

Class of uniform →messages, determines which →data about which →entity types are communicated by a →message belonging to this message type. A message type can belong to a →communication standard.

Synonymous term: Nachrichtentyp (German)

Metamodel

Language for constructing →models of a certain class. A metamodel is the modeling framework which consists of the modeling syntax and semantics (the available modeling concepts together with their meaning), the representation of the concepts (how the objects are represented in a concrete →model, e.g., in a graphical way), and (sometimes) the modeling rules. An example of a metamodel for →health information systems is the →3LGM^2.

Synonymous term: Metamodell (German)

Middleware

Software component of a →computer-based information system that serves for the communication between →application components. One example is a →communication server.

Model

A description of what the modeler thinks to be relevant of a system. In the sciences, models commonly represent a simplified depiction of reality or excerpts of it. Models are adapted to answer certain questions or to solve certain tasks. Models may be developed based on →metamodels.

Synonymous term: Modell (German)

Monitoring

Assessing the development and operation of a →hospital information system with respect to the planned objectives. Monitoring in →strategic information management means continually auditing →HIS quality as defined by means of its →strategic information management plan's directives and goals. Monitoring in →tactical information management means continually checking whether initiated →projects are running as planned, and whether they will produce the expected results. Monitoring in →operational information management means verifying the proper working and effectiveness of all →components of a →hospital information system.

Synonymous term: Überwachung (German)

Multiple usability of data

Condition where →data are captured once but used for more than one task. A prerequisite is →data integration. Multiple usability of data is one important benefit computer support can bring to →health information systems.

Synonymous term: Multiple Verwendbarkeit von Daten (German)

Non-computer-based application component

An →application component where the controlling rules for data processing are not implemented as executable software but as organizational rules.

Synonymous term: nicht-rechnerbasierter Anwendungsbaustein (German)

Nursing management and documentation system

→Application component for nursing documentation, supporting all phases of the nursing process such as nursing patient history, nursing care planning, execution of nursing tasks, and evaluation of results.

Synonymous term: Pflegedokumentationssystem (German)

Object identity

Condition of an →information system where the representation of every entity is uniquely identifiable. In a →health information system, this is especially important for patients and cases because all medical →data need to be assigned to a particular patient and his or her cases. →Patient identification numbers and case identification numbers are used for that purpose. Object identity is an important condition for →integrity within →HIS.

Synonymous term: Objektidentität (German)

Operation management system

→Application component that supports planning and →documentation within operation rooms.

Synonymous term: OP-Managementsystem (German)

Operational information management

One part of →information management. Responsible for operating all →components of an →information system. It cares for its smooth operation, usually in accordance with the →strategic information management plan of a hospital. Additionally, operational information management plans, directs, and monitors permanent services for the users of the information system.

Synonymous term: Operatives Informationsmanagement (German)

Order entry

Process of entering and transmitting a clinical order to a specialized diagnostic or therapeutic service unit (e.g., lab, radiology, surgery) or to another →health care professional. The available service spectrum offered by a service unit may be presented in the form of catalogs.

Synonymous term: Leistungsanforderung (German)

Organizational model

→Model describing the organization of a unit or area. Concepts typically offered are units or roles that stand in a certain organizational relationship to each other.

Synonymous term: Organisations-Modell (German)

Organizational system

A→non-computer-based application component.

Synonymous term: Organisations system (German)

Organizational unit

Part of an institution which can be defined by responsibilities (e.g., the radiology department). Organizational units perform →enterprise functions.

Synonymous term: Organisationseinheit (German)

Outpatient management system

→Application component for outpatient units, supporting, among others, appointment scheduling, medical →documentation, work organization, and billing.

Synonymous term: Ambulanzmanagementsystem (German)

Patient administration

→Hospital function comprising →patient admission, discharge, and transfer (→ADT), and billing. A patient-related (not only case-related) patient administration can be regarded as the center of the memory of a →hospital information system.

Synonymous term: Patientenverwaltung (German)

Patient administration system

→Application component supporting →patient administration.

Synonymous term: Patientenverwaltungssystem (German)

Patient chart system

→Application component supporting documentation and presentation of vital signs, physician orders, procedure documentation, findings, and other clinical information. Central tool for inter-professional communication within the health care professional team.

Synonymous term: (Patienten-)Kurve (German)

Patient data management system (PDMS)

→Application component in intensive care units to automatically monitor, store, and present a vast amount of patient-related clinical →data. In this area, the requirements for the permanent availability of the →application components and their →data is of highest importance to guarantee patient's safety.

Synonymous term: Patientendaten-Managementsystem (PDMS) (German)

Patient identification

Subfunction of patient admission. To determine and record a patient's identity. As a result of patient identification, a unique →patient identification number (PIN) is assigned.

Synonymous term: Patienten-Identifikation (German)

Patient identification number (PIN)

Number for the unique identification of a patient. Should be used in all parts of a →health information system for →patient identification. Is the precondition for the →object identity of the entity type "patient," and for a patient-oriented combination of all →information arising during the patient's previous, recent as well as future hospitalizations. Should be valid and unchangeable lifelong.

Synonymous term: Patienten-Identifikationsnummer (PIN) (German)

Patient record system

→Application component that comprises all →data and documents generated or received during the care of a patient at a health care institution. Document carriers may be paper-based or electronic media. Nowadays, many documents in the paper-based patient record are computer printouts, and the portion of documents created in computer-based form will further increase, which supports the trend towards the →electronic patient record.

Synonymous term: Krankenakte, Patientenakte (German)

Personal health record (PHR)

A patient-owned →electronic health record, with the patient perceived as the primary owner of his/her →data.

Synonymous term: Persönliche Gesundheitsakte (German)

Physical data processing system

A physically touchable object or a simulated physically touchable object being able to receive, store, forward, or purposefully manipulate →data. We denote receiving, storing, forwarding, and purposeful manipulation of →data as data processing. This data processing is controlled by rules.→Physical data processing systems are used to implement computer-based as well as paper-based →application components. They can be human actors (such as the person delivering mail), non-computer-based physical tools (such as forms for nursing documentation, paper-based patient records, or telephones), or →computer systems. Physical data processing systems are also called physical tools.

Synonymous term: Physischer Datenverarbeitungsbaustein (German)

Physical integration

Condition of an →information system where the physical infrastructure for any kind of →data exchange exists.

Synonymous term: Physische Integration (German)

Physical tool

→Physical data processing system.

Synonymous term: Physisches Werkzeug (German)

Physical tool layer

A set of →physical data processing systems in the →3LGM² that are physically connected via →data transmission connections.

Synonymous term: Physische Werkzeugebene (German)

Picture archiving and communication system (PACS)

→Application component that supports the storage, management, manipulation, and presentation of digital images and their communication to attached workstations for the diagnosing specialists or for the ordering departments.

Synonymous term: Bildarchivierungs- und Kommunikationssystem (German)

Planning

One task of →information management is planning the →hospital information system and its →architecture. Planning in →strategic information management comprises →strategic alignment, establishing a →strategic information management plan, and managing →portfolios. Planning in →tactical management means planning →projects and all resources needed for them. Planning in →operational information management means planning organizational structures, procedures, and all resources such as finances, staff, rooms, or buildings that are necessary to ensure the faultless operation of all components of the hospital information system.

Synonymous term: Planung (German)

Plötzberg Medical Center and Medical School (PMC)

Plötzberg ([pløts'berg]) is a hypothetical medical school associated with a tertiary care hospital. Most of the examples in this book are located at the PMC. The PMC is fictitious, but similarities with real hospitals are certainly not just by chance.

Synonymous term: Medizinische Hochschule Plötzberg (MHP) (German)

Portfolio management

Categorizes certain →components of an information system, using criteria to assess the value of these components for the enterprise and to balance risks and returns. Important instrument for strategic →planning of a →hospital information system. Comprises, for example, application portfolio management and project portfolio management.

Synonymous term: Portfolio-Management (German)

Presentation integration

Condition of an →information system where different →application components represent →data as well as user interfaces in a unified way.

Synonymous term: Präsentationsintegration (German)

Process integration

Condition of an →information system where →business processes are effectively supported by a set of interacting →application components.

Synonymous term: Prozessintegration (German)

Project

A unique undertaking that is characterized by management by objectives, by restrictions with regard to available time and resources, and by a specific project organization.

Synonymous term: Projekt (German)

Provider or physician order entry systems (POE)

→Application component for →order entry of diagnostic or therapeutic procedures (e.g., lab examinations) from specialized service units as well as for ordering of drugs.

Synonymous term: Pflegedokumentationssystem (German)

Quality

Degree to which a set of inherent characteristics fulfills requirements. We can typically distinguish three major approaches to quality assessment: →quality of structures, →quality of processes, and →quality of outcome.

Synonymous term: Qualität, Güte (German)

Quality management

All activities of a health care institution's management that ensure and continually improve the →quality of patient care. This includes setting the goals, defining the responsibilities, and establishing and monitoring the processes to achieve these goals.

Synonymous term: Qualitätsmanagement (German)

Quality of data

Integrity, reliability, completeness, accuracy, relevancy, standardization, authenticity, availability, confidentiality, and security of →data.

Synonymous term: Datenqualität (German)

Quality of outcome

Whether the goals of →information management have been reached, or, in a broader sense, to what extent a →hospital information system contributes to the goals of the hospital and to the expectations of different →stakeholders, and how it fulfills information management laws.

Synonymous term: Ergebnisqualität (German)

Quality of processes

→Quality of the information processes that are necessary to meet the user's needs, such as single recording and →multiple usability of data, no →transcription of data, →leanness of information processing tools, efficiency of →information logistics, and patient-centered →information processing.

Synonymous term: Prozessqualität (German)

Quality of structures

Availability of technical or human resources needed for →information processing. It comprises →quality of data, quality of computer-based →application components, quality of →physical data processing systems, and quality of →HIS architectures.

Synonymous term: Strukturqualität (German)

Radiology information system (RIS)

→Application component supporting the management of a radiology department, comprising appointment scheduling, organization of examinations and staff, provision of patient data and examination parameters, creation of reports, documentation and coding of activities, and statistics.

Synonymous term: Radiologieinformationssystem (RIS) (German)

Reference model

A →model is called a reference model for a certain class of systems and a certain class of questions or tasks dealing with these systems, if it provides model patterns supporting either the derivation of more specific →models through modifications, limitations, or completions (generic reference models), or the direct comparison of different →models with the reference model concerning certain →quality aspects (e.g., completeness, →architectural styles) (nongeneric reference models).

Synonymous term: Referenzmodell (German)

Referential integrity

Correct assignment of entities, for example the assignment of cases to a certain patient, or of results to a case. A precondition is →object identity. Referential integrity is an important condition for →integrity within →health information systems.

Synonymous term: Referenzielle Integrität (German)

Remote function call

Synchronous communication between →application components, enabling the execution of a procedure that can run on a remote computer through a process that is running on a local computer.

Return-on-investment (ROI) study

An economic analysis to describe how much an investment in a →component of an information system pays back in a fixed period of time.

Synonymous term: Rendite-Studie (German)

Second-level support

User support unit addressing information processing problems that cannot be solved by →first-level support. It may consist, for example, of specially trained informatics staff in the central →information management department who are usually responsible for the operation of specific →application components. When the second-level support cannot solve the problems, they are handed over to the →third-level support.

Semantic integration

Condition of an →information system where different →application components use the same system of concepts, i.e., they interpret →data the same way, or where different systems of concepts used by →application components are mapped to each other (e.g., using →medical data dictionaries).

Synonymous term: Semantische Integration (German)

Service

A feature provided by an →application component in order to be used by other →application components. Services of similar type can be summarized in a service class.

Service-oriented architecture (SOA)

→Architectural style of →health information systems where an →application component is able to provide →services and/or to invoke →services from other →application components (e.g., by →remote function calls).

Socio-technical system

A (man-made) →system that consists of both human and technical components.

Synonymous term: Sozio-technisches System (German)

Software ergonomics

Comprises suitability for a task, suitability for learning, suitability for individualization, conformity with user expectations, self-descriptiveness, controllability, and error tolerance of a →software product.

Synonymous term: Software-Ergonomie (German)

Software product

An acquired or self-developed piece of software that is complete in itself and that can be installed on a →computer system. Controls computer-based →application components.

Synonymous term: Softwareprodukt

Software quality

Functionality, reliability, efficiency, maintainability, portability, and usability of a →software product.

Synonymous term: Software-Qualität (German)

Stakeholder

Anyone who has direct or indirect influence on or interest in a →component of an information system.

Synonymous term: Interessensgruppe (German)

Strategic alignment

The process that balances and coordinates the hospital goals and the →information management strategies to get the best result for the hospital. Important task of →strategic information management.

Synonymous term: Strategische Anpassung, Angleichung (German)

Strategic information management

One part of →information management. Deals with the enterprise's →information processing as a whole and establishes strategies and principles for the evolution of the →information system. An important result of strategic information management activities is a →strategic information management plan which is aligned with the hospital's business strategy.

Synonymous term: Strategisches Informationsmanagement (German)

Strategic information management plan

Written document that includes the direction and strategy of →information management and the →architecture of a →health information system. Typically, it describes the hospital's goals, the →information management goals, the current →HIS state, the future →HIS state, and the steps to transform the current →HIS into the planned →HIS. Its establishment is an important task of →strategic HIS planning. The strategic information management plan should be written by the →CIO and approved by the hospital management.

Synonymous term: IT-Strategieplan, IT-Rahmenkonzept (German)

Sub-information system

A subset of the components of an →information system and the relationships between them. A sub-information system is a →subsystem of the overall →information system and thus itself an →information system.

Synonymous term: Sub-Informationssystem (German)

Subsystem

A subset of all →components of a →system, together with the relationships between them.

SWOT analysis

Analysis of the most significant *s*trengths (positive features), *w*eaknesses (negative features), *o*pportunities (potential strengths), and *t*hreats (potential weaknesses) that characterize a →component of an information system.

Synchronous communication

Form of communication in which the process in the →application component that initiated communication with another →application component is interrupted as long as response data from the partner are not obtained

Synonymous term: Synchrone Kommunikation (German)

System

Set of persons, things, events and their relationships that forms an integrated whole. We distinguish between natural systems and artificial (man-made) systems. A system can be divided into →subsystems.

Tactical information management

One part of →information management. Deals with particular →enterprise functions or →application components that are introduced, removed, or changed. Usually these activities are done in the form of →projects.

Synonymous term: Taktisches Informationsmanagement (German)

Technical model

→Model describing the →information processing tools used in an enterprise. Concepts typically offered are →physical data processing systems and →application components.

Synonymous term: Technisches Modell (German)

Third-level support

User support unit that addresses the most severe problems that cannot be solved by the →second-level support. It can consist, for example, of specialists from the software vendor.

Three-layer graph-based meta model (3LGM²)

→Metamodel for developing →information system models of →health information systems. It distinguishes three layers of information systems: →domain layer, →logical tool layer, and →physical tool layer. It aims to support the systematic →information management and especially the structural →monitoring of →information processing in health care institutions. 3LGM²-B consists of concepts describing basic elements of a HIS →architecture. 3LGM²-M adds concepts for modeling message-based communication. 3LGM²-S provides additional concepts for modeling →service-oriented architectures.

Synonymous term: Grafisches Drei-Ebenen-Metamodell (3LGM²) (German)

Transaction management

Ensures that every update of →data which have been consistent will lead to another state in which →data are consistent again.

Synonymous term: Transaktionsmanagement (German)

Transcription (of data)

Transfer of →data from one storage device to another storage device, for example, transfer of patient diagnoses from the →patient record to an order entry form, or copy of data from a printout into a computer-based →application component. Transcription is often combined with a →media crack. Transcription usually leads to the duplication of →data.

Synonymous term: Transkription von Daten (German)

Transinstitutional health information system

→Information system of a →health care network.

Synonymous term: Transinstitutionelles Informationssystem des Gesundheitswesens (German)

Utility analysis

Economic analysis that compares costs and consequences of a →component of an information system, taking the staff's personal preferences into account by including weighting factors for each criterion.

Synonymous term: Nutzwertanalyse (German)

Virtualization

One or more →physical data processing systems simulate one →physical data processing system (cluster), or one →physical data processing system simulates one or more→physical data processing systems (virtual machines).

Synonymous term: Virtualisierung (German)

Virtual private network (VPN)

Provides an exclusively used, secure, and trustworthy communication network, based on Internet and encryption technologies. Can be established and used by →health care networks.

Recommended Further Readings

The following list contains some recommended books and journals you may want to use for further reading. Additionally we want to draw your attention to some associations which may on the one hand give you further assistance during education and professional life and on the other hand will give you the opportunity to actively contribute to the field of health information systems.

Selected Books

Chapter 2. Health Institutions and Information Processing

Kohn LT, Corrigan JM, Donaldson MS, eds. *To err is Human: Building a Safer Health System. Institute of Medicine*. Washington: National Academy Press; 2000. http://www.nap.edu/openbook.php?isbn=0309068371.

Committee on Quality of Healthcare in America. Institute of Medicine. *Crossing the Quality Chasm: A New Health System for the 21st Century*. Washington: National Academy Press; 2001. http://www.nap.edu/openbook.php?isbn=0309072808002E.

Chapter 3. Information Systems Basics

Shortliffe EH, Cimino JJ. *Biomedical Informatics: Computer Applications in Healthcare and Biomedicine*. 3rd ed. New York: Springer; 2006.

Chapter 4. Health Information Systems

Commission of the European Communities. e-Health – making healthcare better for European citizens: an action plan for a European e-Health Area. 2004. http://www.eurorec.org/files/filesPublic/com2004_0356en01.doc

Chapter 5. Modeling Health Information Systems

Martin J. *Information Engineering. Book II: Planning & Analysis*. Englewood Cliffs: Prentice Hall; 1989.

Chapter 6. Architectures of Hospital Information Systems

Greenes RA. *Clinical Decision Support: The Road Ahead*. Boston: Academic; 2007.

Van de Velde R, Degoulet P. *Clinical Information Systems: A Component-Based Approach*. New York: Springer; 2003. ISBN 0387955380.

Chapter 7. Specific Aspects for Architectures for Transinstitutional Health Information Systems

Iakovidis I, Wilson P, Healy JC (eds) (2004) E-Health: current situation and examples of implemented and beneficial E-Health applications. IOS Press, Amsterdam. ISBN: 978-1-58603-448-1

Chapter 8. Quality of Health Information Systems

Friedman CP, Wyatt JC. *Evaluation Methods in Medical Informatics*. 2nd ed. New York: Springer; 2000.

Chapter 9. Strategic Information Management

Cassidy A. *A Practical Guide to Information Systems Strategic Planning*. 2nd ed. Boca Raton: Auerbach Publications; 2006.

Hovenga EJS, Mantas J, eds. *Global Health Informatics Education*. Amsterdam: IOS Press; 2004. ISBN 978-1-58603-454-2.

Lorenzi NM, Ash JS, Einbinder J, McPhee W, Einbinder L. *Transforming Healthcare Through Information*. 2nd ed. New York: Springer; 2004.

Weill P, Ross JW. *IT Governance: How Top Performers Manage IT Decision Rights for Superior Results*. Boston: Harvard Business School Press; 2004.

Chapter 10. Strategic Information Management in Healthcare Networks

Blobel B, Pharow P, Nerlich M, eds. *eHealth: Combining Health Telematics, Telemedicine, Biomedical Engineering and Bioinformatics to the Edge*. Amsterdam: IOS Press; 2008. ISBN 978-1-58603-835-9.

Selected Journals in Health Informatics/Medical Informatics

- Applied Clinical Informatics (ACI). http://www.aci-journal.org
- BMC Medical Informatics and Decision Making. http://www.biomedcentral.com/bmcmedinformdecismak
- Hospital Information Technology Europ. http://www.hospitaliteurope.com
- International Journal of Medical Informatics (IJMI). http://www.elsevier.com/locate/ijmedinf

- Journal of the American Medical Informatics Association (JAMIA). http://jamia.bmj.com
- Journal of Healthcare Information Management (JHIM). http://www.himss.org/ASP/publications_jhim.asp
- Methods of Information in Medicine. http://www.methods-online.com

Selected Associations for Health Informatics/Health Information Management/Medical Informatics

International

- Healthcare Information and Management Systems Society (HIMSS). http://www.himss.org
- International Medical Informatics Association (IMIA) www.imia.org

Regional

- Asia Pacific Association for Medical Informatics (APAMI). http://www.APAMI.org
- European Federation for Medical Informatics (EFMI). http://www.EFMI.org
- Latin American and Caribbean Federation for Health Informatics (IMIA-LAC). http://www.IMIA-LAC.net

National

- American Health Information Management Association (AHIMA). http://www.ahima.org
- American Medical Informatics Association (AMIA). http://www.amia.org
- Deutsche Gesellschaft für Medizinische Informatik, Biometrie und Epidemiologie e.V. (German Society for Medical Informatics, Statistics and Epidemiology, GMDS). http://www.gmds.de

Index

A
Access integration, 147
Administrative admission, 81–82
Architecture, hospital information systems
  clinical business processes, 178–181
  domain layer
    archiving of patient information, 97–99
    clinical documentation, 106–107
    coding of diagnoses and procedures, 90–91
    controlling, 100–102
    cost accounting, 100, 101
    entity types, 76–79
    execution of procedures, 88–90
    facility management, 101, 103
    financial accounting, 101, 103
    hospital management, 104, 105
    human resources management, 95–96
    information management, 101, 103, 104
    order entry, 86–88
    patient administration, 97
    patient admission, 79–84
    patient discharge, 91–93
    patient treatment, 83–86
    quality management, 99–100
    reference model of hospital functions, 108, 109
    research and education, 104–106
    scheduling and resource allocation, 95
    supply and disposal management, 93–95
  health information system (HIS), 40–41
  logical tool layer
    all-in-one *vs.* best-of-breed products, 141–142
    architectural styles, 138
    central *vs.* distributed databases, 138–140
    clinical document architecture (CDA), 154–155
    comprehensive application components, 134–135
    consistency, 145–146
    data warehouse system, 129–131
    Digital Imaging and Communications in Medicine (DICOM), 152
    document archiving system, 131–133
    Electronic Data Interchange for Administration, Commerce, and Transport (EDIFACT), 154
    enterprise resource planning (ERP) system, 128–129
    features, 110
    federated database system, 155
    Health Level 7 (HL7) version 2, 149–151
    Health Level 7 (HL7) version 3, 151–152
    Integrating the Healthcare Enterprise (IHE), 153–154
    integration, 137
    interoperability, 137
    ISO/IEEE 11073, 153
    laboratory information system (LIS), 127–128
    medical documentation system, 113–115
    middleware, 156–160
    monolithic *vs.* modular components, 140–141
    non-computer-based application components, typical, 135–137
    nursing management and documentation system, 115–116
    object identity, 144–145
    operation management system, 122–124

outpatient management system, 116–118
patient administration system, 111–113
patient data management system (PDMS), 120–122
pharmacy information system, 133, 134
physician order entry system (POE), 118–119
picture archiving and communication system (PACS), 125–127
radiology information system (RIS), 124–125
referential integrity, 145
spaghetti *vs*. star pattern, 142–143
transaction management, 155–156
types of integration, 146–149
physical tool layer
clients, 169–170
computing centers, 175–176
data process, hospital's computing center, 176–177
infrastructure, 171–172
non-computer-based data processing systems, typical, 170–171
physical integration, 174–175
servers and communication networks, 169
storage, 170
taxonomy, of architectures, 172–174
Asynchronous communication, 157

B

Best-of-breed 141–142, 206, 220
Business processes, 27
Business process models, 49–51

C

Case identification number (CIN), 81, 112–113, 144
CCHIT functional quality criteria, 273
Central *vs*. distributed databases
DB^n Style, 139–140
DB^1 Style, 139
mixed DB^1/DB^n style, 140
Chief information officer (CIO), 251–253, 290
Chief operating officer (COO), 253
Clinical context object workgroup (CCOW), 153
Clinical document architecture (CDA), 154–155, 195
Clinical information system (CIS), 134–135
COBIT, 270, 272–273
Communication interfaces, 59
Communication link, 59
Communication server, 157
Computer-based information system, 26
Contextual integration, 148
Controlled redundancy, 206

D

Data, definition, 25
Data integration, 146
Data models, 48, 49
Data transmission connections, 61
Data warehouse system, 129–131
Digital Imaging and Communications in Medicine (DICOM), 152
Document archiving system, 131–133
Documentation of entity type E, 65, 107
Domain layer, 79–110

E

Electronic Data Interchange for Administration, Commerce, and Transport
Electronic health records (EHR), 38
Electronic patient records (EPR), 38
Enterprise function, 27
Enterprise resource planning (ERP) system, 128–129
Evaluation, definition, 221

F

Federated database system, 155
Functional integration, 148
Functional leanness, 219
Functional models, 45, 46
Functional redundancy, 219
Functional redundancy rate (FRR), 230–235

G

Gesundheitsnetz Tirol (GNT), 193–196
Gross domestic product (GDP), 4–5

H

Health care networks, 36, 286, 287. *See also* Strategic information management
Health care professional card (HPC), 189
Health information system (HIS)
architecture of, 40–41
benchmarking report, 270, 271
certification, 268, 269
challenges for, 38–40
definition, 1, 33–34
electronic health records (EHR), 38
failures, 1
goal of, 34
importance of, 33
modeling

models and metamodels, 43–51
reference model, for domain layer, 70–71
reference models, 68–70
three-layer graph-based metamodel (3LGM²), 51–68
planning, 257
quality
The Baby CareLink Study, 230
balance, information management, 216–221
The Baldrige criteria, 228–229
concepts, 201
evaluation, 221–228
functional redundancy rate, 230–235
management standards of Joint Commission, 229–230
of outcome, 212–216
of processes, 208–212
of structures, 202–207
tasks of, 34–35
terminology, 2
transinstitutional, 36–37
Health institutions. *See* Information processing
Health Level 7 (HL7)
version 2, 149–151
version 3, 151–152
Health Level 7 Reference Information Model (HL7-RIM), 71
Heidelberg quintuplets, 18
HIS. *See* Health information system
Hospital information systems. *See also* Health information system (HIS)
architecture
clinical business processes, 178–181
domain layer, 75–110
infrastructure, 171–172
logical tool layer, 110–168
physical tool layer, 168–177
areas of hospital, 35
definition, 33–34
management areas, 35–36
as memory and nervous system, 7–9
quality of processes, 212
Reference Model for Domain Layer, 70–71
tasks, 34

I

IMIA. *See* International Medical Informatics Association (IMIA)
Information and communication technology (ICT) progress
economics, 10–11
health care change, 11–12
quality of health care, 8–10
Information, definition, 25
Information logistics, 210
Information management, 30
Information management department, 253
Information processing, 1–2
amount of,
eHealth, estimated impact, 21–22
knowledge access, patient care, 17–18
nonsystematic, 18–19
practice, 23
progress, in ICT
economics, 10–11
health care change, 11–12
quality of health care, 8–10
significance, in health care
as cost factor, 4–6
holistic view of patient, 6–7
hospital information system, 7–9
as productivity factor, 6
as quality factor, 3–4
systematic information management, importance of
data sharing, 14
information processing, basis, 16
integrated processing, 15–16
people and areas, affected, 12
processing amount, 13–14
quality raise, 16
The WHO eHealth Resolution, 19–21
Information processing tools, 27
Information system, 26
architecture, 29–30
components, 26–30
data, 25
definition, 25
infrastructure, 29–30
knowledge, 26
management, 30
Integrated health care delivery systems, 36–37
Integrating the Healthcare Enterprise (IHE), 69, 153–154
Integration types
access, 147
contextual, 148
data, 146
functional, 148
presentation, 147
process, 148–149
semantic, 146–147
International Medical Informatics Association (IMIA), 277

Integrated information processing, 15–16
IT Infrastructure Library (ITIL), 249

K

Knowledge, definition, 26

L

Laboratory information system (LIS), 127–128
3LGM²-B
  domain layer, 55–58
  interlayer relationships, 62–66
  logical tool layer, 58–60
  physical tool layer, 60–63
3LGM²-M, 66–67
3LGM²-S, 67–68
Lock-in effect, 288
Logical tool layer
  all-in-one *vs.* best-of-breed products, 141–142
  application components integration, 188–190
  architectural styles, 138
  central *vs.* distributed databases, 138–140
  clinical document architecture (CDA), 154–155
  comprehensive application components, 134–135
  consistency, 145–146
  contextual integration standard, 153
  data warehouse system, 129–131
  Digital Imaging and Communications in Medicine (DICOM), 152
  document archiving system, 131–133
  EHR systems strategies
    independent health banks, 192
    patient-centric, 191
    provider-centric, 191
    regional-or national-centric, 192
  Electronic Data Interchange for Administration, Commerce, and Transport (EDIFACT), 154
  enterprise resource planning (ERP) system, 128–129
  features, 110
  federated database system, 155
  Health Level 7 (HL7) version 2, 149–151
  Health Level 7 (HL7) version 3, 151–152
  Integrating the Healthcare Enterprise (IHE), 153–154
  integration, 137
  interoperability, 137
  ISO/IEEE 11073, 153
  laboratory information system (LIS), 127–128
  medical documentation system, 113–115
  middleware, 156–160
  monolithic *vs.* modular components, 140–141
  non-computer-based application components, typical, 135–137
  nursing management and documentation system, 115–116
  object identity, 144–145
  operation management system, 122–124
  outpatient management system, 116–118
  patient administration system, 111–113
  patient data management system (PDMS), 120–122
  pharmacy information system, 133, 134
  physician order entry system (POE), 118–119
  picture archiving and communication system (PACS), 125–127
  radiology information system, 124–125
  realizations, 161–163
  referential integrity, 145
  spaghetti *vs.* star pattern, 142–143
  transaction management, 155–156
  types of integration, 146–149
Long-term HIS planning, 257

M

Master patient index (MPI), 113, 189
Meal ordering, 211, 212
Medical admission, 83
Medical and nursing care planning, 56
Medical documentation system, 113–115
Message and message type, definition, 66–67
Metamodel, 44
Modeling, health information systems
  models and metamodels
    definitions, 43–45
    types, 45–51
  reference model for domain layer, 70–71
  reference models, 68–70
  three-layer graph-based metamodel (3LGM²)
    aim, 51
    3LGM²-B, 55–66
    3LGM²-M, 66–67
    3LGM²-S, 67–68
    as metamodel, 71
    UML class diagrams, 52–54

Models and metamodels definitions, 43–45
types
business process, 49–51
data, 48, 49
functional, 45, 46
information system, 51
organizational, 46, 48
technical, 46, 47

N

National health information system (NHIS), 197–198
Nonsystematic information processing, 18–19
Nursing admission, 83
Nursing management and documentation system, 115–116

O

Object identity, 144–145
OpenEHR, 190
Operational information management, 241, 246–248
Operation management system, 122–124
Organizational models, 46, 48
Organizational structures, strategic information management
chief information officer (CIO), 251–253
for information management, 253, 254
management department, 253
Organizational units, 56–57
Outpatient management system, 116–118

P

Patient administration system, 111–113
Patient admission, 219
Patient care, hospital functions
admission
administrative, 81–82
aim, 79–80
appointment scheduling, 81
identification and checking, 81
medical, 83
nursing, 83
visitor and information service, 83
decision making and planning, 83–86
order entry
appointment scheduling, 88
preparation, 86–88
Patient-centered information processing, 210
Patient chart system, 135, 136
Patient data management system (PDMS), 120–122
Patient demographics query (PDQ) 189
Patient identification number (PIN), 81, 112–113, 144
Patient record system, 136, 137
Personal health record (PHR), 191
Pharmacy information system, 133, 134
Physical data processing systems, 28–29, 60
Physical integration, 174–175
Physical tool layer, 192–193
clients, 169–170
computing centers, 175–176
data processed, hospital's computing center, 176–177
infrastructure, 171–172
non-computer-based data processing systems, typical, 170–171
physical integration, 174–175
servers and communication networks, 169
storage, 170
taxonomy of architectures, 172–174
Physician order entry system (POE), 118–119
Picture archiving and communication system (PACS), 125–127
Plötzberg Medical Center and Medical School (PMC), 40
Presentation integration, 147
Process integration, 148–149

Q

Quality
balance, information management
computer and non-computer-based tools, 217–218
data security and working processes, 218–219
documentation quality and efforts, 219–220
functional leanness and redundancy, 219
homogeneity and heterogeneity, 217
The Baldrige criteria, 228–229
concepts, 201
evaluation (*see also* Quality evaluation)
methods, 224–227
phases, 221–224
functional redundancy rate, 230–235
management standards of Joint Commission, 229–230
outcome, fulfillment
hospital's goals, 213
information management laws, 215
stakeholders, 213–215
patient care, 212
processes

data transcription, 208, 209
information logistics, efficiency of, 210
information processing tools, leanness of, 208, 210
patient-centered information processing, 210
single recording, multiple usability, 208
structures
architecture, 206
computer-based application components, 203–205
data, 202–203
physical data processing systems, 205
Quality evaluation
methods
qualitative, 225–226
quantitative, 224–225
studies, 226–227
phases
first study design, 223
operationalization, 223
report and publication, 224
study execution, 224
study exploration, 222–223

R

Radiology information system (RIS), 124–125, 203, 204
Reference information model (RIM), 197
Reference models, 68–70
Regional Health Information Organizations (RHIOs), 289–290
Remote function calls (RFC), 159–160
Remote procedure calls (RPCs). *See* Remote function calls (RFC)

S

Semantic integration, 146–147
Service-oriented architectures (SOAs), 160
Short-term HIS planning, 257
Simpson's paradox, 19
Software product, 27–28
Stakeholders
administrative staff, 214
health care professionals, 214
hospital management, 215
patients and relatives, 214
Strategic directing
exercise, 276
methods, 275–276
project management boards, 276
tasks, 275
Strategic information management, 281–283, 290
challenges, 285
computer network failures, 278–279
deficiencies in, 277–278
health care networks
description, 286, 287
types of, 288–289
health information and converging technologies, implementation, 280–281
in hospitals, 243
IMIA recommendations, 277
information management responsibilities, 279–280
IT service and information management, relationship, 248–249
operational, 241, 246–248
organizational structures
centrality of, 286–288
chief information officer (CIO), 251–253
for information management, 253, 254
intensity of, 288
management department, 253
physician order entry system, computerized, 281
planning, directing and monitoring, relationship, 241, 242
planning, hospitals, 259, 260
regional health information organizations (RHIOs), 289–290
strategic, 240, 244
strategic directing
exercise, 276
methods, 275–276
project management boards, 276
tasks, 275
strategic monitoring
CCHIT functional quality criteria, 273
COBIT, 270, 272–273
HIS benchmarking report, 270, 271
methods, 269–270
tasks, 266–268
strategic planning
information management plan, 259–263
methods, 258–259
plan structure, 263, 264
tasks, 256–257
tactical, 241, 245–246, 250
three-dimensional classification, 241, 242

Strategic information management plan
purpose, 259–260
structure of, 261–263
Strategic monitoring
CCHIT functional quality criteria, 273
COBIT, 270, 272–273
HIS benchmarking report, 270, 271
methods, 269–270
tasks
Ad Hoc monitoring activities, 267–268
HIS certification, 268
permanent monitoring activities, 266–267
Strategic planning
information management plan, 259–263
methods
plans, 259–263
portfolio management, 258–259
strategic alignment, 258
plan structure, 263, 264
tasks
business plans and information management, aligning, 256–257
HIS planning, 257
Sub-information systems, 27
System and subsystems, 26
Systematic information management
amount of information processing, 13–14
data sharing, 14
information processing, basis, 16
integrated processing, 15–16
people and areas affected, 12
quality raise, 16
Systematic information processing, 16

T
Tactical information management, 241, 245–246, 250
Technical models, definition, 46, 47
The Baby CareLink Study, 230
The Baldrige criteria, 228–229
The Plötzberg network, 19, 40, 46–50, 163, 178, 211, 248, 251–253, 288
The Tyrolean health care network. *See* Gesundheitsnetz Tirol (GNT)
The WHO eHealth Resolution, 19–21
Three-layer graph-based metamodel ($3LGM^2$)
aim, 51
$3LGM^2$-B, 55–66
$3LGM^2$-M, 66–67
$3LGM^2$-S, 67–68
as metamodel, 71
modeling, 72–73
UML class diagrams, 52–54
Time-motion analysis, 224–225
Transinstitutional health information systems, 36–37
designing, 185
domain layer
additional enterprise functions, 188
hospital functions, aspects for, 186–188
Hypergenes biomedical information infrastructure, 196–197
logical tool layer
application components integration, 188–190
EHR systems strategies, 190–192
The National Health Information System in Korea, 197–198
physical tool layer, 192–193
The Tyrolean health care network, 193–196
VISTA, 196

U
UML class diagrams, 52–54
Unified modeling language (UML), 48, 52

V
Very low birth weight (VLBW) infants, 230
Veterans Health Information Systems and Technology Architecture (VISTA), 196
Virtual private networks (VPN), 192
VISTA. *See* Veterans Health Information Systems and Technology Architecture (VISTA)

CPSIA information can be obtained
at www.ICGtesting.com
Printed in the USA
LVOW01*1131200716
497065LV00014B/185/P

9 781849 964401